Drug Policy and the Public Good

D0556874

Drug Policy and the Public Good

Thomas Babor
Jonathan Caulkins
Griffith Edwards
Benedikt Fischer
David Foxcroft
Keith Humphreys
Isidore Obot
Jürgen Rehm
Peter Reuter
Robin Room
Ingeborg Rossow
John Strang

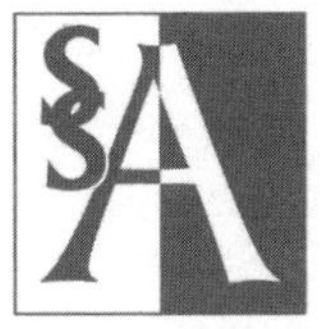

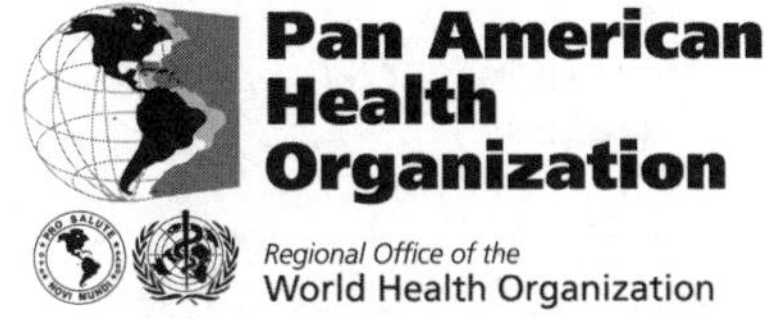

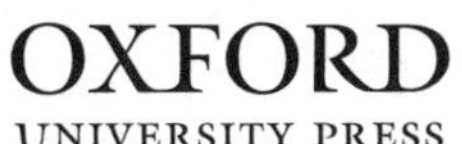

OXFORD
UNIVERSITY PRESS

Great Clarendon Street, Oxford OX2 6DP

Oxford University Press is a department of the University of Oxford.
It furthers the University's objective of excellence in research, scholarship,
and education by publishing worldwide in

Oxford New York

Auckland Cape Town Dar es Salaam Hong Kong Karachi
Kuala Lumpur Madrid Melbourne Mexico City Nairobi
New Delhi Shanghai Taipei Toronto

With offices in

Argentina Austria Brazil Chile Czech Republic France Greece
Guatemala Hungary Italy Japan Poland Portugal Singapore
South Korea Switzerland Thailand Turkey Ukraine Vietnam

Oxford is a registered trade mark of Oxford University Press
in the UK and in certain other countries

Published in the United States
by Oxford University Press Inc., New York

© Oxford University Press, 2010

The moral rights of the author have been asserted
Database right Oxford University Press (maker)

The Society for the Study of Addiction endorses this book on the understanding that the named authors alone are responsible for the views expressed in this publication.

Disclaimer: The designation employed and the presentation of the material in this publication do not imply the expression of any opinion whatsoever on the part of the Secretariat of the Pan American Health Organization concerning the legal status of any country, territory, city, or area or of its authorities, or concerning the delimitation of its frontiers or boundaries. This publication contains the views of the authors and does not necessarily represent the stated policy of the Pan American Health Organization (PAHO).

First published 2010

All rights reserved. No part of this publication may be reproduced,
stored in a retrieval system, or transmitted, in any form or by any means,
without the prior permission in writing of Oxford University Press,
or as expressly permitted by law, or under terms agreed with the appropriate
reprographics rights organization. Enquiries concerning reproduction
outside the scope of the above should be sent to the Rights Department,
Oxford University Press, at the address above

You must not circulate this book in any other binding or cover
and you must impose the same condition on any acquirer

British Library Cataloguing in Publication Data
Data available

Library of Congress Cataloging in Publication Data

Data available

Typeset in Minion by Cepha Imaging Private Ltd., Bangalore, India
Printed in Great Britain on acid-free paper by Clays

ISBN 978–0–19–955712–7

10 9 8 7 6 5 4 3 2 1

Oxford University Press makes no representation, express or implied, that the drug dosages in this book are correct. Readers must therefore always check the product information and clinical procedures with the most up-to-date published product information and data sheets provided by the manufacturers and the most recent codes of conduct and safety regulations. The authors and the publishers do not accept responsibility or legal liability for any errors in the text or for the misuse or misapplication of material in this work. Except where otherwise stated, drug dosages and recommendations are for the non-pregnant adult who is not breastfeeding.

Preface

The production, trafficking and use of illicit drugs, the diversion of prescription drugs to illegal markets, and the harmful effects of alcohol and tobacco use have become central topics of the news, politics at all levels, and concerned families and communities, but relatively little attention has been given to this issue by the Pan American Health Organization (PAHO) in the last decade.

One of the reasons for this vacuum of activity was the lack of scientific and other information to help guide regional responses and technical cooperation with countries. The information available was limited and scattered, and the first attempt to revise and compile it at the regional level came last year with the publication of the technical report "Drug Use Epidemiology in Latin America and the Caribbean: A Public Health Approach" (2009), which provides an overview of the situation and some recommendations for a public health approach, from an epidemiological perspective.

Another central piece of information needed for policy making is to know what has worked and not worked in drug policy around the world, which could help the development of appropriate policies in the countries of our region. This was not an easy task and it took a few years for the group of experts who authored this book to develop criteria for selecting studies; to review hundreds of scientific papers, reports and information available; and to write a document that can shed new light onto the drug policy debate without the need for a definite answer. There is no single solution to the 'drug problem', as it is already difficult to describe what the problem is, given the different types of psychoactive substances, their health and social impacts, and the countries and contexts in which they occur. But non-scientific judgments have driven a substantial part of the debate for many years and PAHO felt the need to support the dissemination of a scholarly review of the literature which could help policy makers think about, discuss and develop a public health oriented approach to illicit drugs.

This book does not reflect the views of PAHO or any specific policy of the Organization, and PAHO staff have not in any way influenced the work of the authors. The support given to the publication of this book, both in its English-language version and its translation into Spanish, is mainly to help disseminate the work of a group of internationally recognized experts who took a public health perspective in their analysis and tried to look at issues from various angles and perspectives, using the highest standards to assess the evidence available. PAHO has also chosen to support this book because it identifies gaps in research as well as limitations in some commonly used but largely unevaluated strategies, such as grassroots coalitions that organize against drug use. Indeed, one of the largest research gaps identified by *Drug Policy and the Public Good* is the small amount of research available from Latin American and Caribbean countries when compared with research conducted in the developed world (most notably Australia, Canada, Europe, Japan, New Zealand, and the USA). And yet, despite this imbalance in research sources, *Drug Policy and the Public Good* strives for a global, multidisciplinary approach to the analysis of drug policy efforts.

A book on drug policy will be inherently controversial as there are different opinions and views no matter what perspective one takes. The work is also not complete, as the available information, by its very nature, is incomplete. However, one of the core functions of PAHO is to shape the research agenda and stimulate the generation, dissemination and application of valuable knowledge. Therefore, it is our duty to help disseminate information even though it may be portrayed or viewed as controversial; otherwise knowledge cannot move forward. We certainly hope this book will help public health policy makers to develop and implement drug policy to the benefit of the public good.

Mirta Roses Periago

Director, PAHO

Author Preface

The Drugs and Public Policy Project was initiated in November of 2004 as a collaborative effort by an international group of addiction scientists to improve the linkages between multidisciplinary research and drug policy. Individual authors' time and travel were funded by multiple sources, listed below, and the central activities were conducted with the support of the UK Society for the Study of Addiction (SSA), in the tradition of its prior support for *Alcohol Policy and the Public Good* and *Alcohol: No Ordinary Commodity*, two books that helped to define the extent of evidence-based alcohol policy on an international level. The authors are grateful to the SSA for its remarkable generosity and its ability to support an independent voice in the pursuit of effective drug policy.

Drug Policy and the Public Good provides an overview of data on the global dimensions of drug misuse, as well as a critical review of the scientific evidence relating to drug policy at the local, national, and international levels. A fundamental aim of this book is to evaluate critically the available research on drug policy, and to present it in a way that informs both the policymaker and the scientific community. The book is meant to address the need for better evidence to inform drug policy, not only in the industrialized countries where significant resources are already invested in drug research but also in the developing world where resources are scarce. The scope of the book is thus comprehensive and international.

The 12 contributors all collaborated in the writing of this book over a 5-year period. Most of the authors have written at least one of the individual chapters, and all have contributed to the chapter revisions. Thomas Babor served as leader of the project. The alphabetical listing of the authors is meant to imply that all authors made relatively equal contributions to the final product. The collaborative writing process consisted of periodic meetings to develop chapter drafts and to discuss the emerging themes of the book. As suggested in the institutional affiliations listed below, the authors represent a broad range of academic backgrounds and professional experience, all relevant to the understanding of drug policy. Disciplinary backgrounds include sociology, political science, psychiatry, psychology, public policy, medicine, criminology, and epidemiology. Institutional affiliations include major universities and university-based research centres in eight countries (Australia, Canada, Nigeria, Norway, Qatar, Sweden, the UK and the USA). Professional experience includes teaching and research in the addiction field as well as consultation (or prior employment) with major policymaking institutions, such as the World Health Organization, the United Nations Office on Drugs and Crime, and the US Office of National Drug Control Policy. Most of the authors have provided consultation to government agencies involved in formulating national drug policies, including the governments of the aforementioned countries plus Denmark and Germany. Nevertheless, nothing in this book should be construed as an official policy position of any agency, organization, or official. Rather, the book is a collective product of authors speaking as individuals.

The authors would like to thank several colleagues who provided invaluable help at various times in the writing and production of this book. First, we thank Jean O'Reilly for her help with the editing and coordination of the drafting process, not to mention her persistence, patience, and good cheer. We also acknowledge the advice provided by Dr Jerome Jaffe and Professor Maria Elena Medina Mora, who contributed to the early planning of the project, and the assistance of Dr Vivek Benegal and Professor Wei Hao at a later stage in the project. Finally, we are grateful to three scholars (Professors Wayne Hall, Alison Ritter, and Ambros Uchtenhagen) who critically evaluated the manuscript before it went to press, and whose timely comments saved the authors from committing various sins of omission as well as commission. Any remaining faults, of course, are the responsibility of the authors.

All of the authors are grateful to their institutional affiliates for the time and resources (including travel funds) provided to support work on this project. In particular, Robin Room acknowledges the support provided by the Centre for Social Research on Alcohol and Drugs (SoRAD), Stockholm University, Sweden; Jonathan Caulkins received support from the Qatar Foundation and his Robert Wood Johnson Foundation Health Investigator Award; Benedikt Fischer was supported by a CIHR/PHAC Chair in Applied Public Health and a MSFHR Senior Scholar Investigator Award; Keith Humphreys received support from the Robert Wood Johnson Foundation and the US Department of Veterans Affairs; Benedikt Fischer and Jürgen Rehm benefitted from salary and infrastructure support to CAMH provided by the Ontario Ministry of Health and Long Term Care (the views expressed in this book do not necessarily reflect those of the Ministry of Health and Long Term Care); and Thomas Babor received a Distinguished International Scientist Collaboration Award from the US National Institute on Drug Abuse to support a sabbatical at SoRAD to work on the book.

By its very nature an interdisciplinary team of authors drawn from a variety of different countries brings to the task a wide range of scientific material, policy views, and practical experience upon which to build a critical analysis of drug policy. This has made the writing of this book an exciting, challenging, and rewarding process. We hope our readers will learn as much from our journey through the complexities of drug policy as the authors have learned in the making of this volume.

The Authors

Contents

Terms and phrases printed in **bold** are defined in the glossary at the end of the book

Section V **Synthesis and conclusions**

Contributors

Thomas Babor, Ph.D., M.P.H.
Professor and Chairman,
Department of Community Medicine and Health Care,
University of Connecticut School of Medicine, Farmington,
Connecticut,
United States of America

Jonathan Caulkins, Ph.D.
Professor of Operations Research and Public Policy,
Carnegie Mellon University, Heinz College and Qatar Campus
Pittsburgh Pennsylvania,
United States of America and Doha, Qatar

Griffith Edwards, D.M.
Emeritus Professor of Addiction Behaviour,
National Addiction Centre, London,
United Kingdom

Benedikt Fischer, Ph.D.
Professor and CIHR/PHAC Chair in Applied Public Health,
Centre for Applied Research in Mental Health and Addictions (CARMHA),
Faculty of Health Sciences,
Simon Fraser University,
Vancouver, Canada;
Senior Scientist,
Section Public Health and Regulatory Policies,
Centre for Addiction and Mental Health,
Toronto, Canada

David Foxcroft, Ph.D.
Professor of Community Psychology and Public Health,
Oxford Brookes University,
Oxford, United Kingdom

Keith Humphreys, Ph.D.
Research Career Scientist, Department of Veterans Affairs and Professor of Psychiatry, Stanford University,
Palo Alto, California,
United States of America

Isidore Obot, Ph.D., M.P.H.
Professor of Psychology,
University of Uyo;
Director, Centre for Research and Information on Substance Abuse (CRISA), Uyo,
Akwa Ibom State, Nigeria

Jürgen Rehm, Ph.D.
Senior Scientist and Co-Head,
Section Public Health and Regulatory Policies,
Centre for Addiction and Mental Health,
Toronto, Canada;
Professor and Chair, Addiction Policy,
Dalla Lana School of Public Health,
University of Toronto,
Toronto, Canada

Peter Reuter, Ph.D.
Professor, School of Public Policy and Department of Criminology,
University of Maryland,
College Park, Maryland,
United States of America

Robin Room, Ph.D.
Professor, School of Population Health,
University of Melbourne,
Melbourne, Australia; Director,
AER Centre for Alcohol Policy Research,
Turning Point Alcohol and
Drug Centre, Fitzroy, Australia;
Professor, Centre for Social
Research on Alcohol and Drugs,
Stockholm University,
Stockholm, Sweden

Ingeborg Rossow, Ph.D.
Research Director,
Norwegian Institute for Alcohol and
Drug Research,
Oslo, Norway

John Strang, M.D.
Professor of the Addictions & Director,
National Addiction Centre,
Kings Health Partners (Institute of
Psychiatry and the Maudsley),
London, United Kingdom

Section I

Introduction

Chapter 1

Framing the issues

1.1 Introduction

An old saying holds that you can't judge a book by its cover. We hope the reader takes this dictum seriously because the simplicity of our title, *Drug Policy and the Public Good*, belies a set of complex truths about global trends in illicit drug use. The use of psychoactive drugs for non-medical reasons is commonplace in many parts of the world, despite the best efforts of policymakers, government officials, public health advocates, and concerned citizens to prevent, eliminate, or control it. If the last century's experience with drugs can serve as a guide, in the future many countries will face periodic drug use epidemics followed by aggressive policy responses to suppress them. In many other countries, continued 'endemic' drug use (i.e. regular and widespread) will generate a patchwork of policy responses that never quite keep up with the problem. These policy responses, or, more specifically, the scientific evidence on their impact, constitute the core of this book. We set out to determine first whether drug policy can be informed by scientific evidence and, if so, how evidence-informed policy can serve the public good. Having stated our goal, the remainder of this chapter outlines the territory that we will cover.

1.2 Why drug policy matters

The use of psychoactive substances dates back to the dawn of recorded history, and may well represent a basic neurobiological process that has contributed to human evolution (Hill and Newlin 2002). The use of drug policy is a more recent development that reflects how governments and societies struggle with substances that can induce pleasure and aid the work of medicine, yet also cause enormous harm. Box 1.1 presents examples of the kinds of drug policy issues that have captured the attention of journalists, the public, and government officials, and which will be the subject of this book. Selected from different parts of the world, these vignettes highlight the individual and societal impact of illicit drugs and drug markets, and draw attention to the need for effective policy measures that reduce drug-related violence, disease, and suffering. They also suggest that policies designed to ameliorate drug-related problems can have unintended consequences that are as serious as the problems they are designed to solve.

Despite the pessimistic picture portrayed in these vignettes, glimmers of hope come from several directions. The examples in Box 1.2 show that when drug policies target specific problems and populations, and when they are informed by sound scientific evidence, they can alter the course of drug use and even drug epidemics. Building on

Box 1.1 Examples of drug policy issues that are the subject of this book

Las Pedras, Puerto Rico. On this Caribbean island located midway between the USA and the heroin- and cocaine-producing countries of South America, about 20% of the drugs in transit remain on the island as a side effect of the trade, 'spawning bloody turf battles, death and addiction'. As described in a news article, a 5-year-old child was killed in 2005 as a result of a gun battle between rival gangs. Also wounded was the target of the attack, a drug dealer at the same housing complex, who had run into an apartment full of children to escape from his rivals (Brown 2005).

Vientiane, Laos. The opium poppy has long bloomed across the mountains of northern Laos, but since 2000 there has been an estimated 73% reduction in opium production, following the implementation of a new programme supported by the United Nations Office for Drugs and Crime. The programme involved the displacement of an estimated 65 000 hill tribe people from the mountains, resulting in increased mortality rates from malaria and dysentery, and greater exposure of the young to 'ya ba' (amphetamines) and heroin, which come across the border from laboratories in neighbouring Burma (Fawthrop 2005).

The Netherlands. In this small European country, the sale and use of smoked cannabis has been de-criminalized since the late 1990s to the point where hundreds of cannabis 'coffee houses' have been allowed to sell cannabis products openly for personal use and consumption on the premises (MacCoun and Reuter 2001a). Although there has been no apparent increase in the prevalence of youth cannabis use, there have been reports of cross-border smuggling into neighbouring countries and of organized crime becoming involved in the cultivation and supply of cannabis. Drug tourism has also emerged, increasing petty crime in Dutch cities. This has aroused community hostility to the coffee house programme.

the cumulative research base relevant to drug policy and the growing capacity to use modern epidemiological methods to monitor drug use trends, the present book examines the extent to which drug policy can be informed by scientific research at the local, national, and international levels.

1.3 What we mean by the term drug policy

As later chapters will elaborate, drug policy as a field of government activity is over a century old. Today governments around the world have developed a variety of laws and programmes intended to influence whether or not individuals decide to use psychoactive substances and to affect the consequences of use for both the individual and the community. That set of laws and programmes constitutes the drug policy of a given nation (Kleiman 1992; Longshore *et al.* 1998). The laws typically prohibit or regulate the possession, use, distribution, and production of these substances and set

Box 1.2 Examples of successful drug policies targeted at specific problems and populations

During the 1950s, Sweden experienced an epidemic of stimulant misuse related to the ready availability of a prescription diet drug called Preludin. The imposition of strict government controls over prescribing practices, combined with restrictions on illegal imports and changing attitudes toward drug use, eventually led to an abatement of the crisis (Edwards 2004).

Facing widespread heroin use in the 1990s, the French government introduced on a large scale a network of treatment programmes that provide synthetic substitutes for heroin (e.g. buprenorphine). Nationwide heroin arrests declined by 75%, as did drug-related deaths, as over 100 000 people enrolled in the treatment programmes (Emmanuelli and Desenclos 2005). There were a comparatively small number of overdose deaths from diverted methadone and buprenorphine (17 cases in 1998; see Auriacombe *et al.* 2001).

In the 1990s, several regions of the USA saw dramatic increases in the use of methamphetamine, a synthetic stimulant produced in small laboratories using materials available from pharmacies and other legal suppliers. Governmental regulatory policies directed at the control of materials used in the fabrication of methamphetamine (drug precursors) contributed to a sharp reduction in hospital admissions and related indicators of harm (Cunningham and Liu 2003).

penalties for violations of prohibitions. The programmes include efforts to persuade children not to try the substances, help heavy users either to stop drug use or to use drugs in less dangerous ways, and discourage producers from making and distributing drugs. They also attempt to control the medical prescription of certain drugs, with penalties for any breach of regulation.

Drug control programmes occur in many different government sectors, including schools, communities, health care, policing, and border control (Reuter 2006). A country's Ministry of Education might provide funds for primary school teachers to deliver drug prevention classes, whereas its Ministry of Health might fund methadone maintenance clinics for heroin-dependent patients. These programmes are frequently embedded in services with broader goals. For example, programmes to improve access to mental health services often benefit people with drug problems, who might be a small fraction of those who use the services. Similarly, increased police patrols, aimed at improving the safety of a neighbourhood, might shift the location of street drug markets to other areas of the city, or to more discreet settings, which in turn could change the need for programmes and services.

Contemporary drug policy therefore constitutes a broad range of administrative actions. These actions comprise three areas, each of which will be covered in this volume: (1) programmes to prevent the initiation of drug use by non-users; (2) health and social service programmes intended to help heavy drug users change their behaviour or reduce the consequences of their drug use; and (3) laws, regulations, and initiatives to control the supply of illegal drugs (as well as the supply of diverted prescription drugs used for non-medical purposes). The latter category typically differs from the other two by having an international as well as a domestic component.

We restrict our review of drug policy to the general area of governmental activity and do not include efforts by individual citizens or organizations, although these may also affect drug use and its consequences. What employers spend on Employee Assistance Programmes to counsel workers with drug problems or what citizen groups do to urge children in their communities to stay away from drugs may have important effects, and actions by the government may either stimulate or hinder these initiatives. However, for analytical purposes, it is useful to restrict the term *drug policy* to the public sector and to view non-governmental organizations either as independent forces or as intervening variables between government policy and the desired outcomes. Our definition of drug policy must be qualified by the fact that in most countries the non-medical use of many psychoactive substances is illegal, thereby denying government the ability to use the policy levers such as regulation and taxation of suppliers that are available for legal substances such as alcohol and tobacco. Finally, drug policy may include government sponsorship of scientific research, programme evaluations, and monitoring initiatives. These activities have grown substantially in the past 25 years as part of the policy response to drug-related problems in many industrialized countries, and will be considered in this book as a part of a long-term solution.

1.4 The need for a global, evidence-informed approach

There are four reasons why a busy policymaker, the general reader, or the less actively involved student of drug policy should invest precious time in perusal of this volume.

The international scope of the book. Drug policy is a complex entity inherently shaped by both national and international trends. The growing globalization of trade, technology, travel, and even criminal activities creates a need to approach drug policy at both levels. Although many high-quality policy books take a single country as their focus, this book attempts to place local and national perspectives in an international context.

The nature of the authorial team. Our use of an international team of authors brings to the task a variety of disciplinary orientations and cultural backgrounds, and increases the range of scientific material upon which the book draws. The team is also unusual because it includes both individuals who have made careers studying drug policy and those who have worked in the development or execution of governmental drug policy. Finally, unlike most drug policy books, the authors here span a wide spectrum of policy views, which we hope will make the book even-handed and of interest to a wide audience.

The focus on evidence. Public policy often does not take into account the scientific evidence available on the nature of the problem being addressed and the likely impact of various interventions. While we do not minimize the right of individual citizens and policymakers to base drug policy on their moral and cultural values, this book offers scientific evidence as an added consideration in the formulation of drug policy. We have reviewed literature from numerous fields including history, epidemiology, psychiatry, psychology, economics, criminology, political studies, and sociology to draw conclusions for policymakers attempting to use different policy levers to produce particular effects.

A 'public good' perspective. To speak of policy is implicitly to ask the question: 'Policy for whom and for what?' Without meaning to appear lofty, we focus our discussion in this book on the 'public good', a concept that comprises public health but is not limited to it. Unlike clinical medicine, which focuses on the cure of diseases in individual cases, one patient at a time, public health is a specialized field of knowledge committed to the management and prevention of adverse health conditions in groups of people, formally termed 'populations'. The value of a population perspective lies in its ability to suggest appropriate interventions that are most likely to benefit large numbers of people at the level of a community or a country. The concept of population assumes that groups of people exhibit certain commonalities by virtue of their shared characteristics (e.g. age, gender), shared environment (e.g. neighbourhood, city, nation), or shared activities (e.g. injection drug use, sex work), and those commonalities increase their risk of disease and disability (Fos and Fine 2000).

Why are these public health concepts important to the discussion of drug policy? During the 20th century public health measures have had a remarkable effect on the health of populations throughout the world. Life expectancy has increased dramatically during this period, owing in large part to the application of public health measures designed to improve sanitation, reduce environmental pollution, and prevent communicable and infectious diseases (WHO 1998). However, even as epidemics of infectious and communicable diseases have receded, health risks associated with lifestyle behaviours and chronic diseases have increased in importance as major causes of mortality, injury, disease, and disability. When policymakers use population approaches instead of, or in conjunction with, individually oriented medical and criminal justice approaches, the overall effects on health, disease, and even social problems are likely to be much more pronounced. As this book will show, public health concepts provide an important vehicle to manage the health of populations in relation to the use of psychoactive substances, partly because these interventions emphasize the need to change the environment as well as individual behaviour.

A public good perspective embraces public health but also goes beyond it. Indeed, a pure public health approach has significant limitations. As has been noted by public policy scholars (e.g. Cook *et al.* 2002), societies do not weigh social problems solely on the basis of public health indicators. For example, when someone is killed in a gun battle between a drug dealer and the police force, people assess the impact of and appropriate response to the death differently depending on whether the person killed was the drug dealer, a police officer, or a bystander. But in a strict public health framework, a death is a death. Another limit of a pure public health approach is that the damage of drug use does not always become apparent in health statistics. When a child comes home from school with friends to find his mother unconscious from drug use, that child's anxiety, sadness, and humiliation may never result in a diagnosable medical illness. Yet most people would concede that the child's suffering has some meaning and importance. Likewise, in a drug-motivated mugging in which no one is injured, the anger and sense of injustice experienced by the victims may warrant a policy response despite the lack of injury. Finally, there may be societies in which belief in individual liberty from government interference is so deeply valued that substantial health harm seems a reasonable price to pay for it.

The views expressed in this book are therefore heavily informed by public health concerns without being limited to them or, even worse, implicitly asserting that health harm is all that a society *should* care about. The idea that societies have every right to care about matters other than health is uncomfortable for some public health purists. But to the authors of this book, concerns about justice, freedom, morality, and other issues beyond the health domain have an important place in drug policy formation and should not be ignored by public health experts.

1.5 **Evidence-informed drug policy. What is it? Is it possible?**

Although most scientific research has policy implications, it was not until the 1970s that scientific investigators began systematically to evaluate specific prevention, treatment, and enforcement policies in the area of illicit psychoactive substances. Chapters 2, 3, and 4 will show that researchers have applied the science of epidemiology with increasing sophistication to study the prevalence of drug use, the distribution of drug problems across population groups, and the underlying causal influences that account for substance use. Current epidemiological research methods, particularly social surveys and the monitoring of vital statistics (called *disease surveillance*), make it possible to estimate the prevalence of drug use with reasonable accuracy, and to describe trends in drug use and drug problems. In addition to the expansion in epidemiological research tools, the necessary infrastructure has grown to support an international cadre of policy researchers focusing on the problems associated with psychoactive drugs (Edwards 2002; Babor *et al.* 2008b). That growth is illustrated by the increasing numbers of addiction specialty journals, career professionals, specialized research centres, and scientific publications relevant to drug policy.

All of these developments make it possible to create a scientific evidence base for the evaluation and implementation of drug policy. As noted in Chapter 7, a variety of scientific methods is available to investigate the effects of different intervention strategies. Saltz (2005) has characterized these methods as falling into three broad categories:

1 Natural experiments: studies of variations in environmental forces, such as the initiation of a new drug enforcement programme, in relation to changes in drug use or its consequences within a population.

2 Efficacy studies: evaluations of interventions that are directly or partially controlled by the investigator, with appropriate comparison groups to account for natural changes over time.

3 Effectiveness research: studies of the effectiveness of a particular intervention in natural settings.

In addition to these general research approaches, researchers have also investigated the effects of drug policies using the methods of historical analysis, economics, sociology, and ethnography (Thoumi 2003; MacCoun and Reuter 2001a). Given the variety of methods available for policy evaluation and analysis, we answer affirmatively the question of whether science can inform the development of drug policy.

We cannot stress strongly enough that the term *evidence-informed* leaves ample room for many other forces to affect public policy. Democratic processes (e.g. voting), religious values, cultural norms, and social traditions can and should affect how societies respond to harmful drug use. Consideration of the scientific evidence rules out none of these other factors, nor is it intended to.

1.6 **A note on terminology**

The choice of words is an important part of communication. Terms that are familiar and colloquial, such as *addict* and *addiction*, lack precision and can be used in diverse and sometimes pejorative ways, promoting miscommunication. Terms such as *psychoactive substance*, on the other hand, may seem overly technical or, worse, represent obscure academic jargon. The authors have attempted to strike a balance between the economy of familiar terms and the precision of science.

Here is what we mean by the most important terms the reader will encounter in this book. Other terms indicated in bold throughout the book are defined as well in the Glossary at the end. The term *psychoactive drug* (or *drug*, for the sake of economy) refers to a substance capable of influencing brain systems linked to reward and pleasure. In general, we use it to mean substances controlled or prohibited by legal regulations, otherwise know as illicit drugs. This definition covers both diverted pharmaceutical agents that may have therapeutic value, such as pain medications, as well as the more common substances prohibited in most countries, such as heroin, cocaine, and cannabis. We use the term *drug use* because it is transparent, neutral, and free of moral judgement: it covers drug taking, of which society may approve or disapprove. Similarly, we use the terms *drug misuse* or *problematic drug use* to describe the point at which psychoactive substances cause problems for the user or for society. We favour these terms over the more familiar term *drug abuse*, which may convey pejorative meanings, because our main purpose is to distinguish use that is relatively free of consequences for a given individual (as when a pain medication is taken as prescribed) from use that causes social, psychological, or medical problems. In other words, drug misuse is synonymous with harmful use.

Another important term, *drug dependence*, refers to a psychobiological syndrome characterized by impaired control of drug use, an acquired ability to tolerate large amounts of the drug, continued drug use in the presence of adverse personal consequences, and the experience of withdrawal symptoms when drug use is stopped. *Drug dependence* has now replaced the term *drug addiction* in formal medical diagnostic terminology. We use the term *drug-related problems* when referring to the social, legal, psychological, and medical consequences frequently associated with use of psychoactive substances.

Finally, whenever we employ drug-related terms in this book, the reader should assume that we are not referring to alcohol or nicotine. Although these psychoactive substances have the potential to cause as much harm to individuals and society as illicit drugs, their legality in most societies creates a major contrast from a policy perspective. For reasons of convenience as well as consistency, we do not deal with these other psychoactive substances except for some important comparisons drawn in Chapter 2.

We do, however, give considerable attention in this book to psychoactive medications, which are typically available in industrial societies only with a doctor's prescription. As we shall discuss, the international drug control system has two aims: to suppress illicit drug markets and to ensure the availability of psychoactive medications for medical use. Though the prescription system strives to keep the market for medications separate from the markets for illicit drugs, there are many points of overlap and considerable blurring of the boundaries between the two markets. It is thus increasingly necessary to take psychoactive medications into consideration when considering policy concerning illicit drugs.

1.7 The structure of this book

The chapters in the first section ('Introduction') provide a conceptual overview of the ways in which illicit drugs can be understood from a public health perspective. The chapters in the second section ('Drug Epidemiology and Drug Markets') describe the extent of drug use throughout the world, significant trends in drug epidemics, and the global burden of disease and disability attributable to drug misuse. This section also includes two chapters on the nature of the drug markets that produce drugs and distribute them as economic commodities. After a brief overview of the rules of evidence necessary to evaluate the scientific basis of drug policy, the third section ('The Evidence Base for Drug Policy') describes the research supporting different strategies and interventions that are part of the policy response to drug use in many countries. These include school-based prevention programmes; attempts to control the supply of drugs; criminal sanctions applied to drug users and drug sellers; health, rehabilitation, and social services for heavy drug users; and ways to prevent diversion of prescription drugs to illicit use. The fourth section ('Drug Policy and System Issues at the National and International Levels') covers three topics: the history, function, and effectiveness of international drug control treaties; the nature and consequences of drug policy variations among countries; and how health, rehabilitation, and social service systems for drug users can be organized to impact population rates of drug problems. The final section ('Synthesis and Conclusions') summarizes the main themes of the book and draws conclusions about the impact of various drug policy options.

1.8 Conclusion

If, as we stated at the outset, you can't judge a book by its cover, how should you judge it? We believe that any review of drug policy should evaluate what it is, how it works, and whether it is effective. The analysis should also discuss why we need drug policy, which is where we begin the scientific part of this book, and what science can tell us that will serve the public good, which is where we end our book. By including a scientific perspective and public health concepts in our analysis of the connection between drug policy and the public good, we challenge the reader to join our search for effective drug policy.

Chapter 2

Matters of substance

2.1 Introduction

Psychoactive substances have assumed increasing public attention in most parts of the world, especially when they are defined broadly to include alcohol, tobacco, illicit drugs, and certain types of legal pharmaceutical agents that have high **dependence potential**. The effects these substances have on individuals and society depend on a variety of factors, including the pharmacological properties of each drug, the way the drugs are ingested, their cultural meanings in everyday life, the reasons for using them, and the harms associated with their misuse. Public discussion of drug policies has too often failed to take these complexities into account. Simplistic views that all drugs are the same and all are equally dangerous not only limit our understanding of drug-related problems but also impair our ability to develop meaningful policy responses. Advances in psychiatry, psychology, neurobiology, cultural anthropology, epidemiology, and a variety of other disciplines have substantially increased our understanding of psychoactive drugs, drug actions, and **drug misuse**. In this chapter we address these fundamental 'matters of substance' in order to set the stage for the chapters to follow.

In this book, we will focus on many, but not all, of the commonly used psychoactive substances, specifically opioids, cannabis, cocaine, hypnotics, sedatives, hallucinogens, psychoactive inhalants, as well as amphetamines and other stimulants. We also give special attention to the misuse of psychoactive substances that are marketed legally under prescription regimes, such as opioid analgesics ('pain killers'), stimulants, and barbiturates. Table 2.1 provides definitions of these substances along with their pharmacological effects.

2.2 Three distinctions

To appreciate the complex nature of drug use as well as the public policy issues associated with different psychoactive substances, three distinctions must be made. The first distinction is whether a particular drug is natural or synthetic. Until the 19th century, almost all of the psychoactive substances were used in their natural form. With the advent of modern chemistry, the active components of these natural products could be identified, and this knowledge led to the production of potent extracts, such as morphine and cocaine. Thereafter, it became possible to create synthetic forms of many psychoactive substances, such as heroin and crack cocaine, and to produce new or more potent substances, such as lysergic acid diethylamide (LSD), the benzodiazepines, and the opioids. As in the case of distilled spirits, the ability to produce

Table 2.1 A compendium of psychoactive substances and their pharmacological effects

Drug class	Related substances	Pharmacological effects
Opioids	Heroin, morphine, codeine, methadone, pethidine, buprenorphine	The generic term applied to alkaloids from the opium poppy, or similar synthetic substances, which have the capacity to relieve pain, produce euphoria, and induce respiratory depression, drowsiness, and impaired judgement.
Cannabis	Hashish, THC, marijuana, bhang, ganja	A derivation of the plant, *Cannabis sativa*. Intoxication produces feelings of euphoria, lightness of limbs, increased appetite, tachycardia, and impaired judgement.
Cocaine	Crack, rock	Feelings of elation, exaggerated feelings of confidence. Acute toxic reactions include hypertension, cardiac arrhythmias, auditory and visual hallucinations, seizures.
Amphetamines/ other stimulants	Dexamphetamine, metamphetamine, methylphenidate, phenmetrazine, diethylpropion	A diverse group of synthetic substances whose effects include euphoria, anorexia, nausea, vomiting, insomnia, and abnormal behavior such as aggression, grandiosity, hyper-vigilance, agitation, and impaired judgment.
Hypnotics/sedatives	Benzodiazepines, barbiturates, methaqualone	A group of substances that induce muscle relaxation, calmness, and sleep.Impairs concentration, memory, and coordination. Other effects include slurred speech, drowsiness, unsteady gate.
Hallucinogens	Lysergide (LSD), dimethyltriptamine (DMT), psilocybin, mescaline, MDMA, phencyclidine	A group of natural and synthetic substances that produce feelings of euphoria/dysphoria, mixed mood changes, altered perceptions, and visual illusions. Adverse effects include panic reactions, flashbacks, and mood disorders.
Psychoactive inhalants	Industrial solvents, glue, aerosol, paints, lacquer thinners, petrol, cleaning fluids, amyl nitrite	Signs of intoxication include belligerence, hallucinations, lethargy, psychomotor impairment, euphoria, impaired judgement, dizziness, nystagmus, slurred speech, tremors, muscle weakness, unsteady gate, stupor, coma.

Source: Babor *et al.* (1994).

highly concentrated forms of natural substances greatly increased their portability and dependence potential.

Another important distinction about psychoactive substances relates to the way in which they are ingested. There are four common ways to ingest drugs: (1) through the mouth in the form of natural substances (e.g. coca leaves) or synthetic products (e.g. pain medications); (2) insufflated across mucous membranes, as when cocaine powder is snorted; (3) through inhalation, as with crack vapour and cannabis; and (4) through injection, as with heroin. Drugs that can be injected into the bloodstream provide rapid delivery, which greatly increases their potential abuse, dependence, and harm.

The third distinction is whether or not a psychoactive substance has an accepted use as medicine. Many of the substances listed in Table 2.1 (e.g. sedatives and opioids) were developed for medicinal purposes and are now restricted in most countries for use only under a prescription system. Some remain available as accepted medicines, but with controls (e.g. morphine, amphetamines and barbiturates); others are no longer regarded as medicine despite their original development (e.g. LSD, cocaine, and heroin in most countries). As described in Chapters 3 and 6, substances with medicinal applications have subsequently been used for purposes and in ways other than stated in the doctor's prescription, or are used in amounts larger than recommended on the medication label. In these cases their use may present the risk of physical, psychological, and even legal problems, which concern those who are interested in drug policy.

Despite the medicinal value of some psychoactive substances, and the social and recreational uses of others, government policies ban many such substances and impose penalties on the user. Throughout history, but particularly since the late 19th century, national governments and local jurisdictions have regulated or prohibited the use, manufacture, and sale of various psychoactive substances, with heroin, cocaine, and cannabis among the most notable examples. At the international level, treaties developed within the framework of the United Nations and the **World Health Organization** coordinate the control of different psychoactive substances. These 'drug control conventions', discussed in more detail in Chapter 13, are designed to prevent diversion of pharmaceutical drugs into illegal markets, combat drug trafficking, and tailor controls to the pharmacological properties and dependence potential of each substance. As noted in later parts of this chapter, the classification of substances within the international conventions reflects historical circumstances and cultural factors as well as scientific evidence. For these reasons, international treaties and national laws may not always be consistent with expert opinion and the scientific evidence regarding the danger or harm associated with a particular substance. For example, many experts consider tobacco products to present greater risk of harm than cannabis, yet the former substance is legal in most countries while the latter is not.

These distinctions are necessary but not sufficient to understand the complex nature of drug use. In subsequent chapters we will also consider the diversity, role, and specific risks of different consumption patterns as well as the effects of drug combinations (e.g. for overdose), of situational risks (e.g. driving home after an exhausting club night, being tired after consuming stimulants), and of behavioural risk taking (e.g. unprotected sex during the high after cocaine use).

2.3 Symbolic meanings and use patterns

The use or non-use of psychoactive substances, and the manner, amount, and type of use, have carried strong symbolic meanings throughout human history. In many traditional cultures, psychoactive substances were intrinsic to medicinal practice and religious ritual. This amounts to saying that in the appropriate cultural context—and particularly in many tribal and village societies—psychoactive substances are involved in matters of life and death and the deep meaning of existence. In such circumstances, the symbolic power of psychoactive substances is very strong.

At the opposite extreme, when a drug becomes a regular accompaniment to everyday life, its psychoactivity is often muted and may even go unnoticed. This is illustrated in recent industrial societies' use of tobacco. Forty years ago, a habitual smoker might well not have regarded cigarettes as psychoactive at all. This pattern of 'banalized use', in which a potentially powerful psychoactive agent is domesticated into a mundane article of daily life, occurs when a drug becomes freely available on the consumer market. The symbolism of the substance as a drug is muted but the drug often retains other symbolic associations. For instance, marijuana became a symbol of rebellion in the 1960s, and a thoroughly accepted substance like coca leaves in the Andean countries of South America seems now to symbolize opposition to US influence (Thoumi 2003).

In between banalized use on the one hand, and use that is restricted to medical or religious purposes on the other, lie a range of secular and non-medical use patterns. Use on any occasion may be light, or heavy, or mixed, and there is great variation also in frequency of use. Intermittent use, for instance only at festivals or on weekends, minimizes the build-up of tolerance to the drug. The drug may be understood by both the user and others as having taken over control of the user's behaviour, and thus explains otherwise unexpected behaviour, whether bad or good. According to this view, normal self-control is expected to return when the effects of the drug have worn off. Given the power attributed to the substance, traditional societies may limit access to it via social conventions; industrial societies by legal restrictions.

Cultural attitudes towards different psychoactive substances have varied greatly from one time or place to another (Courtwright 2001), and their symbolic significance has varied at least as much. What is it about the use of psychoactive substances that makes them so symbolically powerful? There are several answers to this question.

First, psychoactive substances are valued physical goods. Their status as physical goods renders them subject to commodification and, indeed, globalization in use and trade (see Chapter 5 for more discussion of this). Given their positive valuation, the possession and use of psychoactive substances is often a symbol of power and domination (Morgan 1983), or at least of access to resources beyond subsistence.

Secondly, the use of psychoactive substances is a behaviour, and very often a social behaviour with strong symbolic value. Social use of substances often serves to demarcate the boundaries of inclusion and exclusion in a social group (Room 1975). The following self-description from a 23-year-old female heroin user illustrates these points:

> I tell you, I grew up as no one, an abused child, dirt. When I became a heroin addict then I became someone. Being an addict, you're important, feels good, yes. ...You tell a bloke

> and it's like saying to him, 'Oh I've got this important job'. Respect, sort of, and the drug gives you mates who are doing the same thing, all one big club.
>
> (Quoted from Edwards 2004, xxiii)

Thirdly, psychoactive substances have the power to change behaviour, mood, motor coordination, and judgement (Room 2001). This quality is both positively valued and feared, and even the terms used regarding the substances often have a double edge. The words *drug* and *intoxication* have both positive and negative connotations, depending on the context. In many cultural circumstances, people value intoxication positively, as a recreational or social experience, and English and other languages are extraordinarily rich in symbolic language to describe intoxicated states (Levine 1981).

On the other hand, people may regard behaviour when intoxicated as unpredictable and potentially dangerous. The effect of the substance is seen as making the intoxicated person less amenable to reason, to social norms, and to laws. These expectations, and people's behaviour while under the influence of the substance, vary among cultures (MacAndrew and Edgerton 1969).

Fourthly, psychoactive substances are seen as potentially causing addiction or, to use the current technical term, dependence. The core meaning of dependence states that the user has lost the ability to control whether and how much of the substance he or she uses (Edwards *et al.* 1981). In the ordinary understanding of dependence, there is also a second, associated loss of control over one's life—that the user's life has 'become unmanageable', in the words of the First Step of Narcotics Anonymous.

There are, then, multiple properties of psychoactive substances underlying their symbolic power. This power finds expression in the everyday lives of drug users, in the symbolism of tobacco and alcohol advertisements, in how the user behaves during and after ingesting a drug, in what others expect from a drug user, and in how that person's actions during and after using are evaluated. The symbolic powers of psychoactive substances also make them a prime arena for political action. Political movements for psychoactive substance control rely heavily on symbolism. The nascent Communist regime in China in the 1940s and 1950s attained extraordinary success, at least for a generation, in its campaign against opium use because the campaign symbolized the struggle against colonial repression and humiliation (Yongming 2000). In the Cold War era, international narcotics control and the 'war on drugs' became an arena in which Eastern and Western blocs could reach some consensus on denunciations of drugs as a global 'scourge' (Room 1999). A discussion of drug policy therefore cannot focus only on a rational consideration of social engineering; it must also recognize the symbolic dimension (Christie and Bruun 1996; Room 2005b).

2.4 Why people use drugs

It is easy to understand the appeal of drugs. As noted above, what distinguishes psychoactive drugs from other medicinal and nutritional substances is their powerful ability to act on brain mechanisms that affect motivation, thinking, mood, and, perhaps most importantly, the experience of pleasure.

This last characteristic is linked to a fundamental aspect of human behaviour and learning, called reinforcement. One of the major advances in the understanding of drug use comes from research on the social, psychological, and biological mechanisms involved in drug reinforcement (WHO 2004). On the biological level, the immediate psychoactive and rewarding effects of different substances, particularly their ability to give pleasure and relieve pain, help to explain why animals and humans will repeatedly self-administer drugs despite their negative consequences. Although substances differ with respect to the particular types of neural receptors and neurotransmitters they affect in the brain, there are considerable similarities among them (WHO 2004). The neural pathways stimulated by these substances are the same ones affected by other pleasurable behaviours, such as eating a good meal or engaging in sexual activity. Combined with the social reinforcement that drugs provide because of their learned symbolic value, psychoactive substances are especially attractive to young people during the formative period of their growth and development.

Beyond the neurobiological and sociocultural factors involved in drug use, recent advances in psychological research and genetic epidemiology have identified several important mechanisms that help to explain why humans initiate and continue to use these substances. Genetic predisposition and broader familial influences (Merikangas *et al.* 1998b; Agrawal and Lynskey 2006) may increase the risk for some individuals, as do certain personal characteristics such as risk taking, impulsivity, and aggressiveness (Chassin and Ritter 2001). Learning disabilities may lead some adolescents to become discouraged with conventional educational achievement, to be attracted to deviant and drug-using peers, and to experience more intense psychoactive effects from drugs (Lynskey and Hall 2001). The associations among these familial, behavioural, and dispositional factors have led some researchers (King *et al.* 2009) to postulate a general core vulnerability to develop drug-related problems called behavioural disinhibition.

Although drug use is more prevalent among young people who have these risk factors, it is never inevitable. Also, the factors that contribute to the initiation of drug use may not be the same as those that lead some individuals to continue drug use (Rhee *et al.* 2003). As discussed below, chronic use and dependence are part of a complex biobehavioural syndrome that differs according to the nature of the substance and the user's personal characteristics.

Finally, we must recognize that availability has enormous implications for the waxing and waning of drug use. Availability refers not only to the supply of drugs (physical availability), but also to their cost (economic availability), their attractiveness (psychological availability), and their social acceptance within the user's primary reference groups (social availability). In general, the more a drug is physically available, affordable, attractive as both a reinforcer and a social symbol, and accepted by an individual's peers, the more likely it is that it will invite experimentation and continued use.

2.5 **Mechanisms of harm**

It is well known that the use of psychoactive substances involves considerable risk of harm to drug users and to those around them. The risks vary according to the nature of the substance and the pattern of use (i.e. amount and frequency of use), amongst other things.

Figure 2.1 illustrates how different consequences of drug use are associated with drug dose, drug use patterns, and mode of drug administration. Three putative mechanisms of action are shown to account for these associations: (1) toxic and other biochemical effects of drugs; (2) psychoactive actions resulting in intoxication; and (3) dependence.

The figure shows that harm can result from three aspects of drug use: dose, pattern, and route of administration. The first aspect, dosage of the drug, ranges from barely intoxicating to lethal, and is often related to the 'purity' of the drug at the time it is sold. In general, the greater the amount taken on a specific occasion, the more likely the user is to experience acute effects, such as intoxication and overdose. And the greater the amount over time, the more the user is likely to experience toxic effects. The second cause of harm is the pattern of use. Pattern of use refers to the frequency and variability of drug taking. Some people use drugs intermittently, such as on weekends or special occasions, while others use them every day. The third aspect, route of administration, refers to the way in which the drug is ingested, i.e. whether it is smoked, swallowed, snorted, injected, or taken in some other way.

The route and patterns of drug use are related to harm in several ways. First, the amount of a drug ingested on a given occasion can exceed the individual's tolerance level, leading to overdose and possibly death. Secondly, a steady pattern of use, such as daily cannabis smoking, can lead to chronic effects, such as lung disease. In addition to the drug's specific toxic effects, it may also cause problems because of its ability to alter consciousness and impair the user's judgement or psychomotor coordination. The intoxicating effect of a drug, particularly at higher doses, can contribute to

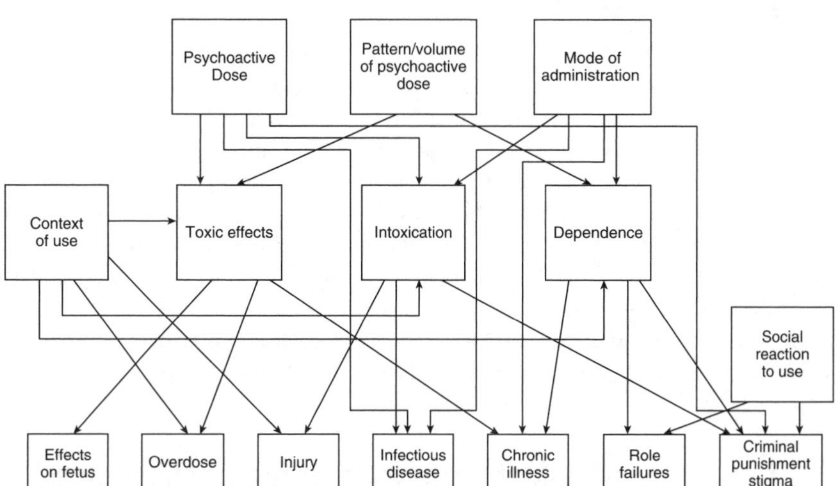

Fig. 2.1 How toxic effects, intoxication, and dependence are related to drug dose, use patterns, and mode of drug administration, and in turn mediate the consequences of drug use for the individual drug user.

injuries, panic reactions, disorientation, violence, and a variety of other medical and psychiatric problems.

2.6 Dependence

One mechanism that contributes to both acute and chronic effects of repeated drug use is dependence, a psychobiological syndrome defined within the International Classification of Diseases (ICD-10). The criteria for substance dependence in ICD-10 include a strong desire to take the substance, difficulties in controlling the onset or termination of use, a physiological withdrawal state after a period of non-use, increased tolerance to the drug's effects, progressive neglect of alternative pleasures or interests in favour of drug use, and persistence of use despite harmful consequences (WHO 1992).

Neurobiological and behavioural research (WHO 2004) has identified a number of biobehavioural processes underlying dependence, including the release of the neurotransmitter dopamine in the nucleus accumbens region of the brain. By activating emotional and motivational centres of the brain, the drug becomes associated with pleasurable feelings, positive attitudes, and focused attention, all of which increase the likelihood that the user will repeat the experience. With repeated exposure, compulsive drug seeking and craving are elicited by the sight, thought, or anticipation of the drug, resulting in a pronounced preoccupation with the substance to the neglect of other important aspects of living, such as family, work, and health.

These general principles of drug dependence do not apply equally to all psychoactive substances, in part because of their differing pharmacological properties. For example, drug dependence does not seem to develop for hallucinogens (WHO 1992; Edwards 2004), and the withdrawal symptoms that precipitate drug self-administration differ according to the drug.

2.7 The influence of context

A drug's toxicity, intoxicating effect, and even dependence potential can be affected by contextual factors such as the set (expectations) and setting in which the drug is used. In a stimulating and supportive setting, for example, LSD may produce enjoyable perceptual experiences, whereas the same drug can produce a panic reaction in an unfamiliar setting or a paranoid reaction in a threatening setting (Edwards 2004).

Thus far we have only described the mechanisms of use-related harms. As noted at the bottom right of Figure 2.1, social reactions to drug use (response-related harms) can also affect the consequences experienced by users. Criminal justice punishment and its associated stigma are a function of societal reactions, not the drug itself. Role failure, such as unemployment and divorce, can result from both the drug itself and society's reaction to drug use. As discussed below, these kinds of harms may be low for tobacco, moderate for cannabis, and quite large for cocaine and heroin.

2.8 The extent of risk or harm from different substances

An important question for public policy is the extent of risk or harm resulting from the use of different substances. Implicit in the development of prevention strategies and intervention programmes is the notion that some drugs are more risky or harmful than others, and as such require more control, resources, and monitoring. For example, international conventions regarding psychoactive substances are based on expert committee recommendations regarding a drug's 'liability to abuse [constituting] a risk to public health', with the various schedules differentiated in terms of the degree of risk for both social and public health problems (WHO 2000, §41). There have been several attempts to characterize different substances in terms of their relative potential for causing harm, taking into account modifying factors, such as route of administration or context of use, that can increase or reduce the dangers (Best *et al.* 2003).

One approach (Hall *et al.* 1999) compares the severity of effects for heavy users of different substances in their most harmful common form. As shown in Table 2.2, alcohol is considered to have the greatest potential for harm, with tobacco, heroin, and marijuana estimated to have fewer adverse effects on health.

Table 2.3 shows four alternative approaches to the issue of dangerousness. The first column shows the likelihood of an overdose based on estimates of the 'safety ratio' of different substances (Gable 2004). According to this scheme, heroin, alcohol, and cocaine have the lowest safety ratios, whereas marijuana has the highest.

Another dimension of dangerousness is the level of intoxication produced by the substance. As noted in one article on this issue (Hilts 1994), intoxication increases the personal and social damage produced by a substance. Taking into account dose, set, and setting, the ratings shown in the second column of Table 2.3 suggest that alcohol has the highest intoxicating effect, followed by heroin, cocaine, marijuana, and tobacco. The final two columns of Table 2.3 show the results of a more global approach to the same general dimensions as reported by a French expert committee (Roques 1999). The committee rated seven substances on general toxicity and social dangerousness. Toxicity includes long-term health effects (such as cancer and liver disease), infections and other consequences of intravenous use, as well as the acute effects represented by the safety ratio. Social dangerousness focuses on aggressive and uncontrolled conduct induced by or associated with use of the drug.

In general, heroin and alcohol rank relatively high on all four dimensions of dangerousness, with marijuana scoring in the lowest range. The other drugs vary according to the criterion employed, with tobacco ranked high on toxicity and low on social dangerousness.

Another dimension of harmfulness is what psychopharmacologists call dependence potential. This term refers to the propensity of a substance, as a consequence of its pharmacological effects on physiological or psychological functions, to give rise to dependence on that substance. Henningfield and Benowitz (cited in Hilts 1994) made comparative ratings of different substances on withdrawal, tolerance, reinforcement, and dependence. Tobacco was considered to have the highest dependence potential, with heroin, cocaine, alcohol, caffeine, and marijuana following in that order.

One of the most comprehensive attempts to estimate the harm associated with the full range of psychoactive substances (Nutt *et al.* 2007) is based on expert ratings of physical damage, the tendency of the drug to induce dependence, and the effect of drug use on families, communities, and society. Figure 2.2 shows the average

Table 2.2 Adverse effects on health for heavy users of the most harmful common form of each of four drugs

Adverse effects	Marijuana	Tobacco	Heroin	Alcohol
Traffic and other accidents	*		*	**
Violence and suicide				**
Overdose death			**	*
HIV and liver infections			**	*
Liver cirrhosis				**
Heart disease		**		*
Respiratory diseases	*	**		
Cancers	*	**		*
Mental illness	*			**
Dependence/addiction	**	**	**	**
Lasting effects on the foetus	*	*	*	**

** = important effect; * = less common or less well-established effect.

Source: Hall *et al.* (1999).

Table 2.3 Ratings of psychoactive substances on different dimensions of 'dangerousness'

	Safety ratio (Gable 2004)	Intoxicating effect (Hilts 1994)	General toxicity (Roques 1999)	Social dangerousness (Roques 1999)
Marijuana	>1000 sm	4th highest	Very weak	Weak
Benzodiazepins (Valium)	nr	nr	Very weak	Weak (except when driving)
MDMA/Ecstasy	16 or	nr	Possibly very strong	Weak (?)
Stimulants	10 or	nr	Strong	Weak (possible exceptions)
Tobacco	nr	5th highest	Very strong	None
Alcohol	10 or	Highest	Strong	Strong
Cocaine	15 in	3rd highest	Strong	Very strong
Heroin	6 iv	2nd highest	Strong (except therapeutic use of opiates)	Very strong

Mode of administration: nr = not rated; sm = smoked; or = oral; in = intranasal; iv = intravenous.

Safety ratio = (usual effective dose for nonmedical purposes)/(usual lethal dose), using the mode of administration specified.

Source: Room (2005b).

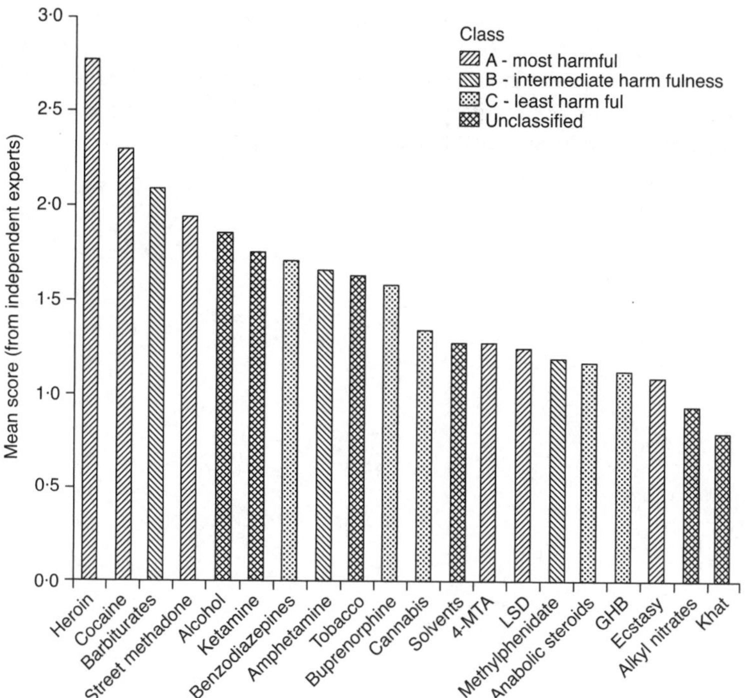

Fig. 2.2 Mean harm scores for 20 psychoactive substances. Classification under the UK Misuse of Drugs Act into three levels of relative harmfulness (class A being the most harmful and class C being the least) is shown by the shading of each bar. Some substances (e.g. khat) are not classified because they were not controlled under the Misuse of Drugs Act. Source: Nutt *et al.* (2007).

harm scores based on all three parameters plotted in rank order for 20 psychoactive substances, both legal and illegal. The results do not support the classification of drugs into high, medium, and low categories of harm currently used as the basis for criminal penalties, policing, prevention, and treatment programmes. While heroin and cocaine rank first and second, alcohol (5) and tobacco (9), both legal substances in most countries, are ranked more harmful than cannabis, solvents, and LSD.

2.9 **Conclusion**

Psychoactive substances vary tremendously in their pharmacological properties, cultural symbolism, and reinforcing effects. Advances in neuroscience and a variety of other disciplines have improved our understanding of how drugs affect brain neurotransmitters, the behaviour of the user, and the adverse consequences of acute as well as chronic use. Rating systems for estimating the dangerousness or risk associated with different substances indicate that legal substances such as tobacco and alcohol are at least as dangerous as many illicit substances. At the same time, the risk associated with each of these substances varies according to the drug's health effects, safety ratio (i.e. lethal dose), intoxicating effect, general toxicity, social dangerousness, dependence potential, the environment/context of use, and social stigma. These considerations suggest that the chemical substance itself, in its pure form, is only one among many factors that determines whether and how much harm occurs. Policies on substance use must reflect the social and pharmacological complexities of psychoactive substances as well as the relative differences among them.

Section II

Drug epidemiology and drug markets

Chapter 3

The international dimensions of drug use

3.1 Introduction

The misuse of psychoactive substances is a global phenomenon, and for a variety of reasons it is important to take a global perspective. No country is immune to the problems associated with the production, trafficking, and use of illicit drugs, although some nations are more affected than others. Countries can learn from one another by studying the growth and decline of drug use. One nation's drug epidemic today could be another nation's drug problem tomorrow. Policymakers especially can benefit from the knowledge and experience gained from other parts of the world, beginning with the growing field of drug epidemiology. Epidemiology is the area of public health research that studies variations in health and disease across population groups, and the causes of these variations according to environmental factors, the 'disease' agent, and the host's characteristics. In the case of drug epidemiology, this chapter will show that significant progress has been made in developing the methodological tools needed to assess variations in **incidence** rates of drug use and **prevalence** trends over time.

As described in Box 3.1, there are considerable challenges to the estimation of illicit drug use in different countries and cultures. Not only is it difficult to find accurate statistics about illicit drug use, but there are also difficulties in using social surveys to ask questions about drugs. First, heavy drug users live very unstable lifestyles, which makes it difficult to find and interview them. Secondly, willingness to report drug use is affected by social intolerance toward drug users, and defensiveness about reporting a stigmatized and illegal behaviour. Thirdly, studies conducted in different countries may use different measurement procedures and methodological approaches, making comparisons difficult or, in some cases, impossible.

Because of these challenges, our knowledge of the epidemiology of drug use is mostly based on studies from Western Europe, North America, and Australia. The limited research in other parts of the world means that a comprehensive perspective on the global dimensions of drug use is necessarily crude. Keeping these considerations in mind, we nevertheless provide a global overview of variations in use and of trends that can serve as a basis for the discussion of drug policies, drawing particularly on estimates by the **United Nations Office on Drugs and Crime (UNODC)**. The prevalence data reported by UNODC are based on various methods and may in many instances be regarded as nothing more than an informed guess (UNODC 2003a).

Box 3.1 Problems with estimating the prevalence of drug use

Prevalence estimates of drug use are typically based on two approaches, each of which has its shortcomings.

1. The estimated proportion of *occasional drug users* in a population is typically based on surveys in general population samples. The estimate may be biased for several reasons. Those who use illicit drugs are less likely to participate in general population surveys, and they may under-report their drug use if they do participate (Rehm *et al.* 2005). This will bias the proportion of occasional users downwards. On the other hand, non-users may for various reasons falsely report drug use, which will bias the proportion upwards (Skog 1992). The uncertainty of the prevalence estimates means that inferences from cross-national comparisons of prevalence rates should be interpreted with caution. Nevertheless, many countries have conducted annual (or frequent) surveys applying the same methodology over time. It is assumed that these surveys provide fairly good indicators of trends in drug use.
2. The number of *problem drug users* in a population is calculated from various data sources, such as mortality statistics, HIV prevalence, treatment admissions, police records, and population surveys. Within a country the prevalence estimate may vary considerably depending on the method applied. The extent to which these methods accurately estimate prevalence varies across countries because of differences in policing practices, provision of treatment services and varying coverage and quality of registers. This means that cross-national comparisons of drug use and drug-related problems need to be made critically and cautiously.

3.2 The current scope of drug use

In 2008, the United Nations estimated that around the globe 208 million people took illicit drugs at least once in the last 12 months, of which 166 million used marijuana and other forms of cannabis, 25 million used amphetamines, and 9 million used ecstasy. Opiate use was estimated at 16.5 million people, of whom some 12 million were taking heroin; 16 million were estimated to be using cocaine (UNODC 2008). As a proportion of the global population, 4% of all adults were estimated to have used cannabis, while the proportion was less than 0.6% for the other drugs.

Cannabis (marijuana and hashish) is thus by far the most popular illicit drug in the world. It was used in 96% of countries that report to the United Nations, followed by opiates (heroin, morphine, and opium) (87%), and derivates from the coca leaf (81%). The use of these natural products is followed by amphetamine-type stimulants (73%), benzodiazepines (69%), various types of solvent inhalants (69%), and hallucinogens (60%) (UNODC 2000).

Consumption of illicit drugs differs significantly among population groups. Whereas a fairly large part of the population may have some experience with illicit drugs, heavy users, who constitute a much smaller fraction of the population, account for a large part of the total consumption. As described in Chapter 2, consumption patterns (e.g. daily or occasional intake), modes of intake (e.g. injection or smoking), and whether more than one substance is taken (i.e. polydrug use), all need to be considered when trying to estimate the health and social risks associated with drug use.

3.3 **Population prevalence estimates**

The UN World Drug Report (UNODC 2008) each year provides for a large number of country-level prevalence estimates for the use of cannabis, opiates, amphetamines, and cocaine. Table 3.1 summarizes these estimates for different world regions according to drug use during the past year. In virtually all countries cannabis is used by a larger fraction of the population than are opiates and amphetamines. The highest prevalence rates are found in the more affluent western industrialized countries. One notable exception to the dominance of cannabis is China, where heroin is the most frequently reported illicit drug (Hao *et al.* 2004).

In many countries a significant proportion of the adult population has had some experience with illicit drugs. For instance, in the USA approximately half of the adult population reports having used illicit drugs (mainly cannabis) at some time (Warner *et al.* 1995; Compton *et al.* 2005b). In the UK and other European countries approximately one-third of the adult population reports having used illicit drugs at some point in their lives (Ramsay and Percy 1997; EMCDDA 2007).

Non-medical use of **pharmaceutical drugs** (i.e. use without or beyond a doctor's prescription) is also of significant concern, although it is not well documented in many countries (Sheridan and Butler 2008). Studies from the USA and Australia show that non-medical use of **psychopharmaceutical** drugs (i.e. medicines with psychoactive

Table 3.1 Annual prevalence of drug use in various world regions in percentage of inhabitants aged 15–64

	Cannabis	Opiates	Of which heroin	Amphetamines	Cocaine
Africa	8.0	0.3	0.2	0.43	0.22
Americas	6.9	0.4	0.3	0.96	1.74
North America	10.5	0.5	0.4	1.27	2.42
South America	3.4	0.3	0.1	0.66	1.05
Asia	2.0	0.4	0.2	0.53	0.01
Europe	5.3	0.7	0.6	0.45	0.73
West and Central Europe	6.9	0.5	0.4	0.61	1.22
South East Europe	2.0	0.2	0.2	0.21	0.08
Eastern Europe	3.7	1.4	1.1	0.24	0.03
Oceania	14.5	0.4	0.1	2.14	1.37
Global	3.9	0.4	0.3	0.58	0.37

Source: own calculations based on data from World Drug Report 2008 (UNODC 2008).

properties) is more prevalent than use of all illicit drugs other than cannabis. The 2006 US National Survey on Drug Use and Health (NSDUH) showed that 2.8% of the population aged 12 years and over reported misuse of prescription-type psychopharmaceuticals in the past month (mainly painkillers but also tranquillizers, stimulants, and sedatives) (SAMHSA 2007). Correspondingly, data from the National Drug Strategy Household Survey in Australia in 2004 showed that 3.8% of respondents 14 years and older reported use of psychopharmaceuticals for non-medical purposes in the preceding 12 months (mainly pain killers and tranquillizers) (Australian Institute for Health and Welfare 2005).

Importantly, only a small fraction of those who have ever used illicit drugs become problem drug users. Data from the European Monitoring Centre for Drugs and Drug Addiction (EMCDDA 2004) indicate that the current prevalence of problem drug use (defined as 'injecting drug use or long-duration/regular use of opioids, cocaine and/or amphetamines') is less than 1% in the age group 15–64 among the 20 European countries included in their monitoring survey. Table 3.2 shows the estimated prevalence of 'problem drug use' among those aged 15–64 in 22 European countries. There is substantial variation across countries, but also within the same country because of different estimation procedures, survey techniques, and sampling procedures.

The **lifetime prevalence** for 'substance abuse' (a term defined by drug use in hazardous situations as well as problems associated with use) is around 6–7% in the North American countries and New Zealand and around 1% in South Korea and Taiwan (Perkonigg *et al.* 1998). One systematic review (Rehm *et al.* 2005) found that in the European Union (EU) countries and Norway the majority of drug use disorders were related to cannabis. For other drugs (opioids, cocaine, and amphetamines) estimates were well below 1%. Other studies have documented a high lifetime prevalence rate of dependence in the USA (7.5%), with lower estimates for Germany (2.1%) and The Netherlands (1.8%), and a considerably lower rate for Mexico, with 0.7% of the adult urban population meeting criteria for drug dependence (Merikangas *et al.* 1998a).

Surveys from six different countries suggest that the proportion of the population who report ever having used an illicit drug (in the range of 10–50%) is some 6–15 times higher than the proportion who report symptoms of drug dependence (Merikangas *et al.* 1998a). Even among current users, a small fraction of heavy users seems to account for most of the drug consumption. For example, it was estimated that one-fifth of current cocaine users accounted for 70% of the total cocaine consumed in the USA in 1990 (Everingham and Rydell 1994).

On a global basis, these geographic variations help to identify factors that contribute to problem drug use. Closeness to the production area and smuggling routes seems to increase the risk of drug use. Hence, the prevalence of cocaine use is high in South America (including Colombia, the main source of cocaine) and in North America compared with most other parts of the world, and cocaine use is estimated to be high in Mexico, which is located on the smuggling route from Colombia to the USA (Brouwer *et al.* 2006). Correspondingly, the prevalence of opiate use is particularly high in some Asian countries close to Afghanistan and Myanmar, the main producing countries (e.g. Thailand and south-western parts of China). Opiate use is also prevalent in some eastern European countries located along the smuggling routes from Afghanistan to Western Europe (e.g. Slovenia) (Prezelj and Gaber 2005). Yet, there are also examples of deviation from such a pattern. Drug use is not very prevalent in The Netherlands, although the country is an important cannabis producer and transfer country for cocaine. Turkey is another exception, despite its role as main entry point for heroin into Europe.

From a global perspective, the prevalence of drug use also tends to be higher in wealthy regions (e.g. Europe, North America, and Oceania) as compared with poorer

Table 3.2 Prevalence of problem drug use (rate per 1000 aged 15–64) estimated by various methods and time periods in 22 European countries

Country and year(s) for which problem drug use rates are estimated	Range of estimates	Estimation method(s)[1]
Austria 2001–2004	3.3–5.4	CR
Czech Republic 2000–2006	1.4–5.2	CR, TM, OT
Cyprus 2004–2006	1.3–1.9	TP
Denmark 1996–2005	4.0–7.5	CR
Finland 2001–2005	0.5–5.3	CR
France 1995–1999	3.8–4.7	CM, MI, OT, PM, TM
Germany 2000–2006	2.1–2.8	MI, PM
Greece 2001–2006	0.7–4.4	CR
Hungary 2005	3.5	CR
Ireland 2000–2001	5.6–5.7	CR
Italy 1996–2006	3.2–8.5	CR, MI, MM, OT, PM, TM
Luxembourg 1996–2000	6.5–8.1	CR, OT, PM
Malta 2004–2006	2.6–6.2	CR
Netherlands 1996–2001	2.6–3.1	CM, MI, OT, TM
Norway 1997[2]	4.2	OT
Poland 2002	1.9	OT
Portugal 1999–2000	6.8–8.5	PM
Slovenia 2000–2001	5.3–5.4	CR
Slovakia 2002–2006	2.1–6.1	MI, OT
Spain 1998–2002	4.0–8 7	TM, OT
Sweden 1998–2003	4.5–4.8	CR
United Kingdom 2001–2005	9.2–10.2	OT

Sources: Summary of EMCDDA report on prevalence of problem drug use at national level (available at: http://www.emcdda.europa.eu/stats08/pdutab102a) and EMCDDA estimates of trends in problem and injecting drug use, 2001–2006 (available at: http://www.emcdda.europa.eu/stats08/pdutab6a).

[1] Estimation methods: CR = Capture Recapture; TM = Treatment Multiplier; HM = HIV Multiplier; MM = Mortality Multiplier; MI = Multivariate Indicator Method; PM = Police Multiplier; OT = Other

[2] Only Injecting drug use.

areas and developing countries (e.g. Africa), except in cases where a particular drug has strong indigenous roots, such as coca chewing in the Andean region, **khat** use in East Africa and the Middle East, and the use of **betel nut** in parts of Asia.

3.4 **Trends in drug use**

Use of cannabis, opiates, cocaine, and amphetamine is not at all a recent phenomenon. Opium was used in China and other South East Asian countries centuries ago. It became widely used in England and in the USA in the 19th century (Courtwright 1982). Coca leaves were chewed for centuries by the people of South America, and cocaine was a popular ingredient in 'patent medicines' in the USA in the late 19th century (e.g. Kandall 1996). Amphetamines were widely used in Japan and in Sweden after the Second World War (Bejerot 1975). The extent of use, modes of intake, and characteristics of the users, have, however, varied significantly when we apply a longer time frame. For instance, in the late 19th century there were probably 200 000 opiate addicts in the USA—the majority of them female—who consumed the drug by smoking, drinking, or eating it (e.g. Kandall 1996). According to Courtwright (1982), the number of opiate addicts in the USA increased during the latter half of the 19th century to more than four per 1000 inhabitants around 1890, a rate that was probably halved during the first decades in the 20th century (Kandall 1996). During this period women constituted a decreasing proportion of the drug users (Kandall 1996).

In more recent times, significant changes in the prevalence of drug use have been reported from various countries, in terms of both increasing and decreasing trends. Global indices show significant increases in use of cannabis, amphetamine-type stimulants, cocaine, and opiates from 1992 to 2003 (based on trend analyses in UNODC member states, UNODC 2005). Although more countries (44% in 2003) report rising levels of drug use than falling levels (25% in 2003), more UNODC member states reported stable or decreasing levels of drug use from 2000 to 2003 (UNODC 2005). In some countries, diversion of psychopharmaceutical products and raw opium from legal production has been linked to increasing trends in both the incidence and prevalence of drug use.

Increases in drug use have been particularly marked in some regions. Whereas opium use had virtually disappeared in China between the early 1950s and late 1970s (McCoy *et al.* 2001), recently there has been a significant increase in heroin use in areas of China close to the 'Golden Triangle', concomitant with the opening of borders, international trade, and economic development (McCoy *et al.* 2001; Li *et al.* 2002; Hao *et al.* 2004). Mexico has over the past decade become increasingly involved in cocaine trafficking and metamphetamine production and trafficking. There has been a dramatic growth of injecting drug use in newly independent states such as Russia and Ukraine since 1990 (Rhodes *et al.* 1999). This has coincided with the globalization of drug markets, transport, and communication networks. Poznyak and co-workers (2002) suggest that the transition period from socialist- to capitalist-oriented economies influenced the dramatic increase in drug use in several ways. Drug supply increased when political, social, and economic factors contributed to an expansion of criminal networks and money laundering, and the social and political turmoil expanded socially deprived groups that are particularly vulnerable to substance misuse. In other Central and Eastern European countries a significant increase in illicit drug use has been reported during periods of political and social change (Moskalewicz 2002). There was a dramatic increase in the number of hospital patients diagnosed with substance use disorders from 1994 to 1999 in the Czech Republic and a 50-fold increase in drug-related criminal offences from 1990 to 1999 (Csémy *et al.* 2002). In Northern Ireland, it appears that political and social changes have been accompanied by an increase in drug use among young people (Higgins *et al.* 2004).

Elsewhere, trends have been more mixed. Cannabis use in The Netherlands (where cannabis has been sold openly in licensed 'coffee shops' since the late 1970s) increased between the 1970s and the early 1990s, but the prevalence rates stabilized thereafter (Korf 2002). The increase thus occurred during a period when cannabis use was decriminalized and an increasing number of coffee shops captured the Dutch retail cannabis market, whereas the stabilization in cannabis use occurred during a period where the number of coffee shops was halved (Korf 2002). However, MacCoun and Reuter (2001a) have shown that lifetime cannabis prevalence for Dutch youth is not very different from that of Norwegian (Oslo) youth, and significantly lower than that for US youth during the late 1970s and 1980s. In both Norway and the USA, possession and use of cannabis are strictly illegal.

In Australia the number of dependent heroin users doubled from the mid-1980s to the late 1990s (Hall *et al.* 2000c; Kaya *et al.* 2004). It has been suggested that the increase could be explained by a substantial increase in availability of pure and cheap heroin as well as an increase in psychosocial disorders among young people (Hall *et al.* 2000c). This period was followed by a marked decrease in heroin availability, after an increase in the price of heroin in early 2001. Degenhardt and co-workers (2005a) reported that there was a concomitant reduction in the frequency of self-reported heroin use among regular injection drug users (IDUs) and a reduction in the number of needles and syringes distributed, as well as a significant reduction in the number of opioid overdose deaths.

In some countries a trend in the use of cannabis is followed by a similar trend in the use of other illicit drugs. Annual data among Swedish male military conscripts (aged ~18) from 1976 to 2005 show a parallel trend in use of cannabis and amphetamines (Centralförbundet for alkohol- och narkotikaupplysning 2007), as do annual data from 1990 to 2005 among Norwegian adolescents with respect to use of cannabis, amphetamines, ecstasy, and cocaine (Norwegian Institute for Alcohol and Drug Research 2008). Data from the USA do not, however, completely conform to this picture. The marked decrease in cannabis use in the USA during the 1980s was followed by an increase in the 1990s. A somewhat similar pattern is seen with respect to use of hallucinogens and opiates in this period, whereas the trend in cocaine use deviated from this pattern (Bauman and Phongsavan 1999).

A more recent trend has been for increased non-medical use of psychopharmaceutical drugs (Compton et al., 2005b; Fischer *et al.* 2006; Fischer and Rehm 2007), particularly morphine, oxycodone, codeine, and hydromorphone. In the USA, Canada, and Australia, this trend may be linked to decreases in the availability of heroin, but, as noted in Chapter 12, increased marketing and availability of a variety of psychopharmaceuticals may also be responsible. For example, as one of the largest producers of licit opium for medicinal purposes, India has become one of the world's largest consumers of illicit opiates due to diversion from licit cultivation (Paoli *et al.* 2009b).

In one cross-national study (Smart and Murray 1983), trends in problem drug use were examined in relation to affluence (e.g. median income), unemployment, and health services. In all five countries studied (Canada, Hong Kong, Sweden, the UK, and the USA), the indicators of drug use were positively correlated with measures of affluence and negatively correlated with unemployment and use of health services. Trends can also reflect cohort-specific changes in drug use preferences in a particular location. Thus, a study of drug use preferences among inner city arrestees in New York City found that changes in norms and preferences affected age of onset and prevalence of problem drug use (Golub and Johnson 1999).

3.4.1 Drug epidemics

In some cases, quite dramatic increases in drug use have been seen, often referred to as 'epidemics' (Golub and Johnson 2005) or 'outbreaks' (Parker *et al.* 1998). For instance, in inner city Chicago the number of injecting heroin users increased dramatically in the late 1940s (Hughes *et al.* 1972), whereas the number of new cases declined markedly during the 1950s. Another example is from Wirral, Merseyside in England where the prevalence of heroin users increased from almost zero to around 4000 over a 6-year period in the early 1980s (Parker *et al.* 1998). A very rapid spread of heroin use as seen in the USA and the UK has been explained by two simultaneous processes: (1) a spread through personal contact between experienced users and novices (microdiffusion) and (2) a supplier and dealer movement to neighbouring areas (macrodiffusion) (Parker *et al.* 1998).

More recent examples of dramatic increases in drug use pertain to countries in Central and Eastern Europe. In the Russian Federation the number of new cases of drug dependence increased from 3 to 51 per 100 000 during the 1990s (Poznyak *et al.* 2002), implying that the prevalence of drug dependence around the turn of the millennium reached a level that was 2–5 times higher in the Russian Federation than in most EU countries. Amongst adolescents the incidence of drug dependence increased 17-fold from 1991 to 2000 (Poznyak *et al.* 2002). A significant although somewhat less dramatic increase in illicit drug use and problem drug use was also observed in the Czech Republic and Slovakia (Csémy *et al.* 2002); in the Baltic states and Poland (Lagerspetz and Moskalewicz 2002); in Hungary, Romania, and Moldova (Elekes and Kovács 2002); and in Slovenia (Flaker 2002).

3.5 Prevalence of drug use by young persons

In most cultures, there is a particular concern about drug use by young people, who are seen as more vulnerable. For this reason, as well as relatively easy access to adolescents through school surveys, there are numerous studies describing drug use in youth populations. The European School Project on Alcohol and Drugs (ESPAD) is a comprehensive collaboration involving 38 European countries (plus comparison data from the USA). School surveys have been conducted at four time points (1995, 1999, 2003, and 2007) applying the same sampling strategies and questionnaires (Hibell *et al.* 2009) in samples of 15- to 16-year-olds. These 2007 data show that cannabis is the drug most frequently used by adolescents (Table 3.3), but that cannabis use varies considerably across countries. Use of inhalants was more prevalent than use of illicit drugs other than cannabis in most of the countries. It is also noteworthy that non-medical use of prescription drugs (tranquillizers) was more prevalent than use of illicit drugs other than cannabis in the majority of countries (Table 3.3). In all countries more than half of the students reported using cannabis fewer than 10 times in their life.

In a review of student surveys reported from 36 countries (Smart and Ogborne 2000), cannabis was the illicit drug most frequently reported. The countries with a high proportion of cannabis use (>15%) included Canada, the USA, Australia, the Czech Republic, and some Western European countries. Surveys from South Africa (Parry *et al.* 2004), Nigeria (see Omoluabi 1995 for a review), Lebanon (Karam *et al.* 2000), and Latin American countries (Dormitzer *et al.* 2004) also show that cannabis is the most frequently used illicit drug. This general trend, however, does not apply to all countries. In several Latin American countries more adolescents reported using inhalants than cannabis or other illicit drugs (Dormitzer *et al.* 2004). A survey among Chinese adolescents (Liu *et al.* 2001) showed that more reported use of heroin and solvents than cannabis.

Table 3.4 shows that there is a significant correlation ($r = 0.70$) across countries between the proportion of students reporting any cannabis use and the mean number of times having used cannabis calculations based on published data from ESPAD. In addition, the proportion of frequent cannabis users (>10 times in life) is very highly correlated ($r = 0.95$) with the proportion of cannabis users. These data imply that adolescents tend to use cannabis more frequently in countries where a larger proportion of their peers have ever tried cannabis. Of course, this could also be explained by differences in prices and in affluence.

There are also significant correlations between the proportion of students reporting lifetime experience with cannabis and lifetime experience with any other illicit drug ($r = 0.75$), and drinking frequency correlates with prevalence of cannabis use ($r = 0.38$) and other illicit drug use ($r = 0.46$). On the other hand, no significant correlations were found between the proportions reporting use of cannabis and those reporting use of inhalants, tranquillizers without prescription, or tobacco smoking (Table 3.4). In other words, the prevalence of all types of illicit drug use tends to be higher in countries where cannabis use is more widespread, and use of cannabis and other drugs tends to be more common in countries where adolescents drink more frequently. In contrast, inhalant use, frequent tobacco smoking, and use of tranquillizers do not vary systematically with illicit drug use across countries (Table 3.4). Comparing data from ESPAD with purchasing power parities in the various countries (excluding the Nordic countries, where use rates are low) demonstrates a significant positive correlation between the two; the higher the purchasing power in a country, the higher the prevalence and frequency of cannabis use.

3.6 Trends in youth drug use

Little is known about why drug use increases and decreases within a population. Data from the four waves of ESPAD data collection from 1995 to 2007, for example, showed

Table 3.3 Lifetime drug use among 15- to 16-year-olds in 36 European countries and the USA

	Cannabis, % used	Any other illicit drug, %	Inhalants, %	Tranquillizers, without prescription, %
Armenia	3	2	5	n.a.
Austria	17	11	14	2
Belgium (Flanders)	24	9	8	9
Bulgaria	22	9	3	3
Croatia	18	4	11	5
Cyprus	5	5	16	7
Czech Republic	45	9	7	9
Denmark	25	10	6	5
Estonia	26	9	9	7
Faroe Islands	6	1	8	3
Finland	8	3	10	7
France	31	11	12	15
Germany	20	8	11	3
Greece	6	5	9	4
Hungary	13	7	8	9
Iceland	9	5	4	7
Ireland	20	10	15	3
Isle of Man	34	16	17	7
Italy	23	9	5	10
Latvia	18	11	13	4
Lithuania	18	7	3	16
Malta	13	9	16	5
Monaco	28	10	8	12
The Netherlands	28	7	6	7
Norway	6	3	7	4
Poland	16	7	6	18
Portugal	13	6	4	6
Romania	4	3	4	4
Russia	19	5	7	2
Slovak Republic	32	9	13	5
Slovenia	22	8	16	5
Sweden	7	4	9	7

Table 3.3 (continued) Lifetime drug use among 15- to 16-year-olds in 36 European countries and the USA

	Cannabis, % used	Any other illicit drug, %	Inhalants, %	Tranquillizers without prescription,%
Switzerland	33	7	9	8
Ukraine	14	4	3	4
UK	29	9	9	2
USA		-		

Source: own calculations based on data from Hibell *et al.* (2009).

n.a. = not ascertained.

that the proportion of students reporting lifetime experience with cannabis increased in some Eastern European countries but remained stable or declined in 11 other countries (Hibell *et al.* 2009).

Extending the time frame for monitoring trends in drug use, data from the US National Household Survey on Drug Abuse show a significant decreasing trend in marijuana use among 15- to 19-year-olds in the USA between 1979 and 1992, which was followed by an increasing trend up to 1998, and then a decreasing trend thereafter (Harrison 2001; Jacobson 2004). Changing perceptions of the risks of drug use have been found to be correlated with changes in prevalence rates (Johnston *et al.* 2003). Annual surveys among 15- to 20-year-olds in Norway show that the proportion reporting use of cannabis increased dramatically in the late 1960s and early 1970s and then remained fairly stable until the mid-1990s, when another significant increase occurred (Skretting 2007; Norwegian Institute for Alcohol and Drug Research 2008). Surveys among Swiss 15-year-olds from 1986 to 1998 showed a significant increase in prevalence of cannabis use (as well as frequency of tobacco smoking and drunkenness) over this period (Kuntsche 2004). Surveys among Greek young adults (18–24 years) covering the period 1984–1998 also showed a significant increase in illicit drug use (Kokkevi *et al.* 2002). Annual survey data from young adult military conscripts in Sweden over the period 1970–2005 show that the proportion who had ever used illicit drugs was fairly stable in the 1970s, decreased in the 1980s, and increased again from the mid-1990s (Centralförbundet for alkohol- och narkotika-upplysning 2007). A similar series of surveys from Israel from 1982 to 2001 show that the lifetime prevalence of illicit drug use decreased during the 1980s, was fairly stable throughout most of the 1990s, and increased significantly from 1997 to 2001 (Neumark *et al.* 2004). Surveys among Dutch adolescents, on the other hand, show a significant increase in the proportion reporting cannabis use from 1988 to 1996, but a stabilization of prevalence rates thereafter (Monshouwer *et al.* 2005).

This review of trend data indicates that assessment of drug use among young people is relatively feasible and fairly common. We may therefore ask whether such data provide a useful indicator of the magnitude of drug use in the entire population. In the UNODC

Table 3.4 Pearson's correlation coefficients showing associations between country estimates of lifetime use of various drugs among adolescents

	Cannabis % used	**Cannabis mean times per student**	**Cannabis mean times per user**	**Any other illicit drug %**	**Inhalants %**	**Tranquillizers without prescription %**	**Drinking frequency mean times per student**	**Frequent smokers (40+ times lifetime) %**
Cannabis mean times per student	0.95							
Cannabis mean times per user	0.70	0.82						
Any other illicit drug %	0.75	0.73	0.61					
Inhalants %	(0.23)	(0.24)	0.33	(0.16)				
Tranquilizers. without prescription %	(0.15)	(0.15)	(0.03)	(0.29)	(–0.23)			
Drinking frequency, mean times per student	0.38	(0.31)	(0.23)	0.46	(0.15)	(–0.11)		
Frequent smokers (40+ times lifetime) %	(0.08)	(–0.10)	(–0.24)	(0.13)	(–0.20)	(0.22)	(0.24)	
Purchasing power parities per capita 2004	0.62	0.72	0.71	(0.44)	0.48	(–0.22)	(0.38)	(0.05)

Source: own calculations based on data from Hibell *et al.* (2004).

Figures in parentheses are not statistically significant.

World Drug Report (2006) data from youth surveys have been applied as the sole basis for calculating the annual prevalence of drug use in the general population in some countries. Data from a number of European countries has shown a fairly high correlation between estimates of occasional drug use in the adolescent and adult populations (UNODC 2006). However, we do not know whether this is the case in other parts of the world.

To what extent is occasional drug use among youth an indicator of problem drug use in a population? Based on data from 16 European countries, we find only a moderate correlation ($r = 0.31$) between the proportion of adolescents reporting any illicit drug use and the rate of problem drug users in the population (this calculation is based on ESPAD data on adolescent occasional drug use and EMCDDA data on prevalence of problem drug use). Trend data on the prevalence of occasional drug use in youth and number of problem drug users also suggest that these are not significantly correlated. For instance, data from Sweden shows that the estimated number of problem ('heavy') drug users increased by 27% from 1979 to 1992 and increased by 37% from 1992 to 1998, whereas the prevalence of occasional drug use among young military conscripts decreased by a third from the late 1970s to the early 1990s, and then increased to reach almost the same level in the late 1990s as in the late 1970s (Centralförbundet for alkohol- och narkotikaupplysning 2007). However, the interpretation of these relationships is complicated by the fact that there is likely to be a time lag of a decade or more between increases in adolescent drug use and concomitant changes in problem rates.

In summary, national surveys show that occasional drug use among young people can vary considerably over time, with cycles of increase and decline lasting for decades or even a generation. Moreover, trends in occasional drug use seem to mirror trends in the adult population, yet they probably do not reflect changes in prevalence of problem drug use over time. Comparisons of long-term trends in occasional drug use among youth across various countries (Figure 3.1) as well comparisons of trends over a shorter period of time (ESPAD data from 1995 to 2003: see Hibell *et al.* 2009) indicate that there is no uniform trend in adolescent drug use. In this respect it seems likely that trends in adolescent drug use in various countries are not only driven by common forces but are also influenced by social, political, legislative, and drug market changes particular to each country.

3.7 **Variations in drug use within populations**

Within populations drug use is unevenly distributed and prevalence rates vary significantly with demographic factors as well as social, behavioural, and mental health conditions. By studying these variations, epidemiologists can provide useful information to guide the development of more informed drug policies for prevention and treatment.

3.7.1 **Gender**

School surveys among adolescents in Europe, North America, and Australia indicate that although the prevalence of illicit drug use is higher among boys than girls, the

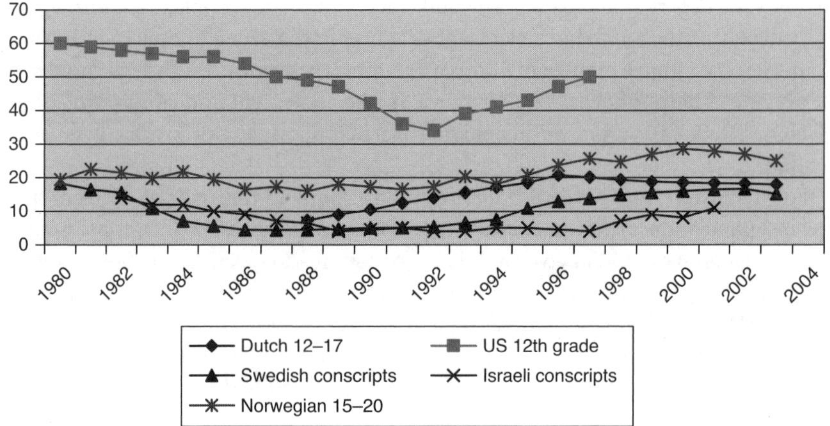

Fig. 3.1 Trends in drug use in various youth populations over time. Percentage reporting life-time use of cannabis by year.

Sources: Dutch 12-17: Monshouwer *et al.* 2005 Swedish conscripts: Central for bundet for alkohol-och narkotikaupplyshing 2007. Norwegian 15-20: Norwegian Institute for Alcohol and Drug Research 2008. US 12th grade; MacCoun and Reuter 2001b Israeli conscripts: Neumark *et al.* 2004.

Notes: Data have been interpolated in the Dutch series (which comprised data points for the years 1988, 1992, 1996, 1999 and 2003). In the Swedish conscripts series (where data were missing for the years 1989, 1990 and 1991) and in the Norwegian series (where data were missing for 1990). In the Israeli series life time prevalence is for illicit drug use. As cannabis is by far the most commonly used drug in this population, it is assumed that the series fairly much reflects the trends in life-time use of cannabis.

gender differences are generally rather small (see for instance Hibell *et al.* 2009 on ESPAD data and Bauman and Phongsavan 1999 for a review). Data from the ESPAD report (Hibell *et al.* 2009) show that the male to female ratio is 1:3 for lifetime prevalence of cannabis use and 1:2 for any other illicit drug use. Nevertheless, significantly higher proportions of males than females report illicit drug use in developing countries such as South Africa (Parry *et al.* 2004). Surveys of adults show larger gender effects than surveys of adolescents in the same population. One study (Perkonigg *et al.* 1998) found that in various countries (e.g. the USA, New Zealand, South Korea, and Taiwan) approximately twice as many adult men as women reported illicit drug use. Similar gender differences have been reported in adult population surveys in China (Hao *et al.* 2002) and in Latin American countries (Medina-Mora *et al.* 2006). Studies of problem drug use also show significant gender differences, with a higher proportion of problem drug users among males compared with females. However, the male to female ratio of problem drug users appears to be lower in Europe, North America, and Australia (around 2:5) as compared with what has been reported from some Asian countries (e.g. Nepal, Pakistan, Turkmenistan, China, and India) and Mexico (Medina-Mora *et al.* 2006). Shrestha (1992) noted that only one in 20 drug addicts in Nepal were women, and similar findings have been reported from Nigeria (Omoluabi 1995).

A review of injection drug use in developing and transitional countries (Aceijas *et al.* 2006) showed that males tended to constitute the vast majority (70–100%).

These gender ratio findings suggest that the risk of transition from infrequent drug use to problem drug use may be higher for males than for females. In line with this, an Australian study (Lynskey *et al.* 2003) showed that among those who had used cannabis by the age of 17, a significantly higher proportion of males developed drug abuse or dependence in young adulthood than females. However, it can also be argued that a narrowing gender gap in infrequent drug use among youth (e.g. Sloboda 2002) reflects a generational change, and may be followed by a smaller male to female ratio in problem drug use when sufficient time has passed for some of these infrequent users to have developed a drug problem.

3.7.2 Age

The age of problem drug users varies across societies and eras. More than a century ago opiates were mainly used by middle-aged and elderly people both in the USA(Kandall 1996) and in South East Asia (Berridge and Edwards 1981). By the latter part of the 20th century, however, drug use had become concentrated overwhelmingly in adolescence and young adulthood (Compton *et al.* 2005b). Regardless of age, most of those who have tried drugs do not continue to use them. Among those who continue, the length of time from onset of use to developing problem use or dependence may be several years, although this tends to vary by type of drug (Wagner and Anthony 2002). As most problem drug users may continue their habits for a number of years, they are generally young or middle-aged adults (e.g. Aceijas *et al.* 2006; Stafford *et al.* 2006). This implies that occasional drug use is concentrated among youth and young adults, whereas dependent use or problem drug use mostly is a young adult to middle age phenomenon.

Research in more recent decades shows that in many countries the average age of problem drug users has increased over time, as has the proportion of middle-aged persons. For instance, in Sweden the number of persons convicted for drug offences more than tripled from 1975 to 2003 and the proportion of these individuals aged 25 or older increased from 33% in 1975 to 64% in 2003 (Centralförbundet for alkohol- och narkotikaupplysning 2007). In Australia the mean age of IDUs increased from 29 in 2000 to 33 in 2004 (Stafford *et al.* 2006), and among IDUs in Oslo, Norway, the mean age increased by almost 5 years over a 12-year period (from 28 years in 1993 to 33 years in 2004) (Bretteville-Jensen 2005).

Three explanations have been suggested to account for these age trends: (1) declining rates of initiation; (2) more drug users continuing their drug use over a longer period of time; and (3) later onset of problematic use. For instance, among Norwegian drug users, the mean age for onset of injection use increased from about 16 years in the 1970s to 25 years after the mid-1990s (Bretteville-Jensen 2005).

3.7.3 Social, behavioural, and mental health characteristics

Frequent and problem users of illicit drugs tend to be burdened by social, behavioural, and mental health conditions of significant relevance for prevention and treatment. A family history of substance use (especially a parent's diagnosis of alcohol or drug dependence) is a major risk factor for drug use disorders in the adult children (e.g. Merikangas *et al.* 1998b). It has been suggested that much of the familial clustering of drug use disorders can be explained by genetic factors (Compton *et al.* 2005b), but genetic epidemiology studies show that specific genotypes only account for a small part of the disorder rates (e.g. Smith *et al.* 2008). This suggests a more complex process of gene–environment interaction throughout the adolescent developmental period. Temperamental features more common in offspring of parents with substance dependence are behavioural/affective undercontrol and negative affect (Hesselbrock and Hesselbrock 2006). The former is evidenced in impulsiveness, hyperactivity, antisociality, emotional lability, frequent boredom, and difficulty in being soothed when upset (by self or others). The latter emerges as a tendency toward worry and sadness. These temperamental features increase the risk that an adolescent will experiment with drugs, and that experimentation will progress into a substance abuse problem. In addition to these temperament factors, some studies suggest that genetically influenced cognitive deficits (e.g. problems with abstract reasoning and memory) may be more common in biological children of parents with alcohol dependence and also increase the risk of developing an substance use disorder later in life (Hesselbrock and Hesselbrock 2006).

Those who initiate illicit drug use are often more likely to be involved in other problematic behaviours, though the direction and patterns of causation are often unclear. Thus illicit drug users are more likely to engage in (other) criminal behaviour and to drop out of school or have poorer academic achievement (Obot and Anthony 2000; Windle and Wiesner 2004). Moreover, **drug use disorders** are strongly associated with mental health problems (mood, anxiety, and personality disorders) (Merikangas *et al.* 1998a; Disney *et al.* 1999; Compton *et al.* 2005b). A systematic review of longitudinal studies of general population cohorts (Macleod *et al.* 2004) showed that use of cannabis and other drugs was systematically associated with early school drop out, poorer mental health, delinquency, and other problem behaviour.

The personal and familial risk factors described above also raise the risk for many other problems parents and policymakers worry about, such as school failure, bullying, violence, depression, and suicide. This means there is no way to identify specifically a group of young people at high inherited risk for substance use who would not also be at high risk for a range of other problems. It follows that if it is possible to modify the impact of these genetically influenced risk factors through prevention programmes, there is every reason to expect that drug use would be only one of the outcomes positively affected.

Studies of environmental risk and protective factors yield a similar conclusion. Research conducted from a range of theoretical perspectives (see Lembke *et al.* 2009) has identified a number of factors that lower the risk of drug use when they are present and increase it when absent: family bonding, parental and teacher monitoring, predictable and safe daily environments, positive role models, non-deviant peer networks, and engagement in prosocial organizations (e.g. religious organizations). These factors predict not just a lower risk for substance use, but also a lower risk of virtually every other problematic outcome young people might experience.

3.7.4 Ethnicity and indigenous populations

Illicit drug use is often found to vary with ethnicity in multicultural societies. This has been most fully documented in the USA. In Chicago, outbreaks of heroin use between 1967 and 1971 occurred more frequently in ethnic minority areas (African-American and Puerto Rican) than in white neighbourhoods (Hughes 1977). On the other hand, surveys among adolescents in the USA show that illicit drug use is reported less frequently by persons of African, Mexican, and Asian descent compared with European-American adolescents (Bachman *et al.* 1991).

Patterson and co-workers (1999) reported that in 1995 the rates of hospital admissions with drug-related problems were almost twice as high among indigenous than non-indigenous Australians. Compared with 15 years earlier, there was a more rapid acceleration of these rates among indigenous than among non-indigenous people. Howard and colleagues (1996) reported that a larger proportion of US war veterans who were Native American were diagnosed with a substance use disorder compared with the total population of veterans. Surveys among adolescents in the USA have shown significantly higher prevalence of illicit drug use (as well as use of other substances) among Native Americans compared with other ethnic groups (Beauvais *et al.* 1985; Wallace *et al.* 2002). It has, however, been argued that such differences reflect the fact that ethnic minorities often live in circumscribed, impoverished areas (Plunkett and Mitchell 2000). Beauvais and colleagues (2004) found that cannabis use among Native American youths was somewhat lower than the national estimates in the late 1970s, but since that time the prevalence rate has been consistently higher than the national estimates. Nevertheless, prevalence rates tended to follow the same national trends.

3.7.5 Inner city and neighbourhood characteristics

Drug use tends to cluster in urban geographic areas and neighbourhoods with certain characteristics. In New York City, Chein and colleagues (1964) observed that the incidence of marijuana and heroin use was higher in areas of relatively concentrated settlement characterized by underprivileged minority groups, poverty, low socioeconomic status, low educational attainment, disrupted family life, and highly crowded housing. Similar observations have been reported in later studies, indicating that problem drug use is more prevalent and more concentrated in inner city areas and in poorer neighbourhoods (e.g. Bourgois 2003). Neighbourhood conditions such as poverty, deprivation, unemployment, and type of housing are associated with high levels of drug use (Parker *et al.* 1987; Storr *et al.* 2004). Studies among street youths, homeless people, and soup kitchen users show that the prevalence of illicit drug use is generally high (Forster *et al.* 1996; Magura *et al.* 2000; Teeson *et al.* 2000; D'Amore *et al.* 2001). A study from Micronesia (Storr *et al.* 2004) showed that the young people were more likely to have been offered marijuana and amphetamines if they lived in more disadvantaged neighbourhoods. However, surveys have found that drug use may be as prevalent in suburban, as opposed to inner city and more rural areas (e.g. Forsyth and Barnard 1999; Saxe *et al.* 2001), and some researchers (Luthar and D'Avanzo 1999) have suggested that experimental drug use may be even more prevalent among affluent suburban youth in certain developed countries.

3.8 Injection drug use

Injection drug use, as compared with other modes of drug administration, implies an increased risk of adverse consequences for two reasons. First, many IDUs share syringes and thereby increase the risk of spreading viral infections (e.g. HIV and hepatitis). Secondly, many IDUs do not know how to avoid, or have little interest in avoiding, health hazards related to drug injecting.

It has been estimated (Aceijas *et al.* 2004) that in 2003 some 13 million adults worldwide (0.3% of the adult population) were IDUs, of which eight out of 10 live in developing and transitional countries. The proportion of IDUs in the adult population was found to vary considerably across countries, the estimated proportions being particularly high (~1–2%) in several Eastern European countries (e.g. Russia, Estonia, Poland, and Ukraine), but generally lower (<0.2%) in most African and Latin American countries. There has been a change in route of administration of opiates in many Asian countries, and many users have turned from smoking or inhaling to injection (McCoy *et al.* 2001). In Central and Eastern Europe as well as Thailand and India, the majority of opiate users are injecting, whereas in China the majority of opiate users are not injecting (McCoy *et al.* 2001; Hao *et al.* 2004). In Nepal the drug scene has been dominated by heroin. During the late 1980s there was a large increase in the proportion of heroin users who inject the drug (Shrestha 1992). Heroin is mainly smoked in South Africa (Parry *et al.* 2002). Within the EU, the proportion of heroin users who inject the drug is relatively small in some countries (e.g. The Netherlands, Spain, and Portugal) whereas in other countries (e.g. Denmark, Sweden, the UK, and several of the new member states) the majority of the heroin users are IDUs (EMCDDA 2005). In the former Czechoslovakia the most prevalent opioid drug, codeine in composite analgesics (sold without prescription over the counter), was mainly used by injection, as was the case with amphetamines (Nerad and Neradova 1991). More recent studies from the Czech Republic and the Slovak Republic suggest that injection is the most common route of administration for heroin and amphetamine (Csémy *et al.* 2002). The reasons for these wide variations in injection drug use are unknown, but are likely to be related to availability of injection equipment, national traditions (e.g. China), and idiosyncratic influences in the drug-using networks.

3.8.1 Polydrug use

It is often found that problem drug users do not consume a single drug, but rather multiple kinds of drugs, often with different psychoactive effects, as for instance heroin and amphetamine. Surveys among adolescents generally show a considerable overlap in use of various illicit drugs (see for instance Macleod *et al.* 2004 for a systematic review). Among problem drug users some drugs are used more or less concomitantly (e.g. Farrell *et al.* 1994; Hafeiz 1995; Gossop *et al.* 2000; Basu *et al.* 2000; Leri *et al.* 2003). For instance, opiate users often report use of benzodiazepines (e.g. Darke *et al.* 2003; Gossop *et al.* 2003), cannabis (Budney *et al.* 1998), and stimulants (Barrio *et al.* 1998; Lawal *et al.* 1998; Hser *et al.* 2003). Of particular relevance for treatment programmes in many countries is the observation that problem drug users are generally polydrug users, with considerable overlap with tobacco and alcohol use.

3.9 Individual trajectories and drug use careers

3.9.1 The gateway hypothesis

Longitudinal studies (both prospective and retrospective) have reported a predictable sequencing of drug use, reflected in the initiation of similar types of drug use over time. Cannabis tends to be the first illicit drug used, followed by amphetamines (or other stimulants) and then other drugs (see for instance Kandel and Davies 1996; Kenkel *et al.* 2001; Novins *et al.* 2001; Kandel and Yamaguchi 2002; Li *et al.* 2002). It should be noted, however, that cannabis use is generally preceded by use of licit substances, mainly alcohol and/or tobacco (Golub and Johnson 2001; Kandel and Yamaguchi 2002), and it has been suggested that alcohol (e.g. Bretteville-Jensen *et al.* 2008) and tobacco (Beenstock and Rahav 2002; Siqueira and Brook 2003) serve as gateways for cannabis use. It should also be noted that most cannabis users do not progress to use of other drugs, as is implied by the global figures showing at least four times as many users of cannabis as of other drugs. Hall and Lynskey (2005) reviewed the evidence on gateway substances, and noted that cannabis use precedes use of other illicit drugs, and that the earlier onset of cannabis use and the more regularly it is used, the higher the probability of use of other illicit drugs. The question then becomes whether cannabis use is a *causal* factor for later use of other illicit substances (e.g. 'hard drugs'). Alternatively, it may be assumed that the observed transitions from one drug type to the next could be due to unobserved common factors that influence the use of several drug types (Fergusson *et al.* 2006; Bretteville-Jensen *et al.* 2008). Several studies have addressed this issue, taking into account a possible 'third factor' explanation, but the results are not consistent. Some studies suggest a modest causal effect (e.g. van Ours 2003; Fergusson *et al.* 2006; Bretteville-Jensen *et al.* 2008), whereas others do not (e.g. Morral *et al.* 2002). It is therefore not clear whether a transition from cannabis to other drugs is due to increased susceptibility to other drugs, or to exposure to users and dealers of other drugs. In either case, most cannabis users do not initiate use of other illicit drugs.

3.9.2 'Natural history' of drug use

This chapter has already noted that the majority of youthful drug users tend to take drugs sporadically, and then desist. If they have avoided adverse consequences from the illegality of the behaviour, most suffer little harm. An analysis of 48 general population longitudinal studies found a lack of evidence of a robust causal relationship between cannabis use by young people and psychosocial harm (Macleod *et al.* 2004).

Little is known about how problem drug use develops and changes over time, especially in response to treatment services or criminal sanctions. Long-term follow-up studies of problem drug users are rare. One study (Hser *et al.* 2001) found that three decades after receiving treatment for heroin dependence, 48% had died. Among the 52% who had survived throughout the follow-up period, almost half were abstinent and one of six were daily drug users. This sample was, however, recruited from a treatment facility, and we do not know how this particular episode of treatment or other interventions affected the course of drug use. Another follow-up study of heroin users (Robins and Slobodyan 2003) found that among war veterans who had used heroin while in Vietnam, the majority (76%) did not use heroin after their return to the USA. What characterized those who relapsed to heroin use back in the USA was deviant behaviour and drug use both before and when they were in Vietnam.

3.10 **Conclusion**

Most of the research on the extent, distribution, and trends in drug use comes from a limited number of affluent countries, primarily those in North America and Western Europe as well as Australia. A global perspective on drug use is hampered not only by this disproportionate concentration of research attention, but also by imprecise estimates of uncertain comparability. Nevertheless, it seems beyond doubt that there are significant differences in the extent of drug use and problem use across countries and regions of the world. These differences at the population level reflect variations in drug markets, drug availability, and legislation as well as political, economic, and social conditions. There is overwhelming evidence from epidemiological research conducted over the past 50 years that adolescence is the period of greatest risk for the initiation of drug use (Compton *et al.* 2005b). However, most of those who have tried illicit drugs do not continue to use them.

Within populations, drug use and particularly problem drug use are unevenly distributed. Problem drug use occurs more frequently among males, and tends to cluster in inner city areas and disadvantaged neighbourhoods. Problem drug users are more likely than others to have a family history of substance use problems, and to manifest delinquent behaviour and mental health problems. Problem drug use is seldom confined to a single substance, but rather is a part of a polydrug use pattern.

Thus, drug use and its related problems do not occur randomly. Some nations and some neighbourhoods are more likely at times to experience high rates of drug use, and some individuals are more likely to initiate and continue heavy drug use. The fact that problem drug use is most often interwoven in a complex network of other social problems, both at the individual level and at the societal level, implies that strategies to prevent drug use or drug-related harms need to address this complexity. Approaches that evaluate the problem in two axes, substance use on one side and problems on the other, and that analyse their inter-relationship in the sociocultural context (Room 1989), can provide a more accurate view of the problem by integrating in the analysis drug supply, individual and contextual variations, social perceptions of the problem, and drug policies.

Chapter 4

Harms associated with illicit drug use

4.1 General principles in assessing harm

For many policymakers, researchers, and ordinary citizens, drug use *per se* is less of a concern than the problems that accompany it: chronic health problems, infectious disease transmission, property crime, and family breakdown, to name only a few examples. This chapter summarizes what is known about the extent of the health risks and social harms associated with drug use. We begin by making four conceptual points.

First, we use the term *associated* advisedly. In science, *associated* means co-occurring and does not necessarily imply that the causal direction of the association is simple, clear, or fully understood. One of the key points of this chapter is that the same kinds of drug use can cause different types of harm, based on the cultural and policy contexts in which drug use occurs. Although in one sense it is logical to assume that a lethal overdose by a heroin injector was 'caused by drug use', at a deeper level the death may have been determined in part by the availability of heroin in the community, recent changes in the purity of the supply, or whether local policies supported **naloxone** availability in all ambulances.[1] These contextual factors have many inputs, but at least one of them is the existing drug policy regime. Therefore, policymakers' choices may influence how strongly drug use is associated with the various harms described in this chapter. Conceptually, harms from the drug use itself can be separated from harms that result from the political and social responses to the drug use (Fischer *et al.* 1997), even if the distinction may not always be so clear in practice.

Secondly, 'harm' is both a subjective and a normative concept that is influenced by social and cultural valuation. A form of harm directly related to illicit drug use that is recognized by one society (e.g., cannabis intoxication in social settings) may not be regarded as a harm in another society because of a different sociocultural context. Policy measures draw such distinctions implicitly, for example by inflicting some harms that are deemed acceptable (e.g. imprisoning a drug dealer who sold a fatal dose of heroin) and by trying to reduce other harms that are viewed as non-acceptable (e.g. muggings and property crimes by drug-dependent criminals).

[1] Naloxone counters the effects of heroin and thus when administered in case of an overdose can prevent death.

Thirdly, we can distinguish *acute* and *long-term* harms. Intoxication, overdose, and drug-related traffic injuries are acute harms, in that they occur immediately after the use of drugs. Consequences such as dependence or endocarditis occur with long-term use or involvement with drug use. Note that some long-term harms, such as HIV or hepatitis C virus (HCV) infection, may also occur after a single occasion of drug use; however, the single occasion is commonly just one of multiple occasions for the individual user who becomes infected. It is empirically documented that time of exposure to drug use predicts the likelihood of such morbidity occurring (Amon *et al.* 2008).

Fourthly, illicit drug users differ tremendously in their drug preferences and patterns of drug use. The data upon which we draw in this chapter do not usually include a breakdown of 'harms' by specific drug. But, as discussed in Chapter 2, drugs differ in their harm potential. For instance, for many outcomes, such as overdose deaths and infectious diseases, cannabis is associated with much less risk than other substances (Hall and Pacula 2003). In analysing broad categories of drugs, one should keep in mind, however, that in many societies polydrug use is the norm rather than the exception. Polydrug use is often linked to more severe outcomes and frequently includes legally available substances as well (e.g. alcohol and benzodiazepines).

As noted in Chapter 1, this book takes a broad, 'public good' perspective on illegal drug use. However, much of the data that we have on harms associated with drug use come from health records such as mortality and morbidity statistics. This necessarily shifts the discussion that follows towards the narrower frame of health harms.

4.2 **Morbidity and mortality**

In the health statistics from hospital records, death certificates, and other sources, many morbidity or mortality outcomes are in some way associated with drug use, but only a few are defined as being 100% attributable to drug use. For outcomes that are not fully attributable to drug use, a drug-attributable fraction (DAF) of the cases must be ascertained. The DAF denotes the proportion of an outcome that would disappear if there had been no drug use. The DAFs are sometimes based on prevalence and intensity of exposure combined with risk relations derived from **meta-analyses** (e.g. English *et al.* 1995), or more often derived directly from meta-analyses of direct measurement of the prevalence of drug involvement (MacDonald *et al.* 2003). The underlying studies have been carried out in a small range of countries, and one cannot assume that DAFs will be the same in different societies, since they are affected by the prevalence and causes of cases with non-drug-related diagnoses as well as by the differing circumstances of the occurrence of drug-related cases. However, the DAFs derived from these meta-analyses are presently the best data we have for estimating drug-related health harm. In the discussion of drug-related morbidity and mortality that follows, we have organized the findings by substantive disease or casualty classes, and according to acute versus long-term consequences of drug use. Comments on the dynamics of association or causality are included where appropriate.

Five classes of morbidity and mortality can be distinguished for the purposes of this chapter: (1) overdose; (2) other injury; (3) non-communicable physical disease; (4) mental disorders; and (5) infectious disease. While the latter three categories are typically long-term outcomes, injury, whether intentional or unintentional, typically occurs during or after a single occasion of drug use. A number of different injuries are associated with illicit drug use (Chermack and Blow 2002; MacDonald *et al.* 2003) and can occur independently of the length or regularity of drug use.

4.2.1 **Overdose**

One type of injury related to illicit drug use is drug poisoning, or overdose. Drug overdoses are prominent among types of drug-related mortality. Although some categories of illicit drugs (e.g. cannabis) present no risk of death by overdose, users of many other illicit drugs have elevated mortality risk (Darke *et al.* 2007). Overdoses related to illicit opioid use are primarily due to respiratory depression, whereas cocaine and amphetamine overdose deaths are typically caused by myocardial infarction or stroke. The major cause of MDMA-related deaths is hyperthermia. Inhalant use may also lead to unintentional injury death.

It has been estimated that between 35 and 50% of IDUs have experienced a non-fatal overdose in their lifetime (Darke *et al.* 1996; Fischer *et al.* 1999; Tobin and Latkin 2003). Most of these overdoses are accidental rather than suicide attempts, and often result from uncertainties about the potency of illegal products as well as the risky circumstances of use (e.g. hurried injecting). For instance, a relatively low proportion (5%) of fatal heroin overdoses that occurred in Australia over a 5-year period were formally classified as suicides (Darke *et al.* 2000a). Similarly, 92% of methadone maintenance patients in another Australian study reported that their most recent overdose was accidental rather than intentional (Darke and Ross 2001). Survivors of drug overdose may suffer from physical complications such as renal failure, cardiovascular complications, lung infections, and cognitive disorders (Darke *et al.* 2000b; Warner-Smith *et al.* 2001).

Several studies have demonstrated elevated mortality rates for so-called 'high risk' drug users (e.g. IDUs), including but not limited to illicit opioid users. In one analysis, Degenhardt *et al.* (2004) estimated the average annual death rate for problem drug users, defined mainly as drug injectors, to be 1.1%. Other studies have identified an annual mortality rate of upto 2.0% among problem drug user populations (Hser *et al.* 2001; Darke and Hall 2003; Darke *et al.* 2007). One meta-analysis (English *et al.* 1995) found that opioid injectors had a mortality risk 13 times higher than the general population.

People who die accidentally from illicit drug overdoses tend to be young adults in their late twenties to early thirties, overwhelmingly male, and with several years' experience of drug use. Most deaths involve daily or almost-daily users. The majority administer drugs by injection (Darke *et al.* 2007). Increased risk of overdose death is associated with poverty, homelessness, concurrent use of other substances (especially co-administration of alcohol, benzodiazepines, or antidepressants), impaired physical health, depression, and a previous history of drug overdose (O'Driscoll *et al.* 2001; Warner-Smith *et al.* 2001; Darke *et al.* 2007). Opiate users who start using again after successful detoxification are at elevated risk of overdose death (Strang *et al.* 2003).

The numbers of opioid-related overdose deaths are increasing around the world (Drummer 2005). There is concern, particularly in the USA, about the greatly increased numbers of overdose deaths in which prescription opioids have been implicated. In 2002 the number of overdose deaths associated with prescription opioids in the USA exceeded the number of both cocaine- and heroin-related deaths (Paulozzi *et al.* 2006).

4.2.2 Other injury: accidents, poisonings, suicide

Drugs impair a variety of skills and abilities (e.g. cognition, vision, psychomotor control, reaction time), and many drugs raise the risk of unintentional injuries of various kinds. The role of illicit drugs in unintentional injury is best documented for motor vehicle accident involvement (Drummer *et al.* 2004; Kelly *et al.* 2004). A recent meta-analysis for cannabis and cocaine (MacDonald *et al.* 2003) found that the proportion of non-fatally injured drivers testing positive for cannabis ranged from 5 to 16.9%, while the proportion testing positive for cocaine ranged from 0.6 to 5.6%. The corresponding percentages for fatally injured drivers were in the same broad range.

Two caveats should be considered in the interpretation of these numbers. First, the underlying studies were conducted in the USA and other developed countries during the 1990s, so the proportions described above reflect the overall pattern of drug use in these countries at that time. Secondly, these findings may not indicate the true rates of accidents *caused* by illicit drugs, as the psychoactive substances in the body must be active and above a certain quantity to cause cognitive and psychomotor impairments. Even at that level, some of the accidents would not be causally related to the use of the drug.

The last type of injury related to drugs is intentional injury resulting from assault or from an attempted or completed suicide. That there is a correlation between drugs and violence is well established. Beneath the correlation, however, are a variety of possible relationships. A classic typology divides the main relationships into three types (Goldstein 1985). *Systemic violence* refers to interpersonal aggression among persons involved in the drug trade. So long as the market is illicit, contracts and agreements cannot be enforced by civil law, and systemic violence is a major alternative means of enforcement. *Economic compulsive violence* refers to violence in the course of criminal activity to obtain resources to support drug use. Although such violence can also result from the act of obtaining legal drugs as well as other goods, it is often noted in the literature that this type of violence applies to all substances for which there is no legal market (Boles and Miotto 2003). *Psychopharmacological violence* refers to causation of violent behaviour (or of victimization by others' violence) by the psychobiological action of the drug. Illegal drugs vary in the extent to which they have been linked to psychopharmacological violence. Those most often linked with it are amphetamines, cocaine, barbiturates, and PCP, while there is little evidence to link heroin, marijuana, or other hallucinogens (Kuhns and Klodfelter 2009). However, recent reviews have concluded that the evidence for psychopharmacological causation is weak even for the drugs most commonly linked (Tyner and Fremouw 2008; Kuhns and Klodfelter 2009).

The rates of completed and attempted suicide among illicit drug users are many magnitudes higher than those in the general population (Hulse *et al.* 1999; Darke *et al.* 2007). Data from five US cities demonstrate that approximately 36% of

IDUs had thoughts of suicide, while 7% attempted suicide in the 6 months prior to being interviewed (Havens *et al.* 2004). Illicit drug users have substantially more risk factors for suicide than the general population, including psychopathology, family dysfunction, and social isolation. In addition, polydrug use has been specifically identified as a risk factor (Darke *et al.* 2007). Drug-related suicide attempts may be a result of stigma, marginalization, barriers to accessing health services, and other factors besides the pharmacological effects of the drug.

4.2.3 Non-communicable physical disease

Adverse health consequences vary with the drug involved, and may reflect the social marginalization of the drug user as much as the drug use itself (Galea and Vlahov 2002). The type of drug, along with the route of drug administration, also affect the severity of disease. For example, chronic use of cocaine and amphetamines may lead to fatal cardiovascular consequences (Darke *et al.* 2007), whereas the rapid heart rate associated with cannabis use is probably not of lasting consequence, as the effect diminishes with tolerance (Hall *et al.* 2001). Although there is some evidence of adverse effects of smoked cannabis on pulmonary function (Aldington *et al.* 2007), its potential contribution to cancer risk is hard to determine because tobacco use cannot be ruled out as a **confounder** (Hall *et al.* 2001). Regarding routes of administration, injection drug use has been associated with higher levels of non-communicable physical disease. Street drug users, including IDUs and oral crack users, have very high rates of long-term health problems. In one study of illegal opioid users in five Canadian cities, 50% of the participants rated their health status to be 'fair' or 'poor' (Fischer *et al.* 2005), about four times the rate found in the general population.

Physical pain is prevalent among many drug users (Rosenblum *et al.* 2003; Peles *et al.* 2005) and may be part of a bidirectional relationship between physical health problems and illicit drug use. Opioid use itself can cause hyperalgesia (increased sensitivity to pain). Further, chronic or severe pain problems (e.g. as a result of injury) can lead to dependence on prescribed opiates preceding illicit drug use, suggesting the possibility that illicit opioid use can be a consequence of untreated or ineffectively treated pain problems. Another possibility is that severe pain occurs in the context of illicit opioid use or even as a consequence of ineffective treatment (Ives *et al.* 2006; Manchikanti *et al.* 2006a).

4.2.4 Mental disorders

Both national and international diagnostic systems define drug dependence as a mental disorder. Thus the drug dependence syndrome itself is recorded as part of the mental health burden. However, only a fraction of drug users are formally diagnosed as dependent (Kendler *et al.* 2000; Lynskey *et al.* 2003). In addition to the diagnosis itself, elevated rates of mental disorders have been widely documented in clinical treatment settings (e.g. Frei and Rehm 2002), surveys of 'street users' (e.g. Wild *et al.* 2005), and general population surveys (e.g. Kessler *et al.* 2005). Frei and Rehm (2002) found that 78% of opioid addicts had at least one co-morbid mental condition, excluding other **substance use disorders.** Co-morbid psychiatric conditions have been found in most groups of illicit drug users. For cannabis use, especially frequent and long-term use, an association with psychotic symptoms has been observed, and cannabis use is suspected to be a causal precipitant in a small number of psychotic episodes (Hall *et al.* 2001; Hall and Pacula 2003).

There is evidence that psychiatric co-morbidity is considerably elevated among psychostimulant users. One study found the lifetime rate of psychiatric co-morbidity in a community sample of crack cocaine users to be substantially elevated, with 36.4% of the sample indicating psychiatric co-morbidity, primarily antisocial personality disorder and depression (Falck *et al.* 2004). A sample of crack cocaine users found that as many as 55% had symptoms of moderate to severe depression (Falck *et al.* 2002).

The association between drug use and mental disorder may have different underlying causal pathways (Meyer 1986); the drug use may be a self-medication of a psychiatric condition (Harris and Edlund 2005). Psychopathology, such as personality disorders, may serve as a risk factor for substance use disorders. Mental disorders can modify the course of a substance use disorder and frequent drug use can cause mental health problems (e.g. paranoid symptoms or drug-induced psychosis). Finally, predisposing factors (e.g. genetic vulnerability) may lead to both drug use and mental disorders, without there being a necessary causal link between the two. The degree of association between drug use and mental disorder depends on the type of illicit drug.

In some discussions, rates of drug-related mental disorder appear very high because the drug dependence diagnosis itself is counted as a mental disorder. Setting this aside, the implications for health services of the correlations found for health policy are not self-evident. Not all drug use is likely to be the sole cause of mental disorder or behaviour problems because many drug users have antecedent personality disorders even before they begin to use drugs. Also, clinical research (Meyer 1986) indicates that many drug-related psychiatric symptoms (e.g. depression and anxiety) remit with abstinence, so that treatment for some putative mental disorders may be unnecessary outside the period of drug withdrawal.

4.2.5 **Infectious disease**

Unsafe injection practices, unsafe sexual contacts, and multiple daily injections increase the risk for infectious diseases, such as hepatitis B virus (HBV), HCV, and HIV infection (Hagan *et al.* 2001; Strathdee *et al.* 2001; Thorpe *et al.* 2002). Prevalence rates for HCV infection among IDUs vary among countries. In many high income countries the majority of IDUs are HCV infected (Roy *et al.* 2002; Fischer *et al.* 2004; Shepard *et al.* 2005; Aceijas and Rhodes 2007). HCV prevalence among young injectors (e.g. fewer than 5 years of injecting) tends to be lower, although numerous studies have demonstrated that the majority of HCV seroconversion occurs within 1–5 years of initiating drug use by injection (Miller *et al.* 2002; Hagan *et al.* 2004; Shepard *et al.* 2005). HIV prevalence rates among IDUs tend to be lower than those for HCV, with prevalence rates ranging between 5 and 30% in many studies, yet those rates also indicate considerable intercountry and inter-regional variability (Hamers *et al.* 1997; Fischer *et al.* 2000; Aceijas *et al.* 2004; Des Jarlais *et al.* 2005; UNAIDS 2006). In addition to the elevated risks for specific infectious disease in IDUs, there is a high rate of co-infection between different infectious diseases, especially HCV and HIV (Alter 2006; Aceijas and Rhodes 2007).

There are two important policy implications to be drawn from these data. First, because infectious disease is prevalent among drug users, clinical and prevention services can benefit not only drug users but also non-users as well (e.g. sexual partners of drug users). Secondly, because virtually all IDUs will carry one or more serious diseases after 5 years of drug use, any efforts to prevent disease must be attractive to younger IDUs and first treatment admissions to be effective.

HIV/AIDS is a global epidemic, in part fuelled by drug use. At the end of 2004 it was estimated that there were 3 million drug users in Russia, and 300 000 cases of HIV (Luo and Confrancesco 2006). About three in four HIV cases in Russia are associated with unsafe drug injection practices. The majority of IDUs in Russia have never been tested for HIV. Most of them lack basic information about the transmission of disease by unsafe drug using practices, and up to 40% of IDUs share non-sterile equipment (Luo and Confrancesco 2006). A similar scenario, though more catastrophic in terms of raw numbers, is occurring in China. Currently there are 840 000 reported cases of AIDS in China, close to half of which are IDUs (Liu *et al.* 2006). Finally, drug use has been contributing to the spread of HIV in Latin America as well (Darke *et al.* 2007).

4.3 **Deaths and burden of disease attributable to illicit drug use: Canada as an example**

Identifying drug-related harms does not address the question of the total health burden from drugs, nor of the relative contribution of drug use to that burden. These questions have now been addressed at national and global levels by studies of how much illicit drug use contributes to the burden of disease. For example, Table 4.1 shows the relative weight of the different disease categories in drug-attributable mortality in Canada for the year 2002 (Popova *et al.* 2006).

Among the deaths caused by illicit drugs, the biggest contributor was death by accidental overdose, as evidenced by coroners' reports. In 2002, there were 733 overdoses for men and 225 for women, totalling 958 deaths. This constituted 56.5% of all illicit drug-related deaths in Canada for the year 2002. Most of these overdose deaths involved the use of multiple drugs, including **psychopharmaceuticals**. For most of the overdose deaths the coroners could not determine which drug caused the death. The second major contributor to drug-attributable mortality was suicide (17.4%; 146 males and 149 females), followed by HCV infection (9.7%; 102 males and 62 females), and then HIV infection (5.1%; 87 deaths: 74 males and 13 females). Overall, the Canadian study shows that illicit drug use resulted in higher fatality rates among men than women. In the age group under 60, the rates were 4.6% in men and 3.0% in women. Similar analyses are lacking for most other countries (see Degenhardt *et al.* 2004 for an overview), but there are indications that the overall proportions of different causes of drug-attributable deaths are comparable for high income countries. Overdose death seems to be the major contributor to drug-related mortality (Darke *et al.* 2007).

Table 4.1 Drug-attributable fractions (DAFs), mean age at death, and number of illicit drug use-attributable deaths in Canada 2002

Disease condition (ICD 10 code)	DAF in % (all ages)	Mean age at death		Number of deaths		
		M	F	M	F	Total
Disease conditions always caused by illicit drug use						
Mental and behavioural disorders due to use of:						
Opioids (F11)	100	52.0	–	1	0	1
Cannabinoids (F12)	100	–	–	0	0	0
Cocaine (F14)	100	34.7	37.0	13	1	14
Other stimulants, including caffeine (F15)	100	–	–	0	0	0
Hallucinogens (F16)	100	–	–	0	0	0
Multiple drug use and use of other psychoactive substances (F19)	100	42.0	43.5	43	25	68
Opiate and cocaine poisoning* (T40.0, T40.5)				733	225	958*
Disease conditions not always caused by drug use (DAF <1.0)						
HIV infection (B20-24)	21.6	44.7	41.0	74	13	87
Viral hepatitis C (B17.1, B18.2)	56.0	58.4	64.3	102	62	165
Viral hepatitis B (B16, B18.0, B18.1)	26.0	58.0	66.3	11	8	18
Acute and subacute endocarditis (I33)	0.14	–	–	1	0	1
Neonatal conditions; Low birthweight (P02.0-2, P04.8, P05-P07, P96.1)	0.3	0	0	1	0	1
Injuries not always caused by drug use (DAF <1.0)						
Cannabis-attributable traffic accidents (Fatal) (V1–V89)	1.4	40.7	45.3	26	13	39
Cocaine-attributable traffic accidents (Fatal) (V1–V89)	0.3	40.4	44.8	6	3	8
Suicide, self-inflicted injuries X60-X84, Y87.0)	8.3	44.0	43.5	146	149	295
Homicide (X85–Y09, Y87.1)	9.0	35.6	35.9	28	13	42
All drug-attributable deaths		42.9	39.2	1193	512	1695

Source: Popova *et al.* (2006).

* This combined total number of overdose deaths was not partitioned by individual drug because most deaths are associated with multidrug use.

4.4 Global burden of disease attributable to illicit drug use

Estimates of how illicit drug use affects health on a global level were generated in recent years by the World Health Organization's Comparative Risk Assessment (CRA; Degenhardt *et al.* 2004), which was part of the Global Burden of Disease (GBD) 2000 study (Ezzati *et al.* 2004). This landmark project focused on the causal role of selected risk factors in order to evaluate how changes in population health and risk exposure affect major disease outcomes. As the CRA restricted itself to an assessment of disease burden, the estimates presented here exclude social harm other than the intentional injury categories captured by the International Classification of Diseases. All estimates were done for the year 2000. The study restricts the definition of illicit drug use to current use of amphetamines, cocaine, heroin or other opioids, and intravenous drug use. Even within that scope, the available data primarily cover the burden of drug overdose deaths and AIDS among injection drug users.

Table 4.2 gives an overview of mortality and burden of disease attributable to illicit drug use. Mortality consists of the proportion of all deaths in 2000 in the population category attributable to illicit drug use. Burden of disease combines years of life lost due to premature mortality and fractional years of life lost due to disability (these are called disability-adjusted life-years or DALYs; see Murray and Lopez 1996). Thus the table shows that 0.8% of the global burden of disease in DALYs was attributed to illicit drugs. Illicit drugs did not rank among the top 10 causes of morbidity and mortality (in DALYs) in either of the developing regions, and ranked eighth among causes in developed regions.

In the year 2000 estimates, mortality attributable to illicit drug use varied according to a country's economic wealth, or the wealth of its subregion, with drug-attributable mortality accounting for the highest fraction of mortality in high income countries. In terms of burden of disease, the same economic gradient occurred, but was even more pronounced. While drug-related mortality is concentrated between ages 15 and 59, the average age for drug-attributable deaths has shifted upwards in many low and middle income countries, but this shift has been slow. Overall, the burden of disease was proportionally higher than the mortality burden, primarily because morbidity from illicit drug use is differentially more prevalent than other illness in younger age populations. Globally, the rates of both mortality and morbidity are about three times higher among men than among women. In developed regions, they are twice as high, which is consistent with male to female ratios for problem drug use noted in Chapter 3.

Table 4.3 gives an overview of the fractions of different disease categories attributable to illicit drugs. This excludes drug use disorders (e.g. overdoses and dependence), for which the attributable fraction is by definition always 100%. In terms of HIV/AIDS attributable to illicit drug use, there are large discrepancies among the different parts of the world. Whereas 43% of the male and 68% of the female HIV/AIDS burden of disease is attributed to illicit drug use in established market economies in 2000, the comparable figure for the poorest countries is less than 1%. It should be noted that the countries of the former Soviet Union are counted in the developed countries in this

Table 4.2 Proportion of illegal-drug attributable mortality and morbidity in 2000, as a percentage of overall mortality and burden of disease, by development status of global subregion and sex*

	High mortality developing regions			**Low mortality developing regions – emerging economies**			**Developed regions**			**World**		
	Africa, poorest countries in Central and South America, poorest regions of Asia including India			**Emerging countries in Central/South America and Asia, including China**			**Europe, North America, Japan, Australia, New Zealand**					
	Male	**Female**	**Both**	**Male**	**Female**	**Both**	**Male**	**Female**	**Both**	**Male**	**Female**	**Both**
Proportion of burden of disease (DALYs)	0.8%	0.2	0.5	1.2	0.3	0.8	2.3	1.2	1.8	1.1	0.4	0.8
Mortality as a proportion of all deaths	0.5%	0.1	0.3	0.6	0.1	0.4	0.6	0.3	0.5	0.6	0.2	0.4

Source: own calculations based on WHO (2002).

* The WHO used standardized child and adult mortality rates to develop a classification system to categorize regions from developing countries into two categories. As mortality is highly correlated with economic wealth, the middle income countries of Asia and Central and South America constitute the low mortality developing countries, whereas the low income countries make up the high mortality developing countries.

Table 4.3 Drug-attributable fractions for particular disorders, by sex and level of development, 2000 (% disability adjusted life years (DALYs) for each cause)*

	World			High mortality developing countries		Low mortality developing/ emerging economies		Developed countries	
	Males	**Females**	**Both**	**Males**	**Females**	**Males**	**Females**	**Males**	**Females**
HIV/AIDS	4%	1%	2%	0%	0%	28%	9%	43%	68%
Unintentional injuries	1%	1%	1%	1%	0%	1%	1%	2%	6%
Self-inflicted injuries	5%	2%	4%	10%	2%	1%	0%	5%	9%

Source: own calculations based on WHO (2002).

* The WHO used standardized child and adult mortality rates to develop a classification system to categorize regions from developing countries into two categories. As mortality is highly correlated with economic wealth, the middle income countries of Asia and Central and South America constitute the low mortality developing countries, whereas the low income countries make up the high mortality developing countries.

analysis, and that the greater part of the HIV/AIDS burden in developing countries is attributable to sexual transmission.

The CRA study team acknowledged that estimates of the disease burden attributable to drug use are not exhaustive and show a high level of uncertainty (Ezzati *et al.* 2004; see also WHO 2002), in part because the main health consequences, especially overdose deaths and HIV infection risk, are linked not only to the substance itself but also to the circumstances of use (e.g. the extent of sharing of needles). In addition, there is a lack of data with which to quantify these socially determined risk relations in different regions of the world. Despite these limitations, the burden of disease attributable to illicit drug use is considerable. But other psychoactive substances cause a substantially higher burden. Globally, smoking and alcohol misuse each cause about five times the disease burden of illicit drugs (see Rehm and Room 2005). Particularly since polysubstance use is typical in most parts of the world, the burden of disease and disability associated with illicit drugs needs to be considered in this broader context.

4.5 **Risk factors for drug-related morbidity and mortality**

Besides drug use itself, a variety of social, environmental, and behavioural risk factors influence the extent to which morbidity and mortality are associated with illicit drug use. These risk factors are important to consider for the development of preventive or targeted interventions aimed at reducing morbidity and mortality among illicit drug users.

One specific example is housing status (e.g. homelessness). Relative to domiciled drug users, homeless 'street' drug users engage in more high risk behaviour (e.g. needle sharing) and are at substantially higher risk for fatal and non-fatal drug overdose, HIV seroconversion, and physical health problems associated with their drug use

(Galea and Vlahov 2002). For example, in a large multisite sample of HIV-infected persons in the USA, the odds of recent drug use, needle use, or sex-for-money exchange were 2–4 times as high among homeless and unstably housed people compared with persons with stable housing (Aidala *et al.* 2005). Several studies have demonstrated that the absence of stable housing is a major risk factor for seroconversion of HIV to AIDS among IDUs (Strathdee *et al.* 1997; Corneil *et al.* 2006).

Incarceration plays a role in drug-related morbidity or mortality. An IDU's incarceration history predicts infectious disease transmission (e.g. HIV) as well as overdose mortality in the period immediately following release from detention (Galea and Vlahov 2002; Hammett *et al.* 2002; Seaman *et al.* 1998). A study of inmates released from correctional facilities in the US State of Washington (1999–2003) indicated that the risk of death among former inmates was over 12 times higher than for other state residents (Binswanger *et al.* 2007).

Injection behaviour is another important risk factor. Frequent 'speedball' injection (combining heroin and cocaine) and engaging in binges of injection drug use were found to be independent predictors of HIV seroconversion (Craib *et al.* 2003). Similarly, studies have also associated speedball use with (non-fatal) overdose episodes in several IDU populations in Canada and the USA (Kerr *et al.* 2007; Ochoa *et al.* 2001).

4.6 **Harms beyond the health domain**

Social harms related to illicit drug use, such as crime, public disorder, and workplace problems affect individuals, the community, and society in different ways. Some of these problems arise from psychopharmacological effects of the drug used, the first category in the Goldstein (1985) typology mentioned above. Problems for others that arise from someone's drug use include injuries resulting from traffic accidents and violence.

Many drug users engage in criminal activities to obtain money to buy drugs, the second of Goldstein's (1985) three categories of drug-related crime. These activities may consist of small-scale drug dealing; property crimes such as shoplifting, theft, fraud, robbery, and burglary; and also sex-work, which in many countries is a criminal activity (Rajkumar and French 1997; Stewart *et al.* 2000; Maher *et al.* 2002). In some countries the proportion of property crimes related to illicit drugs ranges from 50 to 80% (Office of the Auditor General of Canada 2001; Families and Friends for Drug Law Reform 2004). Several factors affect the intensity of criminal activity among illicit drug users, including homelessness (Galea and Vlahov 2002; Manzoni *et al.* 2006), social marginalization, and poverty (Baumer *et al.* 1998; Grogger and Willis 2000; Best *et al.* 2001a). A meta-analysis of 36 studies, over half from the USA, found that compared with non-users, the mean odds ratio for criminal offending was 3.6 for heroin users, 6.2 for crack cocaine users, 2.6 for cocaine users, 1.9 for amphetamine users, and 1.5 for marijuana users (Bennett *et al.* 2008).

Goldstein's (1985) third category of drug-related crime is 'systemic' violence associated with illicit drug markets. Studies have documented an association between illicit drug markets and varying levels of interpersonal violence, including gun violence and homicides (Goldstein, 1985; Blumstein *et al.* 2000; Galea *et al.* 2002). Systemic violence related to drug markets varies considerably across societies, reflecting both the general level of violence and accessibility of lethal weapons. It also varies over time according to whether the market is stable or disrupted.

A fourth category of criminal activity is public nuisance or disorder in public places associated with drug use. Even countries that do not recognize public nuisance as a crime can still regard it as a harm to the public good. Some societies may view the concentration of large numbers of illicit drug users in so-called 'open drug scenes' as a threat to the safety, values, and quality of life of ordinary citizens, visitors, and businesses operating in nearby urban areas (Bless *et al.* 1995; Kübler and Wälti 2001). In addition, many communities regard the unsafe discarding of drug paraphernalia, such as needles or syringes, as a major public disorder problem (Fischer *et al.* 2004; Wood *et al.* 2004).

The frequent use of illicit drugs is associated with reduced earnings, job instability, and receipt of public assistance (DeSimone 2002; Zlotnick *et al.* 2002; Brown and Riley 2005). The association between unemployment and illicit drug use is certainly not unidirectional. Drug use is likely to cause unemployment, but unemployment can exacerbate or lead to drug use. A third scenario, in which an outside cause produces both unemployment and illicit drug use, is also possible.

In North America, Australia, and Europe, random drug testing in the workplace has increased (Verstraete and Pierce 2001; Dolan *et al.* 2004; French *et al.* 2004). Some drug users have difficulties finding or keeping their jobs because of drug testing practices, although this may reduce harm to others (e.g. the passengers in the buses and trains that would otherwise be driven by drug-affected drivers). But heavy drug users have markedly higher rates of unemployment even in countries where employee drug testing is rare or non-existent.

Attempts to estimate the 'total cost' of drug use have gained substantial political importance in many jurisdictions. This is consistent with a 'public good' perspective in that costs are not just limited to expenses in the health area but are also considered in terms of lost productivity related to disability and costs related to criminal justice interventions (Single *et al.* 1996; Wall *et al.* 2000). However, the tradition of 'cost of illness' studies within which they are done has been criticized on a number of grounds, and particularly in terms of who is bearing the cost and of the extent to which the costs, commonly estimated on cross-sectional data, can in fact be saved (Tarricone 2006). For illicit drugs, the issue is complicated by the fact that the costs reflect not only the drug use itself but also a society's drug policy choices (Fischer *et al.* 1997), such as the cost of enforcing drug prohibition (Miron 2003b). Also, a variety of cost estimation procedures have been used, which makes it difficult to compare costs in different countries.

A study of Canada in 2002 estimated the total cost *per capita* for illicit drug use was approximately CDN$262 (Rehm *et al.* 2006), similar to the Australian *per capita* cost of AUS$228 from 1998 (Collins and Lapsley 2002).[2] The respective estimates of total cost *per capita* for the USA for 2002 (US$650, ONDCP 2004a) and for the UK for 2000

[2] In US dollars at the end of June in the respective years, these would be $172 per capita in Canada and $140 in Australia.

(US$450, Godfrey *et al.* 2002) were clearly higher than corresponding estimates for Canada or Australia. This may reflect lower rates of problem drug use in Canada and Australia, as suggested by the lower overdose rates. The lower *per capita* costs also reflect lower law enforcement expenditures in Canada and Australia compared with the USA (Rehm *et al.* 2006). A report of public expenditures on illicit drug use in 16 European countries (EMCDDA 2003a) showed that The Netherlands, Sweden, and the UK (0.66, 0.47, and 0.35%, respectively) expended the highest proportions of Gross Domestic Product (GDP).

It should be noted that these economic cost assessments typically do not consider the illicit use of prescription drugs (e.g. prescription opioids), which now accounts for a substantial proportion of illicit drug use in many countries (Fischer and Rehm 2007), and is also likely to have significant economic consequences as one major form of 'harm' (see Chapter 6).

The overall economic cost for illicit drugs in virtually all societies is typically much smaller than that for legal drugs (alcohol or tobacco). The study of Canada in 2002 estimated that the cost of illicit drug use accounted for approximately CDN$8.2 billion, or 20.7% of the total costs attributable to substance misuse, including alcohol and tobacco. Illicit drug users are less numerous than drinkers and smokers, and the total health burden from illicit drug use is substantially smaller than that for alcohol or tobacco (e.g. Rehm *et al.* 2006). On the other hand, a disproportionate amount of drug-related costs stems from crime and criminal justice expenditures. It is not only that drug users and suppliers engage in high levels of criminal activity, but also that drug use *per se* constitutes illegal activity and is therefore subject to expensive criminal justice interventions (Rajkumar and French 1997).

Because crime and criminal justice responses are such a prominent part of the drug policy response, any interventions that reduce illegal drug use are likely to have a substantial economic benefit (Cartwright 2000; Flynn *et al.* 2003). For example, the co-prescription of medical heroin to chronic heroin users produced cost benefits in Switzerland (Frei *et al.* 2000) and The Netherlands (Dijkgraaf *et al.* 2005) by reducing law enforcement costs and costs of victim damage.

4.7 **Conclusions and policy implications**

Illicit drug use is associated with a marked burden of disease, disability, mortality, criminality, and a variety of other social harms. Although the burden, harm, and costs attributable to illicit drug use are substantial, for most countries they are lower than those attributable to alcohol and tobacco. Only in established market economies is illicit drug use among the major risk factors for the burden of disease. In low and middle income countries, illicit drug use is a minor consideration in the overall burden of disease, but this could change with rising incomes and increasing globalization.

This review of the harms associated with drug use suggests several conclusions that have important policy implications. First, both the specific class of illicit drugs and the pattern of drug administration affect individual and societal outcomes. Opioids, cocaine, and amphetamines entail special risks. Other drugs, such as cannabis, involve less risk, even though their use is substantially more prevalent in most societies.

The highly elevated mortality risk associated with opioids may diminish with the increased prevalence of prescription opioid misuse. With respect to the form of administration, injection drug use constitutes a particular risk of mortality as well as other severe health outcomes. A second conclusion is that many of the harmful consequences are not completely intrinsic to the properties of the drug, but instead are caused by the physical and social environment associated with drug use. Thirdly, a society's drug policy will be more likely to meet its chosen goals if these epidemiological considerations about the distribution of harms are taken into account in the allocation of resources for prevention programmes, treatment, and social services.

Chapter 5

Illegal markets: the economics of drug distribution and social harm

5.1 Introduction

An illegal drug is a commodity. Consequently, it can be produced and distributed in markets. Though the general concept of markets is familiar, and it is widely known that markets can be tracked, predicted, and to a certain extent deliberately influenced, policy discussions show a strange unwillingness to apply this understanding of markets when the commodity is an illicit drug. Large markets for marijuana, heroin, cocaine, and a range of synthetics exist in many nations. Globally, total revenues amount to tens of billions of dollars. Less substantial markets exist as well for diverted **psychopharmaceuticals** and a host of other substances (e.g. LSD, peyote). Some illegal drugs are produced or provided outside of markets, most notably when people consume home-grown marijuana or steal prescription drugs. Likewise, in the early stages of a drug epidemic, drugs may be imported from a distant land or city by an adventurous traveller who then shares the drug with friends with little attention to profit. However, with the partial exception of diverted **pharmaceuticals**, the vast majority of illegal drugs are produced and distributed in markets.

Markets for illicit drugs are of interest for two reasons. First, their existence and characteristics directly affect the success and unintended consequences of drug control efforts. An understanding of these markets underpins this book's consideration of drug enforcement in Chapter 10 and also any intelligent discussion of revising the legal status of currently illegal drugs. Secondly, black markets can harm those engaged in the market (producers, distributors, and buyers) as well as the broader community. The most obvious such harm is violence. The killing of innocent bystanders understandably garners media attention, but the typical victim of drug market violence is a user or seller. That illegal markets are themselves a source of harm, distinct from the drugs they distribute, is a fact that is essentially overlooked by cost-of-illness studies (Miron 2003a; cf. Moore and Caulkins 2005). The severity of the adverse effects depends in part on the drug (e.g. stimulant versus opiate) but also on the country's drug policies (e.g. more or less risky to buy) and general social context (e.g. whether it is a gun-available society, as in the USA or Colombia, or not, as in the UK or Bolivia).

This chapter describes what is known about drug markets and the nature and extent of harms that arise from them. It begins with a brief theoretical discussion about the structure, prices, availability, and product quality of illegal markets. The discussion of harms distinguishes between drug production and international trafficking on the one hand and wholesale distribution and retail marketing of drugs on the other. Each affects a specific set of communities and nations in a particular fashion. But a word of warning before we begin: there is a dearth of studies attempting to measure specific harms. One can only refer to large and small harms in an impressionistic fashion.

Many market-related harms are indirect consequences of prohibition and its enforcement because illegality generates incentives for violence, deception, disorder, and mistrust (MacCoun and Reuter 2001a). That there are adverse effects from prohibition, whether lightly or heavily enforced, does not constitute a final judgement about the desirability of such laws. Also, the extent of adverse effects can vary with the ways in which prohibition is applied, as when laws are lightly or heavily enforced. The symbolic disapproval, reduced availability, and higher prices that prohibition produces may reduce drug use enough to be worth these harms. Chapter 10 discusses the good and bad effects of more or less aggressive enforcement within a prohibition regime.

5.2 The concept of a market

The word *market* has two distinct meanings. The first concept of market is an abstract relationship between buyers and sellers. For example, there is a market in antique musical scores in which buyers and sellers transact through the Internet and rarely meet. There is no place that could be called 'the market', though some transactions occur in various places, such as a Sotheby's auction of an old estate. There are prices, but no single 'price', because the product is highly differentiated. The second concept of a market is a physical place where transactions occur. Indeed we refer to it as a 'marketplace' precisely to make that distinction. A flea market or bazaar is a place where sellers and buyers congregate to trade various goods. It is not a market for something in particular, nor is it a place where all transactions of any category occur. Until the advent of modern communications, all transactions required a place. Now, place and market can be distinguished.

High level drug control agencies aim to curtail the abstract market for drugs. For example, the Australian Federal Police investigate importers and wholesalers in an effort to make drugs more expensive. They do not directly concern themselves with marketplaces.

Local law enforcement agencies tend to think of marketplaces for illicit drugs, rather than the abstract 'markets' for drugs. For example, a study by David Kennedy, *Closing the Market: Controlling the Drug Trade in Tampa* (1991), describes innovative police methods aimed at controlling an open air drug market. The police were not concerned with reducing the number of buyers and sellers, let alone eliminating the drug market in Tampa, Florida, though some reduction could have occurred as a result of making it more difficult for sellers and buyers to come together. Instead, they were concerned about eliminating concentrated drug selling and disorder at a small number of places. The study measured success in terms of the location and associated crime. It did not estimate the impact on the wider market itself.

In the remainder of this book we will refer to *markets* when dealing with the abstract notion and *marketplaces* when the important issue is location.

5.3 Key traits of drug markets

Drug markets have distinctive features. Here we focus on three features that differ dramatically from their legal counterparts and have consequences for drug control and drug-related harm: organizational form, price, and product quality. A fourth, corruption, is discussed more extensively in Section 5.4, along with other harms.

5.3.1 Organizational form

Popular accounts of illicit drug distribution are full of references to cartels, syndicates, and organized crime. Yet the reality is almost the opposite. For example, in 1997 in the USA the vast majority of incarcerated federal and state drug offenders (85.7 and 91.9%, respectively) reported that they were not part of an organized drug group (Sevigny and Caulkins 2004). Likewise, when the Medellin cartel was at the peak of its power, cocaine prices plummeted (ONDCP 2004b). The cartel was organized to defend its members against kidnapping, not to control drug prices, the defining purpose of any true cartel.

The relative absence of large drug-dealing organizations is one consequence of the most fundamental observation about drug markets: illegal market participants have no recourse to the system of property rights and dispute resolution offered by the civil courts and legal system. This has important consequences for the structure, conduct, and performance of drug markets (Reuter 1983). For example, a desirable location for selling, which for legal businesses would be allocated to the highest bidder by whoever currently owns it, goes instead to whichever drug seller can most effectively intimidate the others. This encourages the development of reputations for contingent violence, with at least occasional exercise of violence for reputational purposes (Caulkins *et al.* 2006). As another example, written records, essential to modern businesses, are a source of danger for illegal enterprises since they provide information to agencies aiming to seize assets and incarcerate personnel. The lack of records creates uncertainties in transactions that themselves result in misunderstandings and violence. It also hinders the building of large global enterprises.

Instead of an organization or firm, the more appropriate metaphor for drug markets is a network. Drugs are produced and distributed by the collective efforts of literally millions of individuals and small organizations that operate in a highly decentralized manner. No one is in charge. Indeed, most people in the network only know the identities of those with whom they interact directly. There is a good reason why no one even has a 'map' of this distribution system. Since law enforcement officers constantly arrest and interrogate drug dealers, the less individual dealers know, the better the situation is for all of the other dealers. These networks place many intermediaries between the users and retail sellers (who are most vulnerable to enforcement) and the high level dealers (who sell larger quantities).

Hence, most of the more important drugs (e.g. cocaine, heroin, imported marijuana, and many amphetamine-type stimulants or ATSs) are distributed through long chains of participants. For example, heroin may be bought and sold 10 times in the chain connecting opium production in Afghanistan to retail sale in Rome. The chain starts with the farmer and then moves through local trader, regional trader, heroin refiner, and exporter. There are more sales in both Iran and Turkey, and yet further transactions between import, high level and low level wholesale, and retail personnel in Italy. Each transaction presents both an opportunity for intervention and a potential social problem.

The distribution network has structure. Drugs flow one way, down from their original source to users, and money flows the other way, up. Not all of the drugs reach users; some are lost to seizures. Much less of the money makes it very far back up the network. Most of the money that users spend on drugs compensates retail sellers and low level wholesale dealers.

That does not mean that retail sellers are rich. Another aspect of the network's structure prevents that. In terms of the numbers of participants at each market layer, Figure 5.1 illustrates how the network for cocaine and heroin is shaped like two funnels placed tip to tip, with the broad mouths (indicating many market participants) at the very top and bottom.

Using the example of coca and opium, there are many farmers growing small quantities of each in the producing countries. In Afghanistan it is estimated that as many as 1.9 million persons are involved on at least an occasional basis in opium production (Buddenberg and Byrd 2006). The number of people who buy the raw opium and refine it into heroin is very small by comparison. There are also relatively few smugglers and top level importers (perhaps only a few hundred for heroin in the USA) in consumer countries. Entering the second funnel, there are more wholesale sellers and a very large numbers of retailers. In the USA, it is likely that 1 million persons are at least occasional sellers of cocaine (Caulkins and Reuter 1998). The number who distribute cannabis is most probably considerably greater inasmuch as retail distribution often occurs within friendship networks, frequently not for profit (Caulkins and Pacula 2006).

As compared with most legal markets, there are many sellers relative to the number of buyers for two distinct reasons. From the customers' perspective, individual sellers

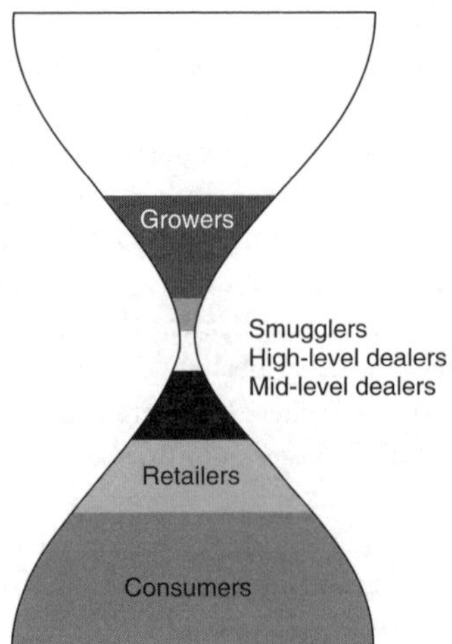

Fig. 5.1 Relative number of market participants at different market levels.

are unreliable because they are not always actively selling, so regular buyers need to have many potential sources. For example, Riley (1997) finds that heroin buyers in the USA each know an average of 10–20 sellers from whom they purchase. Secondly, a substantial share of drug-dependent users have few opportunities to earn money except through drug selling. As a result, many sell drugs at least occasionally, even if only on a part-time basis, as opposed to having a smaller number of higher volume sellers.

The top funnel may not exist, and the distribution chains may be much shorter, for drugs that are diverted from medical use (e.g. by forged prescriptions) or that can be efficiently produced domestically in small batches. This is true of domestically produced marijuana in Australia. Shorter distribution chains with larger branching factors (i.e. more lower level dealers supplied per dealer at the next higher level) may also be expected in cases where enforcement is less stringent (Caulkins 1997).

There are three important consequences of this decentralized network structure, one bad and two good. The frustrating consequence of the network character of drug distribution is its resilience. Eliminating individual players or even entire (inherently small) organizations within a mature, cross-connected drug distribution network has little impact on the ability of the network as a whole to transport drugs from their source to the customers. Incarcerated individuals are easily replaced (Kleiman 1997b), individuals have multiple alternative suppliers, and individual arcs in the network (connections between dealers) can rapidly increase their drug supply to meet increased demand. This adaptability of mature drug distribution networks limits the ability of enforcement authorities to eradicate mass-market drugs, as discussed at greater length in Chapter 10.

The first benefit of decentralization is that even though drug distribution networks are adaptable in the sense of being resilient to enforcement-induced tears or holes in the web, they are not very innovative, at least not with respect to products or marketing. This observation is subtle, but important. Drug dealers, particularly smugglers, may be masters of improvisation, adapting a multitude of tools and tactics to their purpose, but the rate of true invention of new products, product promotions, and production processes is extremely low. A simple explanation for the lack of innovation is that no drug organization is large enough to justify investing in development costs for innovations that could later be copied at little or no cost by other organizations.

Innovation raises consumption, as is evidenced by the occasional exceptions to the lack of innovation rule discussed above (e.g. the development of crack and new methamphetamine synthesis methods). It is fortunate that there are no large-scale, organized, and well-funded programmes under way to invent new **psychoactive substances**, improve the efficiency of coca or poppy cultivation or refining, or invent new ways of bundling current drugs with other products (e.g. breakfast cereal with performance-enhancing amphetamine supplements). The considerable innovation in cannabis cultivation over the past decade and subsequent dissemination of those innovations may be seen as something of a caution about what happens when drug producers feel less pressure to remain secretive.

For typical consumer goods, innovation involves not only performance but also image. Designer dresses are in demand not because they are highly functional, but in many instances because of their brand allure. Branding is common for licit experience goods (i.e. a good whose quality can only be judged after consumption). Consider, for example, the brand recognition strategies of restaurant chains. Meaningful branding is less common for illicit drugs perhaps because of the transience of selling organizations and the inability to create legally binding claims to product quality. Exceptions that prove the rule are branded ecstasy tablets and retail heroin sellers, particularly on the east coast of the USA, who stamp 'brand names' on heroin bags (Goldstein *et al.* 1984). However, Wendel and Curtis (2000, p. 238) note that sellers routinely manipulate quality so that '[u]sers are aware that different stamps do not necessarily mean different heroin and that one of the bags might often be better than the rest.' In contrast, there are systematic differences in tetrahydrocannabinol (THC) content between different types of cannabis products sold (*de facto* legally) in Dutch cannabis cafes (Pjilman *et al.* 2005).

The second benefit of drug distribution's decentralized character is that it is inherently inefficient, providing drugs at far higher cost than they otherwise would be. One source of inefficiency is the need to operate covertly. It costs about US$50 to send a 1 kilogram package by express mail from Bogota to New York, but the price markup for shipping 1 kilogram of cocaine over the same route is about US$13 000 (Caulkins and Reuter 1998).

Another source of inefficiency is the absence of economies of scale. Drugs are produced, refined, packaged, and retailed in very labour-intensive ways. A typical retail drug seller in the USA does well to make 10 sales per day (Caulkins *et al.* 1999). A grocery cashier can scan about 20 items per minute. Even allowing for the fact that scanning is only about half of a check-out clerk's time on task, granting 50% idle time, and presuming the cashier is assisted by a full time bagger, grocery stores still achieve productivity (measured by sales per labour hour) that is over 100 times better than the illicit drug distribution network.

Likewise, dealers pay hired help about 6–10 cents per vial to package crack in 0.1 gram retail containers (Caulkins *et al.* 1999), plus another 2–10 cents per vial for the vials. Restaurants can buy sugar packets (to go with coffee or tea) containing 2.85 grams of sugar for 0.6–0.8 cents per packet. So for the (legal) sugar industry, which takes advantage of mechanization and economies of scale, the cost of packaging, raw materials, distribution, advertising, billing, and return on capital is only one-tenth of what it costs the drug distribution industry just for the labour cost of packaging.

Not all of the high cost of illicit drug distribution stems from such structural consequences of product illegality. Some distribution costs constitute monetary compensation for risks, notably the risks of enforcement. The most popular theory quantifying this risk compensation suggests that dealers demand compensation equivalent to the expected value of the non-monetary risks they face (Reuter and Kleiman 1986). For example, suppose that a certain class of dealers faces a 50% chance of receiving a 10-year prison term, and their willingness to pay to avoid such a prison term is US$500 000. The theory says that a risk-neutral dealer in that market would demand 50% of US$500 000, or US$250 000, over and above the regular compensation for effort, materials, and other traditional factors. A 'risk compensation' payment of that size could greatly increase the cost of distributing drugs and, hence, increase drug prices. That figure would be higher if dealers were, like most individuals, risk averse.

Risk compensation creates winners and losers. To illustrate, imagine that two similar dealers each receive US$250 000 to induce them to offer their drug distribution 'services'. After they have completed their business transactions, one is very happy, having received US$250 000 and no prison term. But the other dealer is very unhappy, since the US$250 000 only offsets half of the pain of the 10-year prison term he has received (even if that money is not seized by the police).

Both the winners and the losers are bad for society. The losers become a burden on society, using taxpayers' dollars while in prison and perhaps never being able to return to legitimate work. The winners may themselves be happy, but they make poor role models for impressionable youth and can demoralize neighbours who work hard at a legitimate job but make much less money. Furthermore, it seems that winning the drug-selling lottery is rarely a vehicle for upward social mobility. While Pablo Escobar bought his way into the Colombian legislature (before being gunned down) (Streatfeild 2003), typical lower level dealers save so little of their money that the vast majority cannot even afford to hire a private attorney when they are arrested (Harlow 2000). Similarly, Levitt and Venkatesh (2000) emphasize that the high returns enjoyed by the leaders of a drug retailing organization induce many young men to work for below minimum wages as street sellers.

5.3.2 **Price**

We can identify two general characteristics of drug distribution that lead to high prices: (1) structural consequences of product illegality; and (2) compensation for non-monetary risks. The best way to appreciate fully just how powerful these two factors are is to look at data on prices for different drugs and different market levels. Illicit drugs are very expensive relative to legal drugs, or indeed to any commodity in regular commerce. At retail, cocaine and heroin in Europe cost six times more per unit weight than does gold (UNODC 2005). Table 5.1 gives data on prices for cannabis and heroin in a number of western markets. The prices are expressed per dose.

There are many ways of scaling these prices. For example, tobacco at the retail level, even with all of the state's taxes imposed, cost only about 21 cents per cigarette in the

Table 5.1 Retail price of marijuana and heroin in various nations, circa 2002

	Heroin (50 mg pure)	**Marijuana (0.3 g)**
Germany	12 Euros	2.2 Euros
Italy	12 Euros	1.8 Euros
United Kingdom	12 Euros	1.5 Euros
United States	19 Euros	2.8 Euros

Sources: Based on the average price reported by EMCDDA and average purity from seizures, where available.

USA in 2006 (Centers for Disease Control and Prevention 2007), with a larger quantity of the natural leaf per cigarette (~2/3 of a gram) than is normally found in a marijuana cigarette (~1/3 of a gram). The marijuana 'joint', on the other hand, costs US$2–4 in most western nations. It is also useful to compare the cost of a year's consumption for an addicted heroin user with that of someone dependent on alcohol. In the UK, a heroin habit might cost US$25 000 per annum (Bramley-Harker 2001), compared with about US$5000 for alcohol. In low income nations along major smuggling routes that have weak enforcement, prices seem to be substantially less high. For example, in Tajikistan, a neighbour of Afghanistan, heroin sufficient for one dose costs less than a dollar (Paoli *et al.* 2009a).

Cocaine and heroin prices are higher in higher income countries, apparently both because the residents are richer and because the countries are, on average, farther from the producing regions (UNODC 2006). There is a strong positive correlation between retail prices and per capita GDP for most drugs, even cannabis. Yet geography matters in and of itself, as can be seen by looking at ratios of cocaine and heroin wholesale prices around the world (UNODC 2005). In the USA, heroin is two and a half to three times more expensive than cocaine. In Asia and Eastern Europe, the ratio is reversed. In Western Europe, prices are much closer to parity.

A high drug price is double-edged. On the one hand, it reduces consumption. Even users who are drug dependent cut back on their consumption when price rises (Grossman 2004), a matter discussed more fully in Chapter 10. On the other hand, the price is likely to influence the amount of crime committed by drug users to finance drug purchases as well as 'systemic crime' related to drug markets and drug distribution (Goldstein 1985).

A striking feature of drug markets is the huge markup from production to final sale. Table 5.2 presents typical figures for cocaine and heroin. In the year 2007, the 10 grams of opium that went into 1 gram of pure heroin cost only 85 cents at the Afghanistan farm gate.[1] By the time it is sold on the streets of London (in 45% pure packages of 100 milligrams) it costs about US$240. Most of the price increase stems from payments to the lowest level distributors. As noted earlier, these retailers and low level wholesalers do not earn large sums, but there are very large numbers of such distributors. High level distributors each earn much larger amounts, but there are relatively few of them, so that in total they account for a modest share of the total cost of distribution.

It appears that the largest proportionate markups usually occur as the drug crosses international borders from the producer countries but the largest absolute price increases occur inside the rich consumer countries. Some of the markup is achieved by the addition of diluents, so that, for example, the ounce of heroin purchased by a wholesaler at 60% purity is then solid in 1 gram units that are only 45% pure as a consequence of the addition of a quantity of paracetamol equivalent to about a quarter of that

[1] This assumes a conversion factor of 10 grams of opium for each gram of heroin. More recent studies suggest that the effective conversion factor might be only seven to one for Afghanistan, the dominant producer. See UNODC (2004, p. 107).

Table 5.2 Prices of cocaine and heroin through the distribution system, circa 2007 (1 kilogram)

	Cocaine				Heroin			
Stage	**Raw price**	**Purity**	**100% Pure**	**Location**	**Raw price**	**Purity**	**100% Pure**	**Location**
Farm-gate	US$800	100%	US$800	Colombia	US$900	100%	US$900	Afghanistan
Export	US$2200	91%	US$2400	Colombia	US$3400	73%	US$4700	Afghanistan's neighbours
Import/wholesale (kilogram)	US$14500	76%	US$19000	Los Angeles	US$10000	58%	US$17000	Turkey
Mid-level/wholesale (ounze)	US$19500	73%	US$27000	Los Angeles	US$33000	50%	US$66000	England and Wales
Retail	$78000	64%	US$122000	USA	US$105000	44%	US$239000	UK

Source: Kilmer and Reuter (2009).

Note: All of these figures are from publicly available sources. All 100% pure figures are based on mid-points for ranges.

diluted heroin. Though the buyer might only be willing to pay half as much per gram as a consequence, there appears to be some degree of 'purity illusion' that benefits the seller, though Coomber (1997) suggests there is less such dilution than is usually claimed.

5.3.3 **Product quality**

Illicit drug markets deliver low quality goods and services, primarily because of the inability to enforce contracts through normal means. A user can hardly complain to a consumer protection agency about receiving substandard heroin. One fascinating consequence of the extreme vertical disaggregation in distribution chains is that drug distribution is almost pure brokerage activity, with sellers at one level acting as buyers at the next level higher in the distribution chain. Hence, sellers themselves often do not know the quality of the product they offer (Reuter and Caulkins 2004), and there are even reports of dealers offering to replace a substandard product they unwittingly sold (Fuentes 1998).

For street drugs in particular, as opposed to diverted pharmaceuticals, the pure quantity of drugs obtained in a purchase of a particular size varies enormously, at least in the USA and Australia (Caulkins 1994; Weatherburn and Lind 1997). Wendel and Curtis (2000, p. 239, citing Strategic Intelligence Section 1996) report that '[a]ssays of street-level heroin in New York City found that among a sample of 40 bags, at least 27 types of adulterants and cuts had been added to produce heroin'. Impurities are not confined to the USA, to heroin, or to retail level transactions; research reports similar findings for Germany, Italy, and the UK (Coomber 1997; Paoli 2000; Pearson and Hobbs 2001). Indeed, studies of markets for relatively new synthetics such as gamma hydroxybutyric acid (GHB) and ketamine have found that a substantial percentage of purchases do not contain any of the expected active ingredient (Winstock *et al.* 2001; Walters *et al.* 2002).

Adulteration can clearly cause harm, and even dilution can harm users if it increases variability in purity (Davies 2005). If someone who is used to injecting heroin that has been diluted to 20% purity unwittingly buys and injects 60% pure heroin, he or she could accidentally overdose. Not all diluents create problems; indeed some appear to help the user to achieve the desired experience. For example, the addition of barbiturates in fairly low concentrations to samples of illicitly produced heroin (both brown base and white salt) is probably an indication of its intended use by smoking. Sublimation of the heroin while **'chasing the dragon'** is much more efficient in the presence of such extra products.

There are other important market-related harms to users. One that receives considerable attention is the lack of provision of safe injection equipment. The inability to protect fixed capital assets from seizure discourages bundling provision of drugs with provision of an associated use-location, the way bars do with alcohol. Likewise, the illegality of drug transactions means that drug sellers rarely face civil or criminal liability for harms the way that bartenders in some countries can be held accountable for harm caused when they serve inebriated patrons who cause fatal traffic accidents.

An obvious but overlooked harm of drug markets for users is impoverishment. The structure and nature of drug markets for many drugs (notably heroin, cocaine, and many ATSs) means that anyone who uses these substances regularly (except perhaps those living in producer or transit countries) will give up a substantial amount of disposable income. Being poor *per se* is a source of health harms (Marmot 2004). Owing money to violent people who have no legal means of debt collection can also be a source of harm.

Purchasing drugs regularly consumes not only money but also a lot of time. Street ethnographers have long described drug-dependent users as leading a busy life, even when they are not holding a job (Preble and Casey 1969; Johnson *et al.* 1985; Taylor 1993). Extended 'search times' to obtain drugs may be a boon to those who want to reduce total drug use (Moore 1973), but they are a real cost to the users. The need of dependent users to make frequent, time-consuming purchases may interfere with their ability to work and meet other responsibilities. Conversely, results from the heroin maintenance programmes in Switzerland suggest that almost half of heroin users who receive heroin on prescription can maintain a regular job (Rehm *et al.* 2001).

5.4 **Effects of production and trafficking on source and transit countries**

Production of some substances, notably cannabis, is widespread, but a small number of nations produce the bulk of the world's raw materials for cocaine and heroin, the two drugs that account for most of the international drug trade (by value). Production of some ATSs is also highly concentrated. For example, The Netherlands is thought to account for a sizable share of ecstasy production (UNODC 2007). However, less is known about effects of ATS production on producer nations, so here we focus on cocaine and heroin production.

According to official estimates by the **United Nations Office on Drugs and Crime** (UNODC 2006), three countries (Bolivia, Colombia, and Peru) account for the entirety of commercial coca production. There are reports of small amounts of coca being produced in Brazil and Venezuela, but nothing that contributes substantially to world production. Afghanistan and Myanmar accounted for over 95% of global production of opium in 2004 (4570 out of 4850 tons). This two-country dominance in opium production has occurred in every year since 1988 (when systematic estimates began), except for 2001 when the Taliban successfully cut Afghanistan's production by over 90% (Paoli *et al.* 2009a). Even in that year, Afghanistan still supplied large quantities of opium and heroin to the world market out of stockpiles. Second-tier opium producers include Colombia, Laos, and Mexico. Pakistan, Thailand, and Vietnam comprise the third tier. Once substantial producers between the 1970s and the early 1990s, these countries now produce insignificant amounts (UNODC 2006).

Table 5.3 displays the global production of dry leaf coca and opium for various years between 1990 and 2005. Most coca is currently produced in Colombia, although Peru was the primary producer a decade ago. Production in Bolivia and Peru declined sharply between 1995 and 2000, but increased Colombian production more than offset those losses. More recently, Colombian production has fallen, with only modest increases in Peruvian and Bolivian production.

It is useful to contrast this pattern of production with cannabis, the other prominent drug that has its source in a natural substance. Many rich nations supply a high fraction of

Table 5.3 Coca and opium production, 1990–2005 (tons)

	1990	1995	2000	2005
Coca leaf production potential				
Bolivia	77 000	85 000	13 400	30 900
Colombia	45 300	80 900	266 200	170 730
Peru	196 900	183 600	46 200	67 900
Total	319 200	349 500	325 800	269 530
Opium production potential				
Afghanistan	1570	2335	3276	4100
Colombia		71	88	28
Laos	202	128	167	14
Mexico	62	53	21	71
Myanmar	1621	1664	1087	312
Pakistan	150	112	8	36
Thailand	20	2	6	
Vietnam	90	9		
Other	45	78	38	40
Total	3760	4452	4691	4850

Source: UNODC (2005).

Missing cells are included in the 'Other' row.

their own consumption. According to the United States Drug Enforcement Administration (2008), much of the domestic supply is apparently grown indoors. Canada may produce all of what it consumes and perhaps more (Bouchard 2008). In Western Europe it is thought that production in The Netherlands accounts for a large share of the cannabis consumed in Europe (UNODC 2007), though this is disputed by the **European Monitoring Center on Drugs and Drug Addiction** (EMCDDA 2007). Morocco and Mexico supply substantial quantities of cannabis resin and cannabis herb to Western Europe and the USA, but they are certainly not dominant, and Australia's cannabis is primarily domestically produced (ACC 2009). Cannabis' exceptional status probably rests on four factors: the absence of economies of scale in processing to prepare the agricultural product for use; the bulkiness per unit value (roughly 10 times the weight per unit value at the wholesale level, ONDCP (2004b)), which raises smuggling costs substantially; the high yield per acre, which makes indoor cultivation possible (Bouchard 2008); and the existence of a boutique market of user/growers interested in developing better breeds of the plant (Navarro 1996).

Synthetic drugs are produced in both developed countries (e.g. ecstasy in The Netherlands) and poor countries (e.g. Myanmar supplies methamphetamine to Korea, China, and Thailand) (Jagan 2003). Some rich markets get their supplies both domestically and from developing nations (e.g. methamphetamine consumed in the USA is produced both there and in Mexico).

There are myriad harms surrounding production. However, the paramount harm for coca and opium production is probably corruption in both the narrow sense (e.g. the paying of bribes) and the broad sense (i.e. undermining the legitimacy of the state).

Growing is done openly in most major coca and opium producer countries, and the farmer is vulnerable to any official who cares to enforce the law (on Afghanistan see Ward *et al.* 2007). Systemic corruption, in which a whole agency is corrupted, is essential to undisguised growing unless the government simply decides to ignore the violations of law and take no action. In other settings, for example the growing regions of Myanmar, quasi-state groups have replaced the central state. Taxing growers then becomes an important part of the tax base for groups such as the Wa United Army (Yawnghwe 2005).

The greater corruption threat comes from processors and traffickers within the producer nations. In contrast to typical dealing organizations in final market countries, these include some of the largest and most organized drug trafficking operations anywhere, such as the Colombian cocaine trafficking groups in the 1980s (Clawson and Lee 1996), Mexican smugglers since 1990 (Cook 2007), and drug lords in Afghanistan. For example, trafficking organizations in Mexico, which handle both Mexican-produced heroin and Colombian cocaine, have corrupted the highest levels of government. In 1997 the Mexican government official serving essentially as drug tsar, a former army general, was convicted of taking payments from a trafficking group (Preston 1997).

Another set of countries, though not producers, generate large incomes from trafficking between producers and consuming countries. Prominent among these nations are Iran and Turkey, long established in these roles, and the nations of Central Asia, which have taken on this role only since the development of the Russian heroin market in the late 1990s (Paoli *et al.* 2009a). In some of these nations the violence and corruption are just as substantial as in the producing countries. However, in general, trafficking (including smuggling) generates corruption of a narrower kind in part because it is less visible and perhaps less continuous.

All of the major coca- and opium-producing and trans-shipping countries have chronic corruption problems, quite apart from those related to drugs. This is not a coincidence. It is easier for drug production to take root in places with a pre-existing culture of corruption. Even if the drug industry only exacerbates pre-existing corruption, the effect can still be very serious. In a few countries, drugs generate a large share of all potential revenues for corrupt officials. That is probably a fair characterization of Tajikistan since the late 1990s, where it is possible that heroin trafficking revenues are equivalent to 50% of recorded GDP and hence may generate a huge share of public officials' earnings (Paoli *et al.* 2009a).

Tajikistan's case also illustrates the problems of corruption in the broader sense of corrupting the society, not just specific individuals. Drug production and trafficking can contribute to political instability and violence. In some nations, the government essentially becomes part of the trafficking system itself (Paoli *et al.* 2007). In Colombia, the left-wing FARC has received much of its funding from the taxation of coca farmers since the collapse of the Medellin cartel in the early 1990s (Thoumi 2003). Powerful warlords heavily dependent on taxation of the opium and heroin industry continue to destabilize Afghanistan (Goodhand 2005). In Bolivia, an organization of coca farmers became a major political force, resisting the central government's efforts to eliminate the industry (Black 2005). Their leader, Evo Morales, came second in the presidential election in 2002 and then won the presidency in 2005.

The list of harms to producer countries readily extends beyond corruption. There are perennial claims that ecological damage from coca growing, processing, and/or eradication can be substantial (e.g. Vargas 2002), though a recent risk assessment questioned the magnitude of the problems related to eradication (Solomon *et al.* 2005). Injuries also stem directly from drug production (Porter and Armstrong 2004). The expansion of import income can generate unfortunate and unintended increases in international exchange rates that hurt the rest of the economy, a version of 'resource curse' or 'Dutch disease' (Ward *et al.* 2007).

However, it is also important to note the economic benefits of drug production. For a very few countries it has become, at specific points in time, a dominant source of wealth. In the middle of the first decade of the 21st century, this seems to be true for Afghanistan. In 2003, Afghanistan, as the consequence of historically very high opium prices, may have generated US$2.8 billion in additional earnings from opium production and heroin trafficking, or as much as 30% of total national legitimate GDP (Byrd and Ward 2004). While such high percentages are exceptional, there are other nations (such as Bolivia, Colombia, and Myanmar) in which drug-based income is occasionally of considerable regional significance.

5.5 **Market harms in rich countries**

We return now to the distinction between markets and marketplaces. Some but not all retail drug selling is place based. 'Street markets' and 'crack houses' or 'tinny houses' (terms used in New Zealand) are physical places where illicit drugs are routinely sold (Jacobs 1999; Wilkins *et al.* 2005). New York City used to be notorious for flagrant street marketplaces that plagued neighbours (Zimmer 1987), but those markets have evolved (Johnson 2003). Now 'beeper sales' are common, with drug users paging their suppliers, or calling them on cell phones, to arrange to meet at a specific location such as a restaurant where drug selling is not routine or flagrant. Edmunds and colleagues (1996) describe such phenomena in British drug markets. Similarly, marijuana seems to be sold primarily through friendship networks, not via arm's length transactions between people who interact primarily as drug seller and buyer (Caulkins and Pacula 2006; Coomber and Turnbull 2007). A study of the ecstasy market in Amsterdam, Barcelona, and Turin found little evidence that a drug scene had developed around the selling of this drug (Massari 2005).

Drug markets generate some harms regardless of whether they are place based, virtual, or social network based, though Burr (1983, 1984) provides descriptions of well ordered opiate markets in London in the 1980s. Prominent among these harms are the diversion of drug sellers' productive time away from school or legitimate labour market activities (Harwood *et al.* 1998), and the accumulation of people (mostly sellers) with criminal records who subsequently find it difficult to re-enter legitimate labour markets even after they 'mature out' of their illicit drug activity (Bourgois 1996).

The extent of these harms may depend somewhat on policy. It may take more sellers to supply a given number of users when enforcement is aggressive, partly because each seller wants to do business with a smaller number of customers and partly because long prison terms may open up selling opportunities for replacement dealers and complicate efforts to rehabilitate convicted sellers. However, it is not possible to make stronger statements about policy, since these harms have been subject to little study. These harms revolve around sellers, not users, and so may be overlooked by health-oriented research. Since the direct 'victims' of these harms are the drug sellers themselves, law and order proponents may view ameliorating those harms as a low priority.

The more prominent market-related harms, however, stem from physical marketplaces. They include, in increasing order of severity, disorder, property crime, and violence. Even 'mere' disorder can be a significant concern (Zimmer 1987). Disorder was a principal reason for Zurich's abandonment of its famous 'Needle park' experiment, when the police tolerated the open sale and purchase of drugs in a park behind the main train station, which resulted in a large increase in the number of users in the downtown area (MacCoun and Reuter 2001a).

It is not clear how much additional disorder is caused by concentrating market participants in specific locations, as opposed to merely making disorderly individuals more visible by bringing them together in one place. Proponents of the 'broken windows' theory (Wilson and Kelling 1982) might argue that visible signs of disorder cause subsequent offenses by signalling to perpetrators that conventional social norms are not enforced (Kelling and Coles 1996), but criminologists have criticized the causal interpretation of the broken windows hypothesis for crime (e.g. Sampson and Raudenbush 1999, though see also Keizer *et al.* 2008). Disorder may still deter business investment and affect migration patterns (Skogan 1990) even if it does not directly promote serious crime. Causal attribution concerning the observed correlation between the presence of dealing and the absence of other businesses (Ford and Beveridge 2004) is also complicated, since places that are already disorderly are a logical focal point around which a place-based market can coalesce (Kleiman 1992).

Concentration of property crime is a near-universal concern about place-based markets for expensive drugs (e.g. heroin, cocaine, and ATSs, as opposed to cannabis). Cost-of-illness studies in Australia and the USA estimate that approximately a quarter of all property crime nationally is committed to finance the purchase of illicit drugs (Harwood *et al.* 1998; Collins and Lapsley 2002). In a recently developed British government Drug Harm Index, which is intended to measure the social cost of illegal drugs, property crimes account for a majority of the harms (MacDonald *et al.* 2006). Presumably, drug-dependent individuals commit additional crime to finance non-drug purchases (food, rent, etc.) because their drug use reduces access to legitimate income (Moore and Caulkins 2005). Given how concentrated dependent drug use is in certain neighbourhoods, particularly those that host drug marketplaces, the crime burden in those neighbourhoods can be very great.

Still, the most notorious and severe consequences of drug markets may be the promotion of violence, at least in countries such as the USA that have widespread gun availability and an underlying culture of violence. As previously described in Chapter 4, it is useful to distinguish three types of drug-related crime (Goldstein 1985): 'psychopharmacological crime' that stems from the drugs' effects on the user (e.g. through intoxication and disinhibition); 'economic compulsive crime' committed to finance drug purchases; and 'systemic crime' related to drug markets and drug distribution (popularly construed as 'turf wars' among dealers but probably more often pertaining to drug deals gone bad). Caulkins and colleagues (1997) estimate that for cocaine in the USA, market-related systemic crime accounts for fully half of all drug-related crime. The proportion can be even higher for lethal violence. Brownstein and colleagues (1992) report that over half of a sample of New York City homicides were drug related, and 74.3% of those were systemic. Just 3.7% were instances of economic-compulsive violence. These estimates are specific to a time and place and the figures may be entirely different in other cities or countries. The New York crack market was at its height in the late 1980s and the city was severely affected by the drug.

Furthermore, Brownstein and colleagues (1992) observe that many homicides that were *not* defined to be drug related took place in drug marketplaces or involved perpetrators and/or victims who were known to have been involved with drugs and drug trafficking. Just as drug dependence can cause property crimes that are not committed specifically to finance a drug purchase, so too can drug marketplaces cause violence that is not directly drug related. There are multiple indirect causal pathways. Blumstein and Cork (1996) identify one: diffusion of firearms among youthful sellers. Youth are disproportionately involved in violence. When those youth are armed because of their drug-selling activity, routine altercations over prices or love triangles are more likely to be lethal.

An underlying culture of violence may be a pre-condition for widespread market-related violence, but it is not a sufficient condition. The relative absence of violence in US marijuana markets may be attributed to marijuana's relatively low cost, but it is noteworthy that even in New York in the 1980s heroin was rarely involved in homicides (Goldstein 1999). The levels of violence in drug markets in other rich countries seem to be much lower than in the USA, but the occasional spate of homicides in European markets do have great public salience (New York Times 1998), as has a more recent homicide in the Sydney airport connected to Outlaw Motorcycle Gangs (Asia Pacific News 2009).

Another harm of place-based markets is increased availability of drugs, both because those markets operate continuously and because most are willing to supply strangers, including novice users (Reuter and MacCoun 1992). The constant availability (and visibility) created by place-based markets may also challenge dependent users in recovery, since recovery rates can depend dramatically on the social milieu (Robins *et al.* 1974).

Corruption is another market-related harm in consumer countries, just as it is in producer and trans-shipment countries. Drug sellers and users are readily extorted by police, who often reflect the ambivalent attitude of the community in which they find themselves and thus are willing to take bribes. Many rich countries have seen recurrent episodes of systemic corruption around drug enforcement, including the New South Wales police inquiry of the late 1990s (Wood 1997), the Dutch scandal of the early 1990s, and the Miami homicide squad in the 1980s (Anderson and Prout 1985).

One might expect corruption to be most acute for place-based markets, but corruption in New York appears to have been a bigger problem in the 1960s than it was during the period of flagrant street markets in the 1980s. The more important factor may be whether enforcement is concentrated in a single agency, implying the need to corrupt only one person or group, as opposed to being distributed across multiple agencies with overlapping jurisdictions. With overlapping agencies, no one group can guarantee protection and any corrupt officer is exposed when his clients are arrested by another agency.

There is a long-standing concern that drug distribution generates a distinctive kind of criminal enterprise called 'organized crime'. The Italian and American Mafia organizations were once very active in the heroin market, both domestically and, in the case of the Sicilian mafia, internationally (Paoli 2003). The Medellin and Cali syndicates that operated in Colombia in the 1980s provide another instance in which drug trafficking was associated with large, powerful, and politically influential organizations. Recent research suggests, however, that these are exceptions. Drug markets in consumer nations are mostly served by small, independent enterprises (Natarajan and Hough 2000; Pearson and Hobbs 2001). That may reflect the imperative and capacity of the modern state to overwhelm organizations that challenge the coercive powers of the government.

Finally, even if place-based markets merely concentrate disorder, property crime, violence, availability, and corruption in certain neighbourhoods without increasing the total amount of harm, that spatial concentration is still important for at least two reasons. First, there are obvious distributional issues associated with concentrating drug-related harms in areas of poverty. Secondly, spatial concentration should make it easier to implement programmes to mitigate or compensate for these market-related harms, in addition to the familiar place-based strategies for addressing use-related harms. That opportunity is not frequently discussed, perhaps because markets are seen to be the domain of law enforcement, and harm reduction the domain of public health, but law enforcement could have a significant role in reducing drug-related harms, even if the market adaptability discussed above sometimes makes it difficult for enforcement to reduce the total volume of drugs distributed through those markets (Caulkins 2002; Curtis and Wendell 2007).

5.6 Conclusion

Chapter 4 documented the global burden of disease associated with drug use. There is not yet a comparable scientific base that quantifies the social and economic burden of drug markets. Yet the total burden is surely a significant part of what troubles society about illicit drugs.

Most of the market-related harms are a consequence of efforts to reduce drug use, most notably the laws and associated programmes prohibiting the production, distribution, and possession of illicit drugs. That means it is worth asking, as we do in a subsequent chapter, whether alternative legal regimes might reduce the combined total harm associated with both drug use and drug markets, but at the same time it does not imply that another regime would better serve the public good. The benefits of reduced use arising from prohibition may well over-ride the market harms that prohibition creates, but that is an empirical question that has not been addressed in any systematic fashion.

We must also be mindful that the level of market-related harm is not an immutable constant. Just as some programmes and policies can aggravate or ameliorate the harms associated with drug use, other programmes and policies can aggravate or ameliorate the harmful consequences of drug markets.

Chapter 6

The legal market: prescription and diversion of psychopharmaceuticals

6.1 Introduction

The previous chapter described what is known about the structure, prices, and products of illegal drug markets, and the nature and extent of harms that arise from them. This chapter describes another drug market, this one consisting of an international pharmaceutical industry that operates legally within the market economies of most countries. There are several reasons to include this chapter in a book on illegal drugs. First, the channelling of **pharmaceuticals** from legal sources to the illicit marketplace or to unintended individuals has become a major source of supply for street drug users in some countries (e.g. Fischer and Rehm 2007). The term **diversion** describes this phenomenon (Inciardi *et al.* 2007). Secondly, legal markets are subject to government regulation and other types of control, thereby providing a possible mechanism to prevent **drug misuse**. This issue will be discussed in Chapter 12. Since the aim of this chapter is to describe an important context for drug supply, our focus here is on the provision and use of **psychoactive pharmaceuticals** (i.e. drugs designed to relieve pain or other mental distress), and not on benefits and harms from their use.

This chapter begins with a historical introduction to the origins of psychoactive pharmaceuticals (also called **psychopharmaceuticals** interchangeably) and the ways in which they are produced and marketed. After describing how the pharmaceutical industry is organized on a global level, we suggest that, with the growth of modern medicine and particularly psychiatry, there has been a substantial growth in prescriptions for mental disorders and distress, and increased comfort with the use of such prescribed medications. This situation has had, in some countries, significant consequences for the illicit drug market. The chapter concludes with a discussion of the question: how separate are the regulated and unregulated markets? The answer is that the two worlds are not separated as much as they might at first appear.

6.2 A brief history of the pharmaceutical industry

In the 19th century, apothecaries and physicians still compounded most medicines in Europe and North America immediately before dispensing, with raw materials for their recipes drawn from plant extracts and a variety of other sources. The production and dispensing of medicines thus still resembled traditional practices in many parts of the world. Pharmaceutical production developed in two main directions out of these traditional practices in Europe and North America. One was the rise of centralized manufacturing of pharmaceutical chemicals, initially in Germany. At first, the raw chemicals were still delivered to the compounding chemist, who made up the pills or the solution to be dispensed at the retail level. The other was the rise of patent medicines, secret preparations of questionable effectiveness sold as remedies for a variety of ailments, particularly in Britain and the USA (Young 1961; Berridge 1999). Patent medicines may be seen as the forerunners of modern pharmaceutical manufacturing and marketing, in that they involved centrally compounded products of fixed composition delivered to the retail level in sealed containers. By the mid-20th century, the compounding chemist was disappearing, as manufacturers compounded most pharmaceuticals into pills or other preparations.

Then, as now, pharmaceutical manufacturing was highly profitable, although the basis for the special profitability has changed. Then, the fact that the formula for a patent medicine was secret gave a popular medicine a monopolistic advantage over less known competitors. Now, the competitive advantage depends particularly on the patent the manufacturer obtains, for either a new drug or a new use for an existing drug, which lasts for a limited number of years.

6.2.1 The global pharmaceutical industry

Over the years, the pharmaceutical industry has become increasingly globalized. Presently, all 50 of the top pharmaceutical companies, ranked in terms of health care revenue, are headquartered in developed countries—22 in the USA, 16 in Western Europe, 10 in Japan, and one each in Israel and Australia (Anonymous 2007). The US dominance in the industry partly reflects the special circumstances of pharmaceuticals in the USA, given the fragmentation of and lack of effective cost control in health care. Partly as a result of this, 45% of the total revenue of the global pharmaceutical industry comes from sales in North America: US$290.1 billion in 2006 out of US$643 billion worldwide (Alva 2007).

6.2.2 The long waves of psychoactive pharmaceuticals

Psychopharmaceuticals have always been a substantial fraction of the products of the pharmaceutical industry, and psychoactive substances were often combined with other ingredients to make up remedies for a variety of illnesses. For example, many 19th century patent medicines contained opium or (by the end of the century) cocaine. At the end of the 19th and the beginning of the 20th centuries, one country or state after another fought long battles to limit availability of such psychoactive medications (Young 1961; Berridge 1999). Along with rising concern about the Chinese opium trade, the indiscriminate use of patent medicines lay behind the rise of international drug control, initially of 'narcotics' (see Chapter 13).

The last century has seen a succession of different classes of drugs in medical favour for the treatment of mental distress (Medawar and Hardon 2004). The era of treatment with opium, alcohol, morphine, and cocaine gave way to an era of treatment with chloral hydrate or bromides, which in turn gave way to the barbiturates in the 1930s. In the 1960s and 1970s, these were succeeded by the benzodiazepines. The 1990s and beyond have been the era of the selective serotonin reuptake inhibitors (SSRIs) or antidepressants. The recurrent history with these waves of new drug classes is twofold, beginning with an initial wave of great enthusiasm, with considerable over-extension of the conditions for which the drugs were prescribed, followed by sobering second thoughts as adverse effects and less than hoped for effectiveness become apparent with wide experience with the drug class. One of the adverse effects of the new drug class has often turned out to be that it fosters its own form of physical dependence. This usually has meant that eventually each class of drugs was brought under international control, as, for instance, the barbiturates and benzodiazepines were eventually brought under the 1971 international treaty on psychotropic substances (see Chapter 13).

As new classes of drugs came to the fore in the treatment of mental distress, drugs from the classes previously in vogue continued in more limited use, often for much narrower indications. One class of drugs that has continued in wide use, however, is the opiates, primarily used for pain relief in a broad range of medical specialties.

Many of the large pharmaceutical firms have long been actively involved in the production of psychoactive medications. For example, the market for such medications accounts for close to one-fifth of the current pharmaceutical market in the USA. In terms of sales, in 2001 the share was 8.1% for antidepressants and tranquillizers, 3.6% for narcotic painkillers, 2.7% for antiseizure drugs, 2.6% for antipsychotics, and 1.6% for antianxiety drugs (National Institute for Health Care Management 2002).

The big pharmaceutical firms have generally stayed away from the opiates market, leaving it to smaller players. One exception to this is Schering-Plough, distributor of buprenorphine in the USA, which is in the second rank of pharmaceutical companies (16th in terms of global revenue). The tribulations of another relatively small firm, Purdue Pharma, maker of **OxyContin**, suggest one reason to stay out of the market. The company and three of its former executives were found guilty of having 'misled doctors and patients when it claimed the drug was less likely to be abused than traditional narcotics', and sentenced by a US court to pay a total of US$634.5 million in fines (Meier 2007). This was a large sum in absolute terms, but only a fraction of what Purdue made from OxyContin. The broader image problem of an association with drug addicts probably also discourages entry by the big firms.

6.2.3 Promoting psychoactive medications

The succession of new psychoactive medications is driven in part by the advancement of science. But there are also other forces at play. As the problems inherent in each new wave of drugs became clearer, a conceptual space developed for the next wave, which in turn could be presented by the industry as a scientific advance unencumbered by the manifest problems of the previous wave. The process was also helped forward by various interests—not only the pharmaceutical manufacturers, but also allopathic physicians, brain-science enthusiasts, and the advertising industry, whose origins as a separate industry can be traced to the marketing of patent medicines

(Young 1961). As the pharmaceutical industry devoted more and more of its resources to sales and promotion (an estimated 36% of its revenues are spent on 'marketing and administration': Angell 2004), it became a force in changing cultural understandings and patterns of behaviour. While patients in mental hospitals may have been the initial focus of psychoactive medications, the industry subsequently broadened conceptualizations of mental distress to take in problems of everyday living.

Until recently, physicians were the ostensible target of the industry's promotional efforts. The lack of direct advertising to the public had been a main distinction between the 'ethical' pharmaceutical industry and the patent medicine industry, and most places prohibited advertising to the public by law or regulation (Conrad and Leiter 2008). As the prohibition frayed, industry marketing efforts took on a two-pronged strategy. On the one side, the industry sought to create patient demand by advertising and by supporting articles for general circulation that identified a particular type of mental distress and stated that there were medicines to control or cure it. Often the condition was given a new, more socially acceptable name. For example, *social phobia* became *social anxiety disorder* along with Smith Kline Beecham's repositioning of paroxetine (Paxil) as a remedy for it (Medawar and Hardon 2004). On the other side, advertising and detailing to doctors promoted the particular company's drug as the remedy to prescribe when patients came in with the symptoms the public information had described for the condition. Eventually, the industry found this approach too indirect, and after a long fight it succeeded in getting approval for direct-to-the-consumer (DTC) advertising in the USA in 1997 (Robinson 2001). Now the industry is pressing hard in the EU (European Public Health Association 2004; SourceWatch 2008) and elsewhere to extend DTC advertising to the global level.

The combination of medical enthusiasm and promotion by pharmaceutical interests can have substantial results in a society. By the mid-1970s, an estimated 10–20% of 'ambulatory adults' in the USA and other western nations regularly used benzodiazepines (Medawar and Hardon 2004). The medicalization of common problems of childhood such as attention deficit and hyperactivity disorder (ADHD) was accompanied in the USA by a sevenfold increase in prescriptions for the stimulant Ritalin (Buckmaster 2005), although current analyses suggest that ADHD involves developmental delay rather than a psychiatric disorder (Carey 2007). Box 6.1 provides another example of how industry promotions, in this case the introduction of a new antidepressant drug, dramatically changed an entire country's diagnostic and treatment practices in the course of a few years.

At a general cultural level, the efforts of the pharmaceutical companies and their allies to promote psychoactive medications for mental states have been quite successful. Nikolas Rose (2007) proposes that the dominance of this idea has turned the USA and Europe into 'psychopharmacological societies' where 'human subjective capacities have come to be routinely reshaped by psychiatric drugs' (p. 146). The idea that mental states can and should be manipulated by psychoactive substances provides a fertile conceptual ground not only for medically approved use of psychopharmaceuticals but also for the diversion of medications and the illicit use of these substances outside the bounds of medical approval.

Box 6.1 Introduction of selective serotonin re-uptake inhibitors (SSRIs) into Japan after 1999

In Japan, the first SSRIs were approved for use in 1999, which was quite late compared with Europe and North America. According to one observer (Applbaum 2006, p. 89), SSRIs had been delayed because international pharmaceutical companies had initially accepted the view of local experts that 'Japanese barely suffer from depression'. One tactic of the companies after the introduction was a campaign 'directed toward increasing *recognition* among the public of how widespread depression, anxiety, panic, bulimia, social phobia, and related disorders are. This enterprise is facilitated by the cooperation of concerned medical practitioners, public officials, and journalists who purportedly recognize the under-diagnosis of depression and anxiety as a social ill that can be remedied by awakening public consciousness to the symptoms and treatability of these disorders' (Applbaum 2006, p. 103). The tactics applied in Japanese circumstances were often reproductions of campaigns elsewhere; 'the marketing director for one of the SSRIs showed me his marketing plan and explained that it was a boilerplate reproduction of the plan that had been used in Great Britain a number of years earlier' (Applbaum 2006, pp. 106–107). The tactics succeeded in Japan. SSRI sales there had quintupled in a 5-year period by 2003, and GlaxoSmithKline alone saw its sales of Paxil increase from (US$) 108 million in 2001 to 298 million in 2003 (Currie 2005).

6.3 **Global patterns of prescribed consumption of psychopharmaceuticals**

Commissioning data runs from IMF, a company that tracks prescriptions globally for pharmaceutical and other clients, Rose (2007) examined the use of psychopharmaceuticals in a selected range of places: the USA, Western Europe (the first 15 member nations of the EU), Japan, South America, South Africa, and Pakistan. Table 6.1 shows the patterns of prescription use in terms of standard dosage units per thousand population in 2001.

For the classes of drugs included in Rose's analysis, Western Europe and Japan are not far behind the USA in total prescriptions per head, although there is some variation by class of drugs, with antidepressants and stimulants more commonly prescribed in the USA, sedatives more commonly prescribed in Europe and Japan, and antipsychotics most commonly prescribed in Japan. But the gap between the USA, Europe, and Japan, on the one hand, and the countries from the 'global South' included in Rose's comparison is huge—about an order of magnitude, indeed. A consumption of 75 000 standard dosage units per thousand population per annum translates to daily use by about 20% of the whole population, presuming use of only one psychoactive medication at a time.

Rose also examined trends between 1990 and 2000 in psychiatric drug prescribing. During this decade prescriptions for the five classes of drugs shown in Table 6.1 doubled in the USA, increased 40% in Europe, and rose 22% in Japan. In Pakistan and

Table 6.1 Psychiatric drug prescribing in 2001, in standard dosage units per 1000 population

	USA	Europe	Japan	South America	South Africa	Pakistan
Tranquillizers	20 361	22 630	28 211	4781	2266	3802
Antidepressants	33 768	19 010	9202	1835	2330	919
Sedatives and hypnotics	7362	15 562	14 721	1299	1701	387
Antipsychotics	6954	8373	14 437	1062	1490	754
Psychostimulants	6488	364	184	47	105	7
Total	74 934	65940	66755	9023	7892	5868

Source: Rose (2007).

South Africa, the number of prescriptions increased by over one-third, while in Latin America it was stable. The trends over the 1990s thus showed little convergence, and if anything increasing divergence between the 'psychopharmacological societies' and the rest of the world.

Rose's analysis does not include the opiates. For this, we must turn to the annual reports of the International Narcotics Control Board (INCB 2007a), which monitors world production and use of opiates and other substances covered by the international conventions (see Chapter 13). The INCB reports show a steady upward rise in the production of opiates intended for medical use. Concerning the main natural alkaloid feedstocks for opiate products, the INCB noted in 2007 that 'manufacture of both morphine and thebaine reached a record level in 2005 [. . .]. Manufacture of codeine, which is mainly obtained from morphine, [. . .] also reached an all-time high' (INCB 2007a, p. 71).

Table 6.2 describes the consumption of 'narcotic' (opioid) medications, primarily in the form of synthetic opioids and morphine, in selected regions of the world. On a per capita basis the USA far surpasses the rest of the world, accounting for 70% of the global market. Canada, Europe, Australia, and New Zealand represent an intermediate level of per capita consumption, with other parts of the world consuming relatively low amounts. The USA consumes about five times as much as the general rate in Europe, and about 170 times the general rate of consumption in the rest of the world.

In 2004, the USA consumed in excess of 200 tons of opium-derived and synthetic opioids (INCB 2006a). Based on ARCOS (Automation of Reports and Consolidated Orders System) data, more than 100 tons of fentanyl, hydromorphone, meperidine, morphine, and oxycodone were dispensed for medical use in the USA in 2002, constituting an extensive base of opioid medications in circulation, much of it in end-users' hands and available for misuse (Compton and Volkow 2006; Kuehn 2007). In comparison, official estimates of pure heroin consumed annually in the US illicit market were less than 20 tons in 2000 (ONDCP 2001a).

It seems highly unlikely that mental distress is distributed globally with such an imbalance toward the USA and Europe as would be implied by the patterns of use of

Table 6.2 Consumption of narcotic drugs* (in defined daily doses; DDD) 2003–2005 by region

Region	Consumption per million inhabitants in DDD	Population in thousand	Relative share of global consumption†
USA	33 532	298 213	70%
Canada	14 133	32 268	3%
European Union‡	6450	461 405	21%
Eastern Europe§	191	215 231	0%
Australia and New Zealand	7284	24 184	1%
Japan	662	128 085	1%
All other countries	116	5 036 513	4%
World	2289	6 195 899	100%

Source: own calculations based on INCB (2006a).

* Narcotic drugs include codeine (2% of total), fentanyl (38%), hydrocodone (7%), hydromorphone (1%), methadone (26%), morphine (11%), oxycodone (5%), pethidine (1%), tilidine (3%), and 'others' (5%).

† Weighted by population (UN).

‡ Also includes Norway and Switzerland.

§ Albania, Belarus, Bosnia & Herzegovina, Croatia, Republic of Moldova, Russian Federation, Ukraine.

psychopharmaceuticals, and that pain is distributed globally with such an imbalance towards the USA, Canada, and Australia as would be implied by the use of opiates. Instead, the differences are presumably driven by a combination of relative affluence, cultural specificities, and the social influence of pharmaceutical marketing. What is notable about this situation is the general parallel between the global imbalance in the use of prescribed psychoactive substances and the imbalance in markets for illicitly produced drugs. This may also be true for markets in medications diverted to non-medical use.

6.4 **Unregulated markets and diversion**

The discussion up to this point has assumed that psychoactive medications are sold in a regulated market to the end-stage user and used under medical direction, usually with a prescription filled by a pharmacist (for discussion of prescription regimes, see Chapter 12). However, much use of psychoactive medications falls outside this framework in one way or another. While this is commonly referred to as *diversion*, presumably from the prescription channels, the broader term used by the INCB in its Report for 2006 (INCB 2007b) is *unregulated markets*. As shown in Box 6.2, the INCB distinguishes among different methods by which unregulated drugs may come onto the market, whether from official sources or otherwise. These include theft, unauthorized sales, prescription fraud, counterfeit drugs, and illicit Internet sales.

Box 6.2 Methods by which unregulated drugs come onto the market

1. Official sources (regulated channels):
   - A. Drugs may be stolen from licensed manufacturers, wholesalers, or retail distributors. Unscrupulous manufacturers may manufacture and sell products for which they have no licence or may sell products in contravention of the conditions of their licence. Drugs that are substandard or recalled by the manufacturer because they have expired or have quality defects may be sold and find their way into the unregulated market.
   - B. Imported drugs or drugs for export may find a way into the unregulated market through theft or unauthorized sales.
   - C. Drugs may be diverted from health care institutions and/or health service providers, again through theft or unauthorized sales.
   - D. Controlled drugs obtained legitimately by retailers or by health care institutions, for example, may be stolen and diverted to the unregulated market; in some cases, individuals who have obtained such drugs using prescriptions may sell them for profit.
2. Other sources:
   - E. Counterfeit drugs may be manufactured or imported or distributed and supplied to the unregulated market, as well as to the regulated market. Unscrupulous manufacturers, importers, exporters, pharmacists, distributors, and brokers have been implicated in such operations.
   - F. Drugs that are stolen from prescription holders may find their way into the unregulated market.
   - G. Through the Internet; even drugs for which prescriptions are required can be obtained relatively easily.

Source: International Narcotics Control Board (INCB 2007b, p. 2).

It is difficult to estimate the relative importance of these different avenues for diversion. The issue is not a new one. In 1965, the US Food and Drug Administration suspected that 'approximately half of the 9 billion barbiturate and amphetamine capsules and tablets manufactured annually in this country are diverted to illegal use' (Anonymous 1965). As described in Box 6.3, there has been little improvement since then in the availability of data.

Regarding theft, there is evidence from the USA that some forms of property crime, with prescription opioids as the property, are one means of routing these drugs towards illicit use. Inciardi et al. (2007) and Joranson and Gilson (2005) document that millions of dose units of various high potency opioids (including oxycodone, morphine, hydromorphone, etc.) were stolen or lost, mainly from pharmacies.

Box 6.3 The inadequacy of reliable information about drug diversion

"Empirical data on the scope and magnitude of diversion, as well as on patterns of diversion associated with specific drugs of abuse, different user populations, and/or other demographic, sociocultural, and psychosocial factors, are largely unavailable and remain absent from the literature. In fact, at a recent meeting [...] on the 'Impact of Drug Formulation on Abuse Liability, Safety, and Regulatory Decisions', representatives from government regulatory agencies, the pharmaceutical industry, and the research community agreed that 1) there are no data on the magnitude of particular types of diversion, 2) there are no systematic data on how the massive quantities of abused prescription drugs are reaching the streets, and 3) there are no empirical data that might be used for making regulatory decisions and for developing prescription drug prevention and risk management plans." (Inciardi *et al.* 2007, p. 172).

Given that prescription drugs are regulated by controlled dispensing through the medical system, prescribers and dispensers have been key sources from which prescription drugs are moved into illicit use. Physicians and pharmacists either make drugs directly available to end-users or else make them available to 'middle-persons' (such as legitimate patients, individuals feigning illnesses, or even fraudulent medical professionals) who eventually (whether knowingly or unknowingly, whether for profit or not) make them available to non-medical users. How important physicians and pharmacists are in making diverted pharmaceuticals available on the illicit market is a matter of much dispute. While several countries, including the USA, Canada, and the UK, have seen much highly publicized disciplinary action against mal-prescribers of prescription opioids (Richard and Reidenberg 2005; Dyer 2004), Hurwitz writes that 'it is unlikely that prescriptions written by dishonest doctors [...] constitute a significant black market supply' since, for example, a 2002 population of 11 million prescription opioid abusers in the USA could not possibly be supplied by a small group of deviant doctors (Hurwitz 2005, p. 157). In the USA, there are more than 1 million registered manufacturers, distributors, pharmacies, hospitals, nursing homes, and physicians who provide controlled prescription substances (Hurwitz 2005).

Street drug users often obtain prescription opioids or other psychopharmaceuticals through 'doctor shopping' or 'double-doctoring', which is the 'fraudulent presentation of disease to multiple doctors and pharmacies' (Martyres *et al.* 2004, p. 212). For example, Martyres and colleagues (2004) examined prescription file data for a sample of 15- to 24-year-old heroin users who had died of a heroin-related overdose between 1994 and 1999 in the State of Victoria, Australia. They found that the 155 subjects received 5860 prescriptions for psychoactive drugs over an average period of just over 5 years; half the sample saw more than eight different medical service providers per year, and the male portion of the sample accessed an average of 35 service providers per year. That number rose to 60 among the females included in the study. The most commonly received prescriptions (43%) were for benzodiazepines; next were prescription opioids (11%). The average number of prescriptions (for any drug) received increased in the 4 years before death, from four per person in the earliest year to a peak of 17 per person in the year prior to death.

Another study (Fountain *et al.* 2000, p. 395) considered diversion of prescription drugs in the UK by those in drug treatment. Noting that 'there are no reports that smuggling, illicit manufacturing and organized crime feature in the distribution of prescription drugs in the U.K.', the authors propose that diversion is a retail-level activity in the UK, and that 'drug users in treatment are the primary diverters'. The authors review the range of motivations they found for purchasing such diverted drugs: to supplement a prescription or, where a prescription is lacking, to replace a prescription not for the preferred drug or formulation, as part of a pattern of polydrug use, as a preference for pharmaceutical over illicitly produced drugs, and as self-treatment.

Inciardi *et al.* (2007) conducted focus groups in Miami with young adult ecstasy users, cocaine and heroin users, methadone maintenance clients, and drug-involved HIV-positive prescription drug diverters. The diversion routes ranged from licit supply channels (e.g. pharmacies) to non-medical use of prescribed drugs. The authors suggest that the contributions of residential burglaries, pharmacy robberies, and thefts to the diversion problem may be understated (Inciardi *et al.* 2007). Miami informants reported a wider range of diversion routes than did the London informants. It is unclear whether this reflects more organized informal markets for prescription drugs in Miami, or that the researchers drew their informants from a wider range of clienteles.

There is also evidence that prescription opioids are sold in 'active street markets' (Inciardi *et al.* 2007). Sajan and colleagues (1998) surveyed a sample of street drug users and dealers in Vancouver, Canada, and found prescription opioids (including the then fairly new controlled-release formulations of opioid analgesics, e.g. MS-Contin) available in great variety and abundance. The authors found that prescription opioids were sold at considerable markups, a factor of 10–40 times their regular retail value, and were either used as substitutes for illicit drugs such as heroin when these were not available or sold to generate funds for more desirable drugs (Goldman 1998; Sajan *et al.* 1998). This phenomenon is of course well known to the special population of patients involved in methadone maintenance for the treatment of opioid dependence, many of whom sell or trade some of their methadone doses in order to obtain more desirable drugs (Fountain *et al.* 2000; Ritter and Di Natale 2005).

Studies such as these, with informants drawn from highly selected populations, may yield results that differ from findings in general population surveys. Experience with non-medical use of prescription medicines is widespread in many general youth populations. For instance, in the US Monitoring the Future survey of high-school students aged 17–18, the experience of using a prescription drug non-medically during the prior year was fairly common (15.4%), taking all prescription drug categories together (National Institute on Drug Abuse 2008). Perceived access to such drugs was very common, as shown in Table 6.3.

Table 6.3 Non-medical availability and use of prescription drugs, US grade 12 students, 2007

	Availability: % saying 'fairly' or 'very easy' to get	**% using in last 12 months**
Narcotics (except heroin, including methadone)	24%	9.2%
Amphetamines	42	7.5
Sedatives (barbiturates)	50	6.2
Tranquillizers	37	6.2

Source: Johnston *et al.* (2008).

Recent studies in student populations in the USA have begun to identify possible sources of prescription drugs used non-medically in the wider population. In a study of youth aged 10–18 in a Detroit public school, 70% of those admitting lifetime non-medical use of a prescription pain drug reported on the source of the drug, with 34% saying they got it from a family member, 17% from a friend, and 14% from a dealer or by theft (Boyd *et al.* 2006). Of the 458 students at a large Midwestern university who reported non-medical use of a prescription stimulant in the last year, 71.4% specified a source, with 67.7% specifying friends or peers, 3.1% a family member, and less than 1% from abroad or a dealer. None reported the Internet as a source (McCabe *et al.* 2006). A weakness of all these studies is that they do not trace drugs across sources, i.e. individuals who get drugs from 'friends' do not know where their friends got them, so a source with a low percentage endorsement may still be ultimately responsible for a large proportion of drugs used.

Viewing the transaction from the other side, 54% of those who had received and filled a medical prescription for a stimulant reported that they had been approached to sell, trade, or give some of the drug away during the last year. Students at a large US public research university reported several sources of non-medical use of prescription opioids, as shown in Table 6.4.

In 2005, the US National Survey on Drug Use and Health asked a general population sample aged 18–25 for the sources of the prescription analgesics they had used non-medically most recently. The mentions included: 'got them from a friend or relative for free' (53.0%), 'bought from a friend or relative' (10.6%), and 'took from a friend or relative without asking' (3.8%), indicating that about two-thirds of the respondents used family or friends as sources for their used prescription drugs non-medically (SAMHSA 2006a). Female respondents were much more likely to have obtained prescription pain relievers from family or friends for free, whereas males were much more likely to have bought them.

Besides stereotypical users or dealers and the more casual drug users identified in population surveys, there is also evidence that some less criminally suspect participants supply illicit prescription drug markets. Inciardi *et al.* (2007) report 'legitimate' patients or Medicaid recipients from a prescription opioid market study in the USA 'selling their prescription drugs for profit or exchanging them for illicit drugs' (p. 177).

Table 6.4 Supply sources of non-medical use of prescription opioids reported by 640 students at a large US public research university in the previous year (multiple responses allowed)

Supply source	Percentage
Boyfriend or girlfriend	7.9%
Room-mate	8.0%
Friend from the same college	27.0%
Friend not from the same college	33.7%
Acquaintance from the same college	3.6%
Acquaintance not from the same college	6.6%
Parent	36.1%
Sibling	5.9%
Aunt or uncle	2.1%
Another family member	3.6%
Drug dealer	3.5%
Abroad	1.0%
Internet	0.2%
Other sources	3.1%

Source: McCabe *et al.* (2007).

In the context of the Canadian OPICAN study, interviewers anecdotally learned from participants that senior citizens, located in certain known bars and pubs, had become a major non-medical source of illicit prescription opioids. They were reported to be easily and credibly able to obtain opioid drugs from the medical system, and they sold them mostly to subsidise their meagre retirement incomes.

Several studies suggest that the Internet has become a substantial and increasingly relevant source for prescription opioids (Compton and Volkow 2006; Forman 2006). While Internet sources for such drugs have been shown to exist in abundance, some researchers have suggested that their use is limited to the more 'socio-economically privileged sections of society' (Littlejohn *et al.* 2005). Others have suggested that the role of the Internet as a source for drugs 'may be overstated' and that many seeking prescription drugs for non-medical use avoid it because of the possibility of theft, surveillance, and the fact that 'prescription drugs are generally cheaper on the street' (Inciardi *et al.* 2007, p. 178).

In the view of the unregulated supply that emerges from these studies, formal illicit markets and direct diversion from the prescription process appear to play a relatively minor part. Most of the supply for those who are casual or occasional users (the dominant category in these student surveys) seems to be derived from a legitimate prescription transaction followed by an exchange through family or friendship relations (though probably not every parent or relative is aware of being a source of supply) or informal exchange. However, we can generalize neither this finding nor the pattern of a more regular market found in the clinical and selected population studies without further studies of other populations and places.

6.5 **How separate are the regulated market and the unregulated market?**

The studies of drugs used non-medically summarized above suggest that it is mainly in the post-retail stage, after the doctor has written a prescription, and the pharmacist has filled it, that diversion occurs, at least in well-ordered developed societies. The production, wholesale, and retail levels of the legal market in medications and the illicit market in drugs such as heroin, cocaine, and cannabis are almost entirely separated. It is easier for the state and for intergovernmental efforts to eliminate outlaw actions from legal than illegal markets, in part because those involved in the legal market—pharmaceutical producers, wholesalers, doctors, and pharmacists—operate under state licence, and the state can easily and effectively threaten their livelihood in case of non-compliance. Further, professional prescribers are strongly influenced by the norms of their colleagues, which discourage careless or corrupt prescribing, making the job of regulation much easier for the state.

However, the state has much weaker powers at the post-retail stage, where its only recourse is criminal law rather than the more flexible instrument of administrative licences and regulations. Punishing those who obtained pills by legal prescription because a young relative raided the family medicine cabinet is not a promising avenue of deterrence. Under most circumstances, the same would apply even to exchange transactions among friends involving an initially legal supply.

The source studies reviewed above suggest that the legal prescription and the non-medical use markets are connected at least by social networks (e.g. friendship or family relations). The connection may often be even closer, in that the patient then uses the drug to excess. An analysis of a large general population sample in the USA found that, even after adjustment for demographics, people who were prescribed opioids for non-cancer pain were three times more likely also to report opioid misuse and six times more likely to report problem opioid misuse (Edlund *et al.* 2007).

The main division between customers of the two markets may be, or at least may traditionally have been, in terms of age. Though it is not usually thought of in this way, a prescription system delegates to the doctor the state's power to control access to a potentially valued commodity. Among doctors, reflecting general social attitudes as much as anything specifically medical, a patient's claim of ill-defined pain will probably be viewed more sympathetically when it comes from an older adult than from a younger adult. Thus Kentucky opiate addicts of the 1940s found it much easier to get a legal opiate supply from a doctor, thereby staying on the right side of the law, as they aged (O'Donnell 1969). For many other psychoactive substances, the presumptive age gradient in the doctor's mind may now be less clear. Given current best practice for ADHD, for instance, the doctor may be less inclined to dismiss peremptorily the teenager in search of a stimulant who also presents with symptoms of ADHD. In part, the process of building 'psychopharmacological societies' may have weakened the prescription system's *de facto* age grading of access to psychopharmaceuticals, which served to keep the legal and non-medical markets more separate.

6.6 **Conclusion**

The use of psychoactive substances as medications extends back to human pre-history, but became strongly established in western medicine about 150 years ago. In the wealthier parts of the world, a wide variety of medications are used under prescription to relieve pain, to cure or counter mental illness, and to reduce distress. Psychoactive substances are an important part of modern allopathic medicine, primarily distributed through and controlled by a prescription system which we discuss later in Chapter 12.

Diversion from this system for non-medical use is a substantial part of the illicit drug market in many places. While there is certainly considerable theft and other criminal diversion, it is apparent that much of the leakage from one market to the other happens more informally, often at the consumer/patient end of the distribution chain. The separation between the markets is, in fact, much less clear in practice than is often presented in theory.

The legal market for psychoactive substances is important to a discussion of illicit drug use in ways which extend beyond being a source for diversion. In societies with substantial use of psychoactive medications, there are strong interests and ideologies that sustain ideas that psychoactive medications are potent in the relief of distress and the pursuit of well-being. Drug-using subcultures in such societies are well aware of the parallel in ideas with their own constructions of drug use, appropriating such phrases as 'better living through chemistry' and 'mother's little helper' to express ironically the convergence of world views.

Section III

The evidence base for drug policy: research on strategies and interventions

Chapter 7

Strategies and interventions to reduce drug use and related harm: section overview

7.1 Introduction

As described in Chapter 1, drug policy is broadly defined as any targeted effort on the part of governments to minimize or prevent drug use and drug-related harm to both individuals and society. The chapters in this section of the book describe research on strategies and interventions that are relevant to the formulation of drug policies. As such, Section III represents the core of any attempt to develop a rational set of drug policies based on scientific evidence. To set the stage for this section, this chapter discusses the context of addiction science as an aid to policy formation and implementation. It also explains how the scientific evidence for policy options was reviewed and organized, the rules that guided our presentation and interpretation of the evidence, and, finally, what topics the chapters cover.

7.2 Advances in policy-relevant research

Section III reviews an extensive body of research likely to be of great value to policymakers. Nevertheless, as an evolving and relatively new endeavour, drug policy evaluations and other research relevant to policy are incapable of providing definitive answers to many of the most pressing policy questions in the worldwide policy arena. Most notably, addiction research is rarely conducted outside the developed world. Most research derives from the USA. The remainder is concentrated in Europe, Japan, Canada, and Australia. It must be candidly admitted that findings from the developed countries do not necessarily apply to the rest of the world. A more nuanced point to bear in mind is that even within one country, research findings may not generalize from one historical era to another because that country's drug problem and its political and social environment can change dramatically from one generation to the next.

As the authors drafted the chapters in this section, we were at once impressed with the growing amount and quality of research evidence about treatment and prevention research and discouraged by the inadequacy of the evidence for many of the most costly policy options, such as crop substitution and interdiction. If progress is to be made on the prevention and treatment of drug problems, new quantitative and qualitative research methods need to be applied in large population areas, methodologies that do not conform readily to traditional experimental and evaluation designs.

This is less a criticism of the state of drug policy research as it is an honest recognition of the inadequacy of traditional research designs to answer meaningful policy questions in the context of complex intervention approaches. New models are needed that combine different but complementary social science methods within interdisciplinary collaborative teams exploring important policy issues simultaneously from the perspectives of history, economics, epidemiology, political science, sociology, ethnography, and psychology. With respect to supply reduction programmes, the problem is not only the lack of systematic research studies, but also the difficulty of collecting adequate data to monitor and evaluate changes in drug policies.

7.3 **Rules of evidence**

With the growth of addiction science, a variety of methodological approaches have been used to assess the impact of drug policies as well as the effectiveness of policy-relevant prevention programmes, treatment strategies, and related efforts. These include experimental studies, survey research, analyses of mortality and morbidity statistics, and qualitative research. The glossary at the end of the book provides definitions of relevant methodological terms used in drug policy research that are not otherwise defined in the text.

Experimental studies typically use the randomized control design, in which research participants or groups of participants (e.g. classrooms) are randomly allocated to either an intervention condition (e.g. a drug education lecture) or a control condition (e.g. a regular history lecture), and changes in knowledge, attitudes, or behaviour are measured after the lectures are delivered. When a large number of **randomized controlled trials** have been conducted, they are typically reviewed to determine whether there are consistent effects across studies. **Cochrane reviews** are comprehensive and systematic assessments of the effects of health care interventions, focusing on randomized controlled trials. Critics of the Cochrane approach argue that there is an over-reliance on the randomized trial for the burden of proof, and that well-conducted cohort or non-randomized controlled studies will provide similar estimates of effectiveness and are more practical for some research questions. While several analyses have suggested that in some instances well-conducted **quasi-experimental studies** provide similar estimates to randomized controlled trials (Benson and Hartz 2000; Concato *et al.* 2000; Cook *et al.* 2008), other research suggests that quasi-experimental studies may find benefit where randomized controlled trials have found none (Chalmers *et al.* 1977; Sacks *et al.* 1982; Hulley *et al.* 1998; Pocock and Elbourne2000; Gotzsche and Olsen 2000).

Randomized trials of prevention and treatment programmes can be difficult to conduct because of political, ethical, and cost considerations. For these reasons, researchers often exploit **natural experiments** for scientific information, using quasi-experimental research designs that make it possible to make inferences about causes and effects. Such studies have credibility insofar as they are conducted under real-world conditions rather than as part of a contrived experiment, but we cannot draw causal inferences as confidently from them as we can from randomized controlled trials. This type of research typically involves before and after measurement of a group, community, or other jurisdiction that is exposed to an intervention, and if possible similar measurement is conducted in comparable groups or communities where no intervention took place. Natural experiments have played a large role in this literature. For example, when increased enforcement is implemented in one jurisdiction and not in an adjacent one, the relative impact of the policy can be examined over time through comparative analysis of archival data such as HIV infection rates or drug overdoses. When consecutive measures are available during a period when a policy is being implemented, **time series analysis** can be conducted to determine how a change on one series correlates with a change on the other (with other factors, called **confounders**, controlled statistically).

The appropriateness of any research methodology for drug policy evaluation depends on the phenomena under study, the current state of knowledge, the availability of valid measurement procedures, and the ways in which the information will be put to use (McKinlay 1992). The most direct evidence in drug policy research comes from studying what happens when the intervention is applied or removed, in comparison with another time or place when there is no change in the intervention. When intervention studies are planned in advance, careful consideration can be given to the collection of the most appropriate kinds of evaluation data. Where possible, those data should include population surveys before and after the change; the compilation of event data on cases coming to the attention of health, police, and other agencies; and qualitative observations of social processes in the period of change. However, researchers can often produce a useful evaluation even in the absence of planning, when the political process unexpectedly provides a natural experiment. In this case, the researcher typically matches post-intervention data with data that were collected for other purposes prior to the change.

Studies of what happens when there is a change (e.g. an intervention is implemented or discontinued) provide the most valuable evidence on the effects of drug policy. Yet one can also learn from cross-sectional studies comparing sites where different policies are in effect. Given the potential sources of **confounding**, data from such studies cannot provide definitive evidence of effectiveness.

The various methods of data collection used in drug policy research have different advantages and drawbacks. Social surveys, for example, generally measure attitudes and behaviours through the direct questioning of individual students or adults. Studies based on survey data tend to be descriptive, correlational, and subject to the limitations of self-report methods. Data collected by social and health agencies (e.g. police statistics, hospital discharge data, mortality records) give a good picture of drug problems in an area, but the available data also reflect cultural perceptions, agency priorities, and recording practices.

Researchers can complement quantitative research methods such as social surveys with qualitative studies, such as ethnographic interviewing, participant observation, case studies, and focus group discussions. As long as researchers apply standard scientific principles of confirmation, refutation, causal inference, and generalizability, qualitative research can provide an additional different form of evidence that can inform drug policy development. Combinations of these methods in a single study are not uncommon. The value of combining different methods is that the strengths of one approach compensate for the shortcomings of another. For example, a focus group of experienced drug users coupled with a population survey offers both in-depth information from a small number of people and less detailed information on a larger group.

Policy evaluation research provides a useful but often underutilized benefit to decision makers. Should resources be devoted to less costly programmes that have at best a modest effect? Or should they be directed to more costly programmes that are likely to have a more substantial impact? Decisions about which strategies to implement, phase out, or modify should be informed by findings from systematic evaluation.

Evaluation research is an applied inquiry process for collecting and synthesizing evidence about the value of a service, programme, or policy. The purpose of evaluation research is to measure the effects of a programme or policy against the goals it set out to accomplish. Evaluation research uses the same experimental and quasi-experimental methods as other research; what distinguishes it from clinical and other scientific research is its practical purpose. Evaluation research is necessary in order to measure whether the policy has any impact, and to provide a 'reality check' to the high expectations often attached to promising new initiatives. Evaluation also needs to be ongoing. Evidence from one time period may not be applicable to situations emerging in another era. And evidence from high income countries may not be applicable to low income countries. Furthermore, communities and countries often want locally based evidence to justify their interventions, rather than relying on findings from other times and places.

In addition to studying whether and how a policy works, it is also valuable to evaluate a policy's effectiveness and societal benefits in relation to its costs. The two most widely used forms of economic evaluation are cost–benefit analysis (CBA) and cost–effectiveness analysis (CEA). In CBA the evaluation examines the relationship between benefits and costs of a policy when both variables are expressed in monetary terms. This makes it possible to determine whether the monetary benefits of a particular policy (such as a drug education programme) exceed its costs. In CEA, the evaluation focuses on the least costly way to achieve the benefits of a policy. Typically, this form of economic analysis compares alternative policies or programmes that could be used to achieve the same objective (e.g. buprenorphine versus methadone maintenance), with the results expressed as net costs needed to produce a unit of a health outcome, such as a life saved, or years of life saved from a drug overdose. Both approaches provide useful information to the policymaker.

In summary, the most reliable way to identify the causal effects of a drug policy is through planned experiments. But in many cases where policies, interventions, and treatments are being evaluated, experimental evidence is not available. To reach sound conclusions under these conditions, it is best to assume that no one research approach, and no one study, will provide conclusive evidence. Using evidence derived from several different populations, methodologies, and contexts is often the best and the only way to proceed, as will become apparent in the chapters to follow in this section. In addition to comparing relevant outcomes, policies can also be evaluated in terms of their costs and benefits.

7.4 **Types of interventions and strategies relevant to drug policy: an analytical framework**

To guide our review of the literature, we divide drug policy options into five categories: primary prevention; services for chronic drug users; supply control; regulations and prescription regimes; and the use of criminal sanctions. For the purposes of this book, what matters most to the policymaker is not the programme's label but its likely effect.

Prevention programmes are designed to delay or prevent either the initiation of drug use or the probability of progressing from experimentation to regular drug use. The most common approaches are those based on information, persuasion, and alternative activities (e.g. school-based drug education programmes, family and community activities, mass media campaigns).

Services for drug users are designed to reduce drug use and/or its consequences among experienced users through a range of programmes that have been developed and evaluated in many countries. These include drug counselling, methadone maintenance, medical care, social services, and needle exchange programmes. Regardless of whether these services are labelled 'treatment', 'rehabilitation', or 'harm reduction', they are considered here as parts of a broader approach to drug-related problems that targets the individual drug user in a non-punitive way.

The *supply control* approach includes law enforcement and alternative development programmes aimed at growers of coca and poppy. The vast majority of resources go to law enforcement, which can be classified into two general types: programmes aimed at producers, traffickers, and dealers, which attempt to reduce the physical and economic availability of drugs by limiting their supply and raising their price; and programmes aimed at users and retailers, which attempt to raise the transaction costs of buying drugs (i.e. time, inconvenience, and risk).

Laws and regulations determine which substances are legal and illegal, for whom, and under what conditions. Examples include complete prohibition of a drug, allowing distribution of a drug only in particular systems (e.g. from licensed pharmacies), and giving only particular individuals the right to use or prescribe drugs (e.g. terminally ill patients in otherwise unmanageable pain can use morphine; specially licensed general practitioners in the UK can prescribe heroin).

Punitive (e.g. criminal) sanctions with the aim of deterring drug use through the threat of punishment or removal of the drug user from the community is the final category of drug policy options considered in this section of the book. In the past half-century, most countries have passed laws to penalize use, possession, or home production of different psychoactive substances. A more recent trend in some countries has been to reduce or eliminate criminal penalties, particularly in the case of cannabis. In both cases, there have also been changes in enforcement practices concerning penalization of possession or use.

Although this five-part classification covers many governmental actions that are official drug policy, these are not the only policy approaches that influence drug problems. Many social programmes, such as health education, infectious disease surveillance systems, and general policing have much broader objectives than drug control, but may be equally important in reducing drug problems (Boyum and Reuter 2001). As with programmes that specifically target drug problems, non-targeted programmes may generate benefits in more than one area.

Table 7.1 lists major programme types according to their specific aims and broader goals. The labels, while useful for classification purposes, impose a level of precision that may be deceiving. As noted above, treatment programmes provide many harm reduction messages; for example, reminding heroin injectors that their tolerance will be lower as a result of treatment should they relapse into heroin use is harm reduction *par excellence* done in the context of treatment. Similarly, when police officers warn heroin users to beware of batches of bad fentanyl, then the enforcement budget is being used for harm reduction goals. Enforcement differs from treatment in many respects, but the boundaries can blur when drug users are given a choice between treatment and prison. And with increasing misuse of psychoactive drugs manufactured by the pharmaceutical industry, it is necessary to include new policy options directed at the regulatory regimes that have evolved to govern the distribution of prescription drugs.

Table 7.1 Categorization of strategies and interventions by policy area and broader policy goals

	Policy area	**Broad policy goals**
Prevention	Drug prevention programmes Mass media campaigns Reducing access for youth through policing	Change attitudes, improve health literacy, and prevent drug use
Services for drug users	Methadone maintenance Counselling, therapeutic communities Coerced abstinence through probation/parole supervision Needle exchange programmes	Reduce use, improve health, reduce crime and overdose deaths, prevent spread of blood-borne viruses, and treat psychiatric disorders
Supply control	Arrest traffickers/dealers Force suppliers to operate in inefficient ways	Keep prices high and reduce availability
Prescription regimes	Regulate pharmaceutical companies, pharmacists, and physicians	Allow psychoactive substances to be consumed for approved purposes and prevent use for non-approved purposes
Criminal sanctions	Increase penalties for drug possession and use Decrease penalties for some types of drug use (e.g. cannabis)	Deter drug use; prevent normalization and contagious spread of drug use. Prevent negative effects of criminalizing less harmful forms of drug use

7.5 **Making sense of the science base**

One of the most useful tools for policymakers in many areas of public health and social problems has been the integrative literature review, which typically consists of a systematic evaluation of the evidence from a range of scientific studies bearing on a particular health or social problem. Using the five-part classification described above, the strategies and interventions discussed in this section of the book were systematically evaluated on the basis of the following rules of evidence. First, the authors reviewed and critically appraised the world literature on each area, with other experts serving as external reviewers. Special attention was given to developments during the last two decades, in part because of the dramatic increase in research during this period. Reviews of the literature were either commissioned as background papers or conducted by the authors themselves. The emphasis was on studies with better research designs (e.g. experimental or quasi-experimental designs with control groups or comparison conditions). The variety of approaches, wide scope of the literature searches, and expert involvement have led to detailed evaluations and careful weighting of the existing evidence. Still, potential biases may be present due to missed studies and selectivity of inclusion.

Given the origins of the scientific literature in the drug field, most of the research reviewed in this section of the book originated in English-speaking countries. To compensate for the relative lack of research in other parts of the world, the authors gave careful consideration to the cross-national generalizability of findings from particular studies. Finally, the authors held a series of meetings to review and critique the contents, findings, and conclusions of each chapter, and to develop a consensus about the conclusions presented in the final chapter. In addition, the authors worked collaboratively on an extensive summary of the strategies and interventions reviewed in Chapters 8–12, which is presented in the Appendix at the end of the book.

7.6 **Overview of chapters in Section III**

The policies, strategies, and interventions discussed in the next five chapters cover the most currently favoured policy options where there is a related research base capable of review. Chapter 8 focuses on strategies aimed at young people in school, family, and community settings. There has been an improvement in the evidence base over recent years and there is now convincing evidence for family-oriented and classroom management prevention efforts, although this is based on a relatively small number of studies from the USA. Chapter 9 examines research conducted on treatment and harm reduction strategies, showing that there is cause for optimism regarding the modification of continued drug use and the minimization of drug-related problems. Chapter 10 deals with a broad range of strategies aimed at supply control activities, primarily enforcement against producers and dealers. It discusses efforts aimed at production/refining, international trafficking, high-level domestic enforcement, and retail enforcement. Because research has been neglected in this area, the most striking finding is perhaps the fact that so little is known about some of the most costly and ambitious approaches to drug policy and policy implementation. Chapter 11 reviews policies designed to deter drug use through criminal sanctions on the possession and use of psychoactive substances. Finally, Chapter 12 examines how well laws and regulations governing prescription drug regimes perform their role of allowing psychoactive substances to be consumed for approved purposes, while preventing their misuse for non-approved purposes.

Drawing on an extensive literature involving both original research and integrative literature reviews, the chapters in this section provide evidence not only of a wide variety of effective strategies that can be translated into drug policies, but also of ineffective policies that consume scarce resources without any apparent impact. Moreover, they point to gaps in knowledge and a surprising lack of commitment to evidence-based policy, conclusions that cannot be ignored if substance-related problems are to be addressed in the future.

Chapter 8

Preventing illicit drug use by young people

8.1 Introduction

Preventing people from becoming illicit drug users is a broadly shared goal among policymakers. When focused on young people, prevention programmes enjoy broad popular support as well. This chapter summarizes research on programmes designed to delay or to prevent entirely the use of illicit drugs and the problems connected with them. The focus on young people is chosen because the volume of research in this population is much larger than for prevention in adults (e.g. workplace programmes) and because, as highlighted in Chapter 3, adolescence is the period of life in which drug use is most likely to begin. There is a broad array of prevention options available within the ambit of youth-focused prevention, comprising both distinct strategies (e.g. mass media campaigns, community-based family strengthening programmes) and dozens of variations on particular strategies (e.g. the many putatively distinct forms of school-based drug prevention).

There are two important limitations of research on youth prevention programmes. First, researchers have studied a fairly narrow band of strategies. Some commonly used strategies, such as supporting grassroots coalitions that organize against drug use, have rarely been evaluated, leaving scientists with no reliable conclusions to draw for policymakers. School-based interventions have the largest evidence base; not coincidentally, they operate at a unit of analysis (the classroom) for which it is easier to administer randomized controlled trials than for community-based or mass media interventions. Secondly, while drug prevention programmes are used throughout the world, programme **evaluation research** has been limited except in the USA. Indeed, about 90% of prevention programme evaluations have been conducted in that country (White and Pitts 1998). Later in the chapter, we will discuss whether conclusions drawn primarily about US-based prevention programmes can be generalized to other countries.

Historically, the prevention field has passed through a succession of conceptual models (a few of which could fairly be called fads) that are based on different theoretical assumptions about how prevention is supposed to work. Early programmes often highlighted the dangers of drug use. One might argue they worked for a time, inasmuch as drug use was relatively rare before the 1960s. But as drug use, or at least cannabis use, became more prevalent, it became harder for prevention campaigns to convince a population with extensive first-hand experience that drug use invariably led to serious harm. The next conceptual approach was to provide accurate but not exaggerated information about the dangers of drug use. Although such programmes sometimes affected students' knowledge about drug use, they generally had no effect on drug use itself. The next idea in the history of prevention was that low self-esteem left youth vulnerable to drugs. This assumption led to the development of interventions designed to improve self-esteem. Whereas these programmes may have helped youth feel better about themselves, they apparently had no meaningful effect on drug use.

A subsequent theory held that most youth generally do not want to use drugs but rather fall into drug use in an unplanned way owing to peer pressure. This gave rise to *resistance skills* approaches in which students role-played ways of 'saying no' to such offers without losing status in the eyes of their peers. That wave of programmes advanced the field of prevention science by embracing active learning methods (role-playing) and recognizing the importance of decision making within a social context (as opposed to an abstract rational choice ideal). However, the peers encouraging youth to try drugs are often not bullies in the school yard making one-time offers but close friends with whom the individual has ongoing contact. The resistance skills idea thus evolved into a more general *social influences* approach that emphasized the importance of social and psychological factors in the onset of drug use, including both peer and parental influences. Those ideas are still seen as relevant and useful, but other tactics were introduced in the late 1990s, when it became popular to speak of *comprehensive* approaches. These programmes supplemented social skills training with other tactics such as *norm setting*, which provided objective information derived from school surveys to persuade young people that the use of alcohol and drugs was the exception, not the norm. Alongside this largely drug-specific prevention programming, other prevention approaches have come to the fore over the last 20 years, largely influenced by theories from developmental as well as social psychology. These approaches have a broader, non-drug-focused goal: to impact positively on antisocial behaviour, criminal activity, health, and well-being as well as drug use and misuse by influencing the early social development of children and adolescents.

Table 8.1 provides brief descriptions of some of the typical school, family, and community programmes guided by these general theories. Contemporary school-based drug prevention programmes that focus on social influences or social skills include three major components—psychological inoculation, normative education, and resistance skills training (Botvin 2000)—and so are often called comprehensive programmes. Media programmes have generally followed the more traditional theories (e.g. emphasizing dangers), but they also seek to create associations at a more reflexive level (e.g. sports heroes endorsing a drug-free lifestyle) or work indirectly (e.g. television messages targeted at parents, encouraging them to spend more time with their children). Family-based interventions tend to draw on problem behaviour models that stress the importance of protective factors (e.g. parents spending time with children) and risk factors (drug-using peers) that suggest ways to prevent the development of drug use. For example, a programme might try to increase family cohesion and its ability to manage emotions and conflict. These interventions also include social skills components. Community programmes, on the other hand, are typically based on theories of community organization and participation. They are often multicomponent interventions that target schools, families, peers, and the wider community in an effort to shape drug use norms.

Table 8.1 Drug prevention programmes reviewed in this chapter

Key	Prevention programme
ALERT (Ellickson *et al.* 2003)	Project ALERT (revised): seeks to change students' beliefs about drug norms and consequences and help them to identify and resist prodrug pressures. Eleven lessons in 7th grade (aged 12–13 years) and three in 8th grade, using interactive teaching methods (question-and-answer techniques and small group activities).
CBI (Snow *et al.* 1992)	Cognitive Behavioural skills Intervention: familiarizes students with the basic concepts of effective decision making to promote role flexibility, increase students' abilities to recognize and manage peer pressure, and enhance students' ability to seek information and support when faced with decisions. Teaching techniques include presentation, brainstorming exercises, discussions, and role-plays. Forty-minute sessions once per week for 12 weeks.
CC (Furr-Holden *et al.* 2004)	Classroom-Centred intervention: curricular enhancements, improved classroom behaviour management practices (using the 'Good Behaviour Game'), and supplementary strategies for children not performing adequately. An interactive read-aloud component was added to increase listening and comprehension skills. Strategies employed with respect to academic non-responders include individual or small group tutoring and curricular modifications to address individual learning styles.
CP (Biglan *et al.* 2000)	Community Program (CP): a funded community coordinator (full time for 1 year, 0.75 for 2 years) is charged with implementing a media advocacy module, youth antitobacco module, family communication module, and ACCESS module (designed to stop stores from selling tobacco to minors).
DARE, DARE+ (Perry *et al.* 2003)	Drug Abuse Resistance Program Plus: DARE curriculum plus peer-led sessions, extracurricular activities, and neighbour-hood action teams organized by community organizers. Community organizers create and facilitate youth action teams to conduct extracurricular activities. Neighbourhood action teams led by the same community organizers address issues of drug use and violence.
FoF (Catalano *et al.* 1999)	Focus on Families, with children of methadone-using parent(s): parental skills training plus home-based case management for 9 months; 53 hours of training in groups of 6–10 families. One five-hour 'retreat', 32 90-minute meetings twice weekly. Delivered to families (12 sessions) or parents (20 sessions), with 6–10 families per group.

(continued)

Table 8.1 (continued) Drug prevention programmes reviewed in this chapter

Key	**Prevention programme**
GBG (Kellam *et al.* 2008)	Good Behaviour Game: the game is a way of managing whole classes during lessons. It aims to socialize children to the role of being a school pupil and to reduce aggression or disruptive behaviour, which are known to be related to later drug abuse, dependence, and antisocial behaviour. Children are divided into teams that can win prizes depending on the good behaviour of the team as a whole.
LST (Botvin *et al.* 1995, 2001; Spoth *et al.* 2006)	Life Skills Training: teaching drug resistance skills and antidrug norms, and facilitating the development of personal and social skills. Skills taught using a combination of teaching techniques including group discussion, demonstrations, modelling, behavioural rehearsal, feedback, reinforcement, and behavioural homework assignments.
MCI (Wu *et al.* 2002)	Multidimensional Community Intervention in China. Includes community, clinic, family, and school education elements. Groups of village leaders, parents, youth, militia women, and former drug users formed to mobilize community members to participate in drug prevention activities, including videos on drug and HIV prevention, two 2–3 hour knowledge training sessions for villagers, evening classes for school dropouts, and drug/HIV prevention in schools.
NASCI (Schinke *et al.* 2000)	School plus Community Intervention with Native Americans: community efforts include media releases about benefits of substance abuse prevention efforts; flyers and posters distributed to schools, churches, and businesses; health, and social services agencies; and information meetings held at schools for parents, neighbours and teachers.
PDFY (Spoth *et al.* 2004, 2006)	Preparing for the Drug Free Years: substance abuse education, parenting skills, peer resistance skills (for children); one 2-hour session per week for 5 weeks: one session of child plus parents, four sessions with parents only. Group size of approximately 10 families (16 people) plus two leaders.
SCI (Flay *et al.* 2004)	School plus Community Intervention: parent support programme to reinforce parenting skills and promote parent–child communication; school staff and school-wide youth support programmes; community programme to forge links between school, parents, and community; and school task force to implement programme components, propose changes in school policy, develop school–community liaisons, and solicit community organizations to support drug prevention programme.

SFP10-14 (Spoth *et al.* 2004, 2006)	Strengthening Families Program for youth aged 10–14 and their parents/carers, also known as the Iowa SFP: parenting skills including providing love and setting limits, communication, sanctions, having fun, and (for children) peer resistance and peer relationship training; one 2-hour session per week for 7 weeks, the first hour with parents and children separately and the second hour together. Group size 3–15 families, average 20 people plus three leaders.
SMI (Slater *et al.* 2006)	Social Marketing Intervention: in-school and community media campaign (Be Under Your Own Influence) that seeks to reframe substance use as an activity that impairs rather than enhances personal autonomy. Valued items include a series of school-delivered posters as well as promotional items such as book covers, tray liners, T-shirts, water bottles, and rulers. Community campaign media materials include brochures, press releases, ideas for special events, posters, and radio public service announcements.
TND (Sussman *et al.* 1998)	Towards No Drug abuse: conducted with continuation high school students who are unable to remain in the regular school system for functional reasons, including substance use when reaching high school age. Nine sessions with a health motivation–social skills–decision making approach, covering pro-health programming, effective listening, chemical dependency issues, alternative coping skills, and non-drug-use choices.

8.2 What works? Evidence on effectiveness

As discussed in Chapter 7, researchers have used a variety of research methods to study the effectiveness of drug intervention strategies and programmes. Among these the **randomized controlled trial** is considered the highest standard for demonstrating effectiveness. When a sufficient number of trials have been conducted, they are typically reviewed critically to identify systematic trends or inconsistencies. In this chapter, we will focus on the general conclusions of these reviews, giving special attention to reviews sponsored and published by the Cochrane Collaboration, an independent group of scientists who evaluate the evidence from research on health care interventions.

8.2.1 School-based drug prevention programs

The authors of one **Cochrane review** of school-based drug prevention concluded that some programmes deterred early stage drug use (Faggiano *et al.* 2005), whereas other programmes did not. Specifically, programmes that teach social and coping skills reduce drug use slightly relative to normal classroom instructional activities. In contrast, programmes that simply convey didactic information about drugs and their effects have no effect on drug use relative to normal classroom instructional activities. Based on this review and subsequent studies, Figure 8.1 provides estimates of the ability of skills-based programmes to reduce lifetime prevalence over the short term (1–3 years) and longer term (6–7 years). Combining results across studies of different programmes (Life Skills Training (LST), Project ALERT (ALERT), a Classroom-Centred (CC) intervention, a Cognitive Behavioural Intervention (CBI) and a programme called 'Towards No Drug abuse' (TND)) provided an estimate that cannabis initiation is somewhere between 1 and 23% less likely, over the shorter term, when students are exposed to skills-based prevention, compared with usual classroom activities. As with Faggiano's review, the pooling of different studies and the further analyses presented here assume that the interventions are similar (i.e. that they are all variations of social skills training).

Lifetime prevalence is the proportion of people who have ever used a substance. If lifetime prevalence is reduced for several years but not permanently, drug use initiation is said to be delayed. For example, some people who would have initiated soon after the programme was conducted (say, when they were 14) did not do so until later, perhaps when they were 17, which reduces lifetime prevalence measured at age 15 but not at age 18.

Policymakers and the public will differ in how much they value delays in cannabis initiation. For those who consider less cannabis use among the young a good in itself, there is a case for skills-based prevention programmes from the studies just reviewed.

Other stakeholders may take the view that because cannabis use in the teenage years accounts for a very small share of all drug-related social costs, the effects described in Figure 8.1a are of little importance unless they translate into additional effects later. Whether delayed initiation accrues large benefits later in life has not been determined. Because doing so would require studies of very large samples of young people followed up for decades (Gerstein and Green 1993), the long-term impact of skills-based

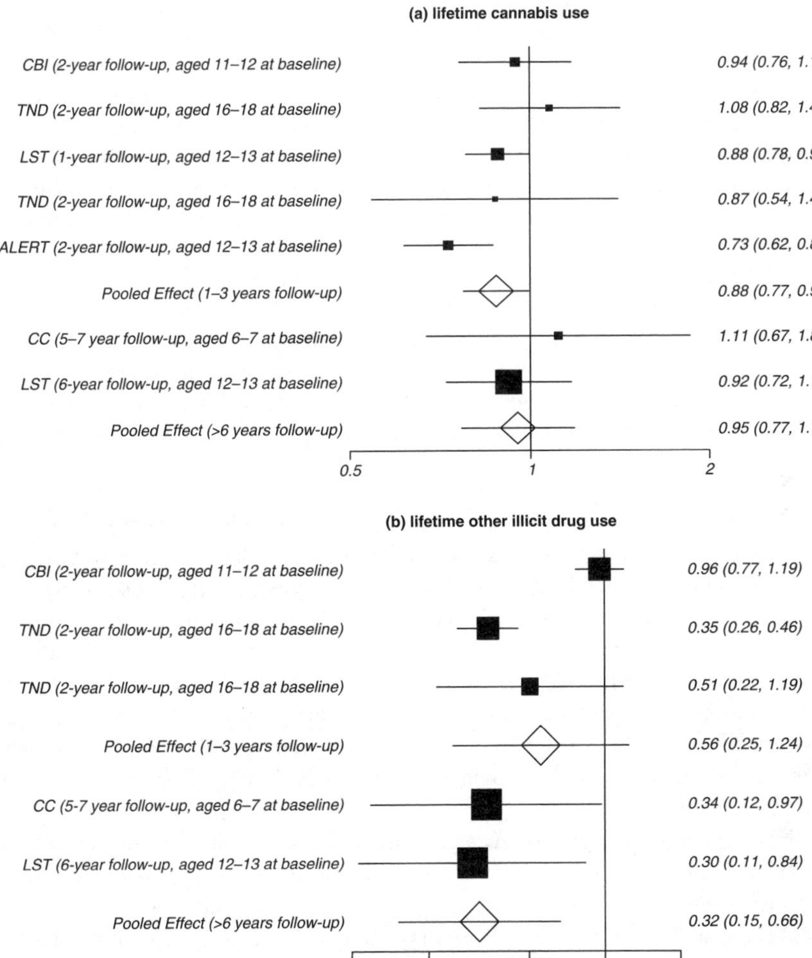

Fig. 8.1 Forest plots with random effect pooled odds ratio estimates of (a) lifetime cannabis use and (b) lifetime other illicit drug use for skills-based school prevention programmes.

Note: Pooled results from separate studies tend to be presented in a fairly standard pictorial form, known as a 'forest plot' of the results from randomized controlled trials where each trial compared a similar prevention programme with a control group, and examined impact in terms of drug use prevented. In Figure a and b the horizontal line corresponding to each of the trials shows the odds of drug use in young people randomized to the prevention intervention compared with young people randomized to a control group. The square 'blob' in the middle of each line is the point estimate of the difference between the groups (the best single estimate of the benefit in drug use prevented by exposure to the prevention programme rather than inclusion in the control group), and the width of the line represents the 95% confidence interval, or precision, of

(continued)

(continued from previous page) *this estimate. The black line down the middle of the picture is known as the 'line of no effect' and in this case represents the levels of drug use in the control group with an odds ratio (OR) = 1.0. If the confidence interval of the result (the horizontal line) crosses the line of no effect (the vertical line), that can mean either that there is no significant difference between the prevention programme and the control group or that the sample size was too small to allow us to be confident where the true result lies. The diamond shapes represent the pooled data across different trials of similar interventions, with a new, typically narrower, confidence interval, and are interpreted in the same way as single effects except for the fact that the result reflects not just one, but several trials. For example, the pooled effect over the shorter term is 0.88 (0.77, 0.99) which means that prevention reduced the odds of drug use initiation by 12% of what they were in the control group. For technical reasons we have used odds rather than risks, even though these are less intuitive to understand than risk ratios. However, in this case the odds ratios are a close approximation of the relative risk reduction, so in the text, for convenience and understanding, we interpret the odds as relative risks (Davies et al.), e.g. a 12% reduction in the risk of drug use, with a precision around this of 1–23%.*

prevention programmes is likely to remain uncertain. In other research, age of cannabis initiation is strongly correlated with a host of drug-related outcomes, including likelihood of using other drugs, amount of other drug use, and likelihood of needing treatment. But such correlations can occur in the absence of a causal link, and therefore cannot directly resolve the issue. Some findings suggest caution. For instance, although Sweden has much lower rates of youth trying cannabis (5% in the last year) than many other European countries (15.5% as an average of 13 countries), the Swedish rate of 'problem drug users' (4.5 per 1000 aged 15–64) is not very different from rates elsewhere in Europe (4.8 in the 13 countries; Tables EYE-5 and OPDU-1 in EMCDDA 2008b).

These conclusions are based on cannabis use, which along with alcohol and tobacco are the primary focus of prevention research because they are the substances most commonly reported in youth surveys. The picture for illicit drugs other than cannabis is different, albeit with fewer studies upon which to draw (Figure 8.1b). In these studies, drug use was measured as having ever used any of a range of substances other than cannabis, including cocaine, hallucinogens, stimulants, inhalants, steroids, heroin, and PCP. For the CBI and the two TND studies, the pooled effect for other illicit drug use could only be estimated over the short-term (1–3 years). Over the longer term, the pooled effect for CC (heroin, crack, cocaine) and LST (methamphetamine) prevention programmes was quite marked. Participants in skills-based prevention programmes were between 34 and 85% less likely to have used an illicit drug (other than cannabis) 5–7 years post-intervention, compared with students exposed to the standard classroom curriculum.

Some will consider such reductions in youth drug use significant and valuable. Others will wonder what these results mean in terms of the impact of these programmes on lifetime drug use and drug-related problems. Results pertaining to other illicit drugs would seem to be more policy-relevant than are results for cannabis because most drug-related harms stem from these other illicit drugs. However, because most people who try a drug other than cannabis do not progress to problematic use, extrapolation to lifetime effects is challenging.

It is also worth considering alternative explanations for the rather surprising finding that in the evaluations considered in this chapter, preventive programmes appear to produce larger reductions in the use of other illicit drugs than they do in cannabis use. A sceptical hypothesis is that because other illicit drugs are more stigmatized, their self-reported use is more susceptible to reporting bias than cannabis. A more credulous explanation is that because other illicit drugs are less available, young people have less experience with them and so are more easily discouraged from using them than the more widely available and socially tolerated drug cannabis.

Faggiano's review suggests that on average, modern school-based prevention programmes can delay or prevent the initiation of drug use, although effects on frequency of drug use are not so clear. Average effects are important, but not every programme is average; some programmes are below average (i.e. have no benefits) and others are above average (i.e. have more than a small benefit). A prominent example of the former is DARE (Drug Abuse Resistance Education), which is implemented in more than 70% of elementary and middle schools in the USA and in 44 other countries as well (Brown 2001). Despite DARE's widespread adoption, **meta-analyses** of outcome evaluations showed that the programme is ineffective (Ennett *et al.* 1994; West and O'Neal 2004).

8.2.2 Changes in classroom management and the school environment

An authoritative review conducted by the US National Research Council (Manski *et al.* 2001) found that programmes that altered the classroom or school environment were more effective than those that tried to change individual behaviour. Such programmes focus on improving school discipline and climate and strengthening teachers' classroom management skills. For example, although the Cochrane review (Faggiano *et al.* 2005) has listed the Good Behaviour Game (GBG) as a component of a skills-based intervention (the CC curriculum mentioned above), much of the focus of the GBG intervention is on improving classroom behaviour management at grades one and two. In a longer term follow-up study (Kellam *et al.* 2008) the GBG reduced lifetime drug abuse by up to 50% in males 14 years after exposure to the programme; a statistically significant effect, with even stronger effects seen in boys identified at age 6 as highly aggressive and disruptive. There was, however, no effect on females, nor were the results so clear cut in a second, replication, study over the same time period (Kellam *et al.* 2008).

This programme includes no discussion of drugs; rather, it targets changes in the school environment that promote consistency and reward positive social interactions instead of social disruption and social withdrawal. Yet its long-term effects would seem to compare well with the best school-based programmes aimed specifically at drug prevention. As has been noted above, illicit drug use does not exist apart from other aspects of a young person's life. Studies show that factors that predict the development of a drug problem are also predictive of school failure, social isolation, aggression, and other problems. The implication is that programmes that have no drug-specific content can nonetheless reduce drug use because they create a more broadly positive developmental context for young people. In other assessments, such programmes have been shown to impact on a broader set of mental, emotional, and behavioural disorders as well as drug use (O'Connell *et al.* 2009).

8.2.3 Drug testing in schools

The majority of school-based prevention programmes use 'education and persuasion' approaches (Paglia and Room 1999). There are, however, other school-based approaches that focus on school drug policies, such as drug testing for student athletes, defining a drug-free zone around school grounds, and punishment or counselling for students found to be drug users. Such policies have not been extensively evaluated (Paglia and Room 1999; Evans-Whipp *et al.* 2004). Drug testing in schools, whether random or on suspicion, is more common in the USA than in other countries, albeit in a minority of schools. One American study (Yamaguchi *et al.* 2003) found that among 8th, 10th, and 12th graders, students' drug use did not differ between schools with and without drug testing, but one might expect that only schools with significant drug problems would adopt such intrusive measures. A later review of school-based programmes (McKegany 2005) found no convincing evidence to support random drug testing in schools. The report also speculated that such programmes could have negative effects, such as reduced trust between pupils and staff.

8.2.4 Prevention of illicit drug use via families and communities

A recent Cochrane review reported on the effectiveness of the prevention of illicit drug use among young people outside of school lessons, covering family- and community-based prevention efforts (Gates *et al.* 2006). There were not enough studies to allow the authors to carry out a meta-analysis and pool results across similar interventions, though significant effects were detected in individual studies of family interventions but not in multicomponent community interventions.

For family-based prevention, one intervention showed prevention effects on cannabis and methamphetamine use. The Strengthening Families Program (SFP10-14) is a brief, seven-session intervention that focuses on promoting family relationships, communication, behaviour, and conflict management. In a randomized trial (Spoth *et al.* 2004) the SFP10-14 was evaluated alongside the Preparing for the Drug-Free Years (PDFY) skills-based intervention and a normal control group, and there was a marked reduction in lifetime cannabis use after 6 years in those young people exposed to the family programme (SFP10-14) compared with PDFY and normal control groups. After 6 years those young people who received the SFP10-14 intervention were less than half as likely to have ever used cannabis (Gates *et al.* 2006). Two randomized studies have also looked at the effectiveness of the SFP10-14 for preventing methamphetamine use (Spoth *et al.* 2006). Combining the results from these two studies suggests that 6 years after the intervention methamphetamine use is reduced by around two-thirds. The impact of the SFP10-14 on other illicit drugs is less clear, though effects on other mental, emotional and behavioural disorders have been highlighted (O'Connell *et al.* 2009).

The Cochrane review found five randomized studies that evaluated multicomponent community interventions, all described in Table 8.1. Four of these studies (Biglan *et al.* 2000; Schinke *et al.* 2000; Perry *et al.* 2003; Flay *et al.* 2004) looked at whether a community component provided any added value over and above school-based prevention efforts. For three studies (Schinke *et al.* 2000; Perry *et al.* 2003; Flay *et al.* 2004) no clear effects were identified over and above school-based prevention efforts. A fourth (Biglan *et al.* 2000) found a marginally significant effect on cannabis use, but the difference after 4 years was small—less than 2% between the community prevention and the school-based prevention comparison group. In a study without a school comparison (Wu *et al.* 2002), a community intervention in China was compared with no intervention. Although the author reported a large reduction in new drug users in intervention villages compared with control villages, the re-calculated result in the Cochrane review does not support this conclusion. Overall, and from a scientific viewpoint, a small group of studies yielding consistent findings of no or little effect suggests that community-based programmes are ineffective as a general class of preventive interventions.

8.2.5 **Mass media and social marketing approaches**

The World Health Organization (Hawks *et al.* 2002) undertook a thorough analysis of mass media approaches for the prevention of psychoactive substance use. This analysis brought together 13 review papers, three of which provided information relevant to developing countries. The authors concluded that the use of mass media alone, particularly in the presence of other countervailing influences such as a prodrug club culture, prodrug music, drug-using role models, and exposure to images of drug use, was not an effective way to reduce psychoactive substance use, although media campaigns in some cases were capable of raising awareness of the negative consequences of use.

Subsequent to the World Health Organization review, a large-scale study reported an evaluation of the US National Youth Anti-Drug Media Campaign (1999–2003) (Orwin *et al.* 2006). This campaign included television, radio, and other advertising media complemented by public relations efforts including community outreach and institutional partnerships. The campaign addressed young people directly as well as indirectly through their parents and other adults, who were encouraged to control youth access to drugs. In addition, the final year of the programme included a specific marijuana initiative. The evaluation showed no effects on youth drug use, either for the specific marijuana initiative or for the campaign as a whole, despite achieving significant exposure of youth to campaign messages. These findings are discouraging, given the campaign's intention to delay onset of drug use.

In contrast to mass media approaches, social marketing programmes are designed to bring about social change using concepts from commercial advertising and marketing. Its advocates argue that such techniques have the potential to increase participation in particular treatment or prevention initiatives, such as smoking cessation services (Hastings and McLean 2006). The way to do this is to make services more consumer oriented and thus more suitable to individual needs. One evaluation of a Social Marketing Intervention (SMI) reported a significant effect on lifetime cannabis use (Slater *et al.* 2006); cannabis initiation was between 10 and 72% less likely 2 years after exposure to the SMI programme, compared with control communities that did not receive the programme. Unfortunately, the results from just one US study with wide confidence intervals can only be interpreted as suggestive in the absence of replication.

8.3 Other key questions policymakers have about prevention

The prevention literature focuses on answering the question 'Does it work?' We have considered this question above and can provide a qualified answer that *some* prevention programmes do appear to work, but the effects are modest and the evidence is on the whole fairly sparse. We also concluded that there are some types of prevention programmes that clearly do not work. Going forward, we consider several other questions that policymakers may ask about prevention.

8.3.1 Are prevention programmes adopted and implemented as intended?

According to one prevention authority, 'the bridge between a promising idea and its impact on students is implementation; however, innovations are seldom implemented as planned' (Berman and McLaughlin 1976). Given the number of promising prevention programmes that have failed to show effects in rigorous replication studies, there has been concern to promote adoption of evidence based interventions with high fidelity (i.e. implementation as intended by the programme developer). A study of school districts in evidence based 11 US states (Hallfors and Godette 2002) found that despite a requirement to select research-based programmes, many school districts select other programmes, and when research-based programmes are selected they are often not implemented with fidelity. Sometimes political considerations confer certain programmes with privileged positions or dedicated funding, as has occurred with DARE. At other times a desire to make programmes culturally congruent requires customization to local circumstances. That such adaptations make the programme more welcome is often taken as sufficient evidence that they also make the programme as effective, but this is by no means guaranteed.

Yet even in the context of rigorous field trials, a programme is often not implemented in line with curriculum objectives (Dusenbury *et al.* 2003). The significance of implementation fidelity is pointed out by Brown (2001) and Gorman (2002). In a 6-year evaluation of LST (Botvin *et al.* 1990, 1995, 2001), students in groups that received less than 60% of the programme (low fidelity) not only reported more marijuana use than the high fidelity group but also reported more drug use than the control group, though such high versus low fidelity comparisons are difficult to interpret because the low fidelity group is probably in some way different, on average, compared with the control group (Foxcroft *et al.* 1997). This creates a selection bias and seriously compromises reports based on this type of subgroup analysis.

8.3.2 Will effective US prevention programmes work in other countries?

At this chapter's outset we highlighted the dominant place that the USA has in the evaluation of prevention activities. This is borne out in the Cochrane review evidence, in which studies highlighted as worthy of replication were all evaluations of US prevention programmes. This raises the question of whether prevention programmes shown to be effective in the USA would work in other countries and cultures, where language and social contexts can be very different (Allott *et al.* 1999; Cuijpers 2003; Foxcroft *et al.* 2003). The USA has relatively high rates of teenage drug use in international comparisons. So would US programmes be relevant or able to show significant effects where the rates of use are considerably lower? The answer may depend on the extent to which a prevention programme can be revised to be culture specific. One study from Phoenix, Arizona (Hecht *et al.* 2003) has shown that a multicultural version of a substance use prevention programme tested in middle schools was at least as effective as culturally targeted versions of the same prevention programme. This is an important finding because culture-specific programmes are difficult to deliver in culturally diverse settings. However, it is naïve to think that prevention programme materials developed for one setting can be adopted in their entirety without making any sort of cultural accommodation. The challenge is to adapt materials and formats without compromising theoretical and conceptual integrity and therefore potential effectiveness (Sue 1998; Tanaka-Matsumi *et al.* 2002; Draguns 2004). Also, even countries that are culturally close to the USA may have goals for school education that differ from the US consensus (Midford *et al.* 1998), which may well raise questions about the applicability of a US-derived prevention programme.

8.3.3 Are programmes targeted at high risk youth effective?

The Traditional Public Health approach (Blane 1976) involves two prevention levels, each determined by current drug use. Primary prevention targets current non-users and involves projects directed toward reducing the incidence of drug use by stopping non-users from becoming users (Staulcup *et al.* 1979). Secondary prevention involves early identification and intervention with existing drug users (Staulcup *et al.* 1979), with the goal of arresting a problem before it becomes fully developed (Blane 1976).

The traditional model of prevention, however, does not account properly for the different forms that drug prevention programmes typically take. First, programmes delivered at the population level do not necessarily distinguish between young people who have already started using drugs and those who have not. Secondly, programmes aimed at high risk groups are not straightforwardly classified as secondary prevention because the increased risk may be environmental (e.g. parenting problems) rather than someone who has already started to take drugs. Consequently, an emphasis on meeting the needs of specific groups or individuals has led to a refinement in the classification of prevention interventions into three categories: universal, selective, and indicated (Cuijpers 2003; EMCDDA 2003; Crome and McArdle 2004). Universal interventions are aimed at the general population level, not at those who are identified on the basis of individual risk factors. Interventions may address an entire school population through drug education lessons, or parents through parenting programmes, or communities through community-wide prevention efforts, all with the aim of preventing, delaying, or reducing drug use and related harms at a general population level. Selective prevention interventions target specific individuals, families, or groups who have increased risk of drug use and associated problems (e.g. children of parents with substance-related problems, or young people living in areas of high risk). Such approaches target the entire group regardless of the degree of risk of any one individual in the group. Indicated prevention programmes are designed to address the multiple and complex risk factors of families considered to be dysfunctional. Examples of problems requiring referral to such programmes include extensive drug use by the young person, exclusion from school, and contact with the criminal justice system, as well as neglect, abuse, or other issues related to poor parenting.

So far we have mainly considered universal strategies that address a whole population, with the aim of shifting the whole statistical distribution of a particular behaviour or risk factor—including its tail—in a favourable direction (Rose 1992). Such population strategies are called for whenever it is difficult to identify and intervene with those at higher risk, or whenever risk is widely diffused through the whole population (Rose 1985). We know that the risk of drug use is widely diffused through the whole population of young people for certain drugs, especially cannabis and the so-called club drugs. Evidence from the Cochrane reviews (Faggiano *et al.* 2005; Gates *et al.* 2006) reported earlier suggests that universal interventions may affect initiation of drug use. On the other hand, selective and indicated programmes may in principle be useful when those at higher risk can be targeted with specific prevention interventions, for example where neighbourhoods are characterized by drug use, where families are known to have particular vulnerabilities, or at 'rave' parties where the use of club drugs is a particular problem. However, there is only a limited amount of high quality evidence that reports on the effectiveness of selective and indicated programmes that target those at higher risk.

A number of programmes that target groups of high risk youth (e.g. in schools or neighbourhoods) as well as individuals (e.g. adolescents with conduct disorders or early onset of drug use) have been evaluated. A review of this literature (Roe and Becker 2005) comprised 16 good quality studies of effectiveness based on short-term follow-up, all from North America. Seven studies reported on the effectiveness of school-based programmes (life-skills training) among at-risk adolescents, some demonstrating positive effects and others demonstrating no effects. Results from studies of the effectiveness of counselling services for young people at risk were mixed: some studies showed favourable results, others unfavourable results, and still others no effect at all. Similar mixed results were reported with respect to multicomponent interventions involving such services as family support, after-school activities, and mentoring. In one study, less drug use was reported among programme participants than controls at 1 year follow-up, whereas another multiple-component intervention study found increased marijuana use among programme participants.

Universal programmes may be most effective for young people who have not already initiated drug use. In *post hoc* analyses in a small number of studies, prevention programme effects appear to be stronger (Hansen *et al.* 1988; Ellickson *et al.* 1993) for this group, leading some to suggest that universal programmes may have little or no impact on those who are at most risk because they have already initiated drug use (Manski *et al.* 2001). This is held up by some as an argument for more targeted prevention programmes with high risk individuals (Manski *et al.* 2001) but it is also reasonable and clearly preferable that universal interventions should be delivered earlier, before the onset of drug use in those higher risk individuals.

8.4 Are small prevention effects worth the effort?

There is fairly persuasive evidence that some prevention programmes can delay drug use initiation. Historically, age of initiation is correlated with many other outcomes of interest. However, because the most serious consequences of drug use occur many years after prevention programmes are typically delivered, scientists will probably never be able to measure with certainty the extent to which, for example, less cannabis use in the teenage years translates into reduced cocaine abuse, HIV infection, and overdose deaths years and decades later.

This will not disturb those policymakers who see preventing youthful cannabis use as a good in itself. However, there are other policymakers who wish to prevent cannabis use primarily because they hope it signals a correlated effect on later illicit drug use and consequences. What more can one tease out of the scientific literature to inform policymakers that adopt this perspective? On the optimistic side, one does not need to accept a 'gateway' assumption (i.e. that use of one substance leads inevitably to another) in order to believe that delayed cannabis use signals reductions in subsequent use of other substances. All one has to believe is that both youthful cannabis use and later use of other substances are driven by common unobserved traits (e.g. social skills or norms about drugs more generally) that are affected by the prevention programme.

On the pessimistic side, we do not know whether programmes, when effective, mainly affect initiation by those who would have become infrequent drug users or whether they also affect initiation among those who would otherwise have become frequent and potentially more problematic drug users. Some studies (e.g. Ellickson *et al.* 2003) suggest that although social skills interventions may delay initiation of cannabis use, they do not affect current or regular cannabis use. On the other hand, the results discussed earlier show better results for other illicit drugs, although replication studies are needed.

A report from the RAND Drug Policy Research Center in the USA (Caulkins *et al.* 2002) attempted to answer the question: 'Are prevention effects large enough to be worth the effort?' Analysing the costs and effectiveness of several established drug and alcohol prevention programmes, the report concluded that the investment may be worthwhile even when a universal prevention programme has a relatively small impact on lifetime prevalence, provided the causal effect on subsequent lifetime use approaches the level suggested by historical correlations between age of initiation and lifetime use.

The authors' mathematical model combined 10 factors to provide an assessment of the benefits of school-based drug prevention programmes in terms of health care costs and wider societal costs (e.g. loss of productivity) that were avoided due to cases prevented. This assessment was then set alongside the cost of providing the prevention programme, and a straightforward comparison was made. The report's conclusion—that the health and social benefits per participant stemming from reduced drug use

(US$840 from tobacco, alcohol, cocaine, and cannabis) substantially exceed the economic costs of running the programmes (~US$150 per participant)—was robust in the face of a fairly wide-ranging sensitivity analysis. Thus, even if the prevention programme merely delays rather than prevents initiation, the benefits could still outweigh the costs over the longer term if effects on long-term use are similar to those historically observed between early and later initiators.

The mathematical model provides these projections for lifetime use of tobacco, alcohol, cocaine, and cannabis. The projections suggest that the major benefit derives from reductions in the use of tobacco and alcohol, accounting for approximately two-thirds of the effect. Thus the cost and benefit are much more evenly matched if only prevention of illicit drug use is considered: even if heroin and methamphetamines are added to the model, the conclusion remains that prevention programmes may avert more social costs associated with licit rather than illicit substance use.

Overall, this model suggests that effective drug prevention programs are worthwhile (at least in the USA, as US data form the basis for the model). However, the model does not tell us which drug prevention programme provides the best value in particular settings. One prevention programme may be four times as effective as another, but at three times the cost. Policymakers should consider alternative prevention programmes, and the opportunity costs of implementing one over another, to determine which programme provides the best value for a particular situation.

8.5 **Conclusion**

The Appendix following Chapter 16 summarizes the main findings of this chapter regarding different kinds of prevention programmes. The interventions that have the largest effect share two characteristics: they focus on early intervention with the proximal social environment, either the classroom or the family, and they address issues other than drug use by focusing on social and behavioural development. Equally worthy of comment are the number of nil ratings in the table, including the ratings of some widely used programmes. None of the programmes has a particularly high cost per recipient. This may make tolerable to policymakers the modest ratings of effectiveness.

The key conclusion drawn by this chapter is that evidence-based school- or family-oriented prevention programmes are on average a relatively low cost activity that can yield modest, but potentially important, benefits. This general conclusion concerning modest effects is qualified by the observation that some prevention programmes have no evidence of benefit, whereas others have evidence of some effectiveness. The conclusions we draw about what makes programmes more effective are that prevention programmes that provide an early intervention within the proximal social environment, either the classroom or the family, and that focus on positive social and behavioural development, are potentially important for delaying use and limiting harm. On the other hand, programmes that only provide drug-relevant information or try to boost self-esteem are not likely to be effective.

An interesting question is why we persist with information-based or other ineffective prevention programmes. Part of the answer may be that the most important audience for these programmes is not the young people who are their putative beneficiaries, but concerned adults, especially parents of adolescents, who wish to see something being done that they think is likely to be effective. Hence we end up with programmes that send the messages that parents think most appropriate for their children, rather than programmes that may be of use to young people.

Societies tend to make a small investment in prevention and, on average, they reap a small return. Poor choice of programmes can result in no benefit; even the wisest choices will not generate an enormous one. The science base lacks definitive information on a number of areas of prevention, but the information provided in this chapter ought to help policymakers use prevention resources more effectively than they could without reference to the evidence base.

Chapter 9

Health and social services for drug users

9.1 Introduction

This chapter describes services designed to change the behaviour of drug users, with the aim of benefiting them and those people around them. The goals of such services are diverse, and may include initiating or maintaining abstinence from drugs, reducing the amount or frequency of drug use, or changing behaviours other than drug use (e.g. criminal activity, needle sharing). This chapter focuses on the outcomes of various types of health and social services. In a subsequent chapter on service systems (Chapter 15) we consider how the interventions discussed here are organized within communities and nation states and their more general impact at the population level.

Some drug policy analysts attempt to divide drug-related health and social services into two non-overlapping categories, namely those that focus on eliminating drug use *per se* and those that focus on reducing the amount of suffering drug use causes to the user and society. We intentionally do not adopt this distinction for two reasons. First, all drug-related health and social services intend to reduce the damage of drug use. Professionals who strive to reduce clients' drug use are as committed to reducing human suffering as are those who strive to change clients' drug-related behaviour, and it would be incorrect to imply that only the latter group is concerned about the harms of drug use. Secondly, the daily reality of the interventions discussed in this chapter is often a blend of these two allegedly distinct approaches (Hall 2007). For example, significant numbers of individuals who access needle exchange programmes (which target infection risk rather than drug use *per se*) are referred by programme staff to services designed to reduce drug use (US General Accounting Office 1993). In like fashion, someone who permanently ceases heroin use after joining Narcotics Anonymous certainly reduces the amount of drug-related consequences they and others around them will experience.

Accordingly, the evidence reviewed in this chapter covers health and social services that attempt to reduce drug-related harm through reducing drug use *per se* and/or through changing drug-related behaviours that are independent of the amount of consumption (e.g. safer injection-related behaviours). We limit our scope to programmes that are intended to help, rehabilitate, or assist drug users rather than solely coerce or punish them. Although the types of services vary widely within and across societies, all drug-related interventions explicitly or implicitly assume that rehabilitative services can produce individual-level changes (e.g. in coping responses, relapse prevention skills, attitudes, and moral values) that will translate into lower rates of drug use, drug-related infections, overdose deaths, unemployment, and criminal activity. We restrict our review mainly to those services on which a significant number of scientific studies have been done, which will limit our discussion of recently developed programmes that have not been extensively evaluated, such as the distribution of drinking water at 'raves' and modafinil treatment for methamphetamine dependence.

9.2 Types of interventions and their effects

This section discusses the strength of evidence to support the assertion that different services change drug users' behaviour. Our review covers direct benefits to users as well as beneficial effects that radiate beyond them (e.g. reductions in crime and in infectious disease transmission) and are therefore of significant policy interest to a wide range of stakeholders.

Systematic knowledge about the 'natural history' of drug use and dependence is lacking for many drugs, but it is safe to say that changes in level of use independent of intervention are not uncommon. One sort of change is widely recognized: the volume, frequency, and health risks of drug use usually intensify significantly during the development of drug dependence. The opposite change, in which individuals dramatically reduce or entirely stop drug use or a drug-related behaviour in the absence of receiving services, has received far less attention from addiction specialists. The existence of such individuals poses a problem for many outcome studies because, in the absence of non-intervention comparison groups, the interventions evaluated may receive credit not only for genuine successes but also for an unknown number of **natural recoveries**. We will return to this point as we discuss different programme evaluations.

9.2.1 Interventions focused primarily on users of heroin and other opioids

Opioid substitution therapy (OST)

These services are typically provided on an outpatient basis, often in the context of stand-alone clinics, and offer both psychosocial services and a substitute agonist medication. OST clinics primarily target heroin users, but they also may serve individuals dependent on morphine, opium, and prescribed analgesics. Daily, orally administered methadone is far and away the most widely disseminated of the multiple forms of OST. There is a diverse array of other opioid agents and routes of administration that are available as OST around the world, including sublingual buprenorphine, and slow-release oral morphine tablets, injectable methadone, inhalable heroin, to name just a few.

OST has stronger evidence of effectiveness than any other intervention for drug use (Uchtenhagen *et al.* 2004; see also Box 9.1). One major review (Amato *et al.* 2005) concluded that heroin users enrolled in OST programmes are more than twice as likely to cease heroin use as untreated users. Individual studies described in Table 9.1 indicate that this benefit is not due to a placebo effect; higher doses of methadone are, on average, more effective than lower doses. In addition, it has been found that

Table 9.1 Selected studies of opiate substitution therapy

Topic and study	Participants per group	Intervention	Outcome
Maintenance versus detox (Newman and Whitehill 1979)	$n = 50$ patients with heroin dependence	Methadone maintenance (100 mg) versus methadone dose reduction (decreased by 1 mg/day from 60 mg start)	After 32 weeks, 72% of maintenance patients were still receiving services versus only 10% of the dose-reducing group. Only the maintenance group showed reductions in heroin use.
Maintenance versus detox (Sees *et al.* 2000)	$n = 88$–91 patients with opioid dependence	Ongoing psychosocial services with methadone as a maintenance versus detoxification treatment	Methadone maintenance patients were retained longer (438 days versus 174 days) and showed double the opioid abstinence rate (42% versus 20%) relative to medically managed withdrawal patients ($P < 0.01$).
Dose (Ling *et al.* 1976)	$n = 142$–146 VA patients with opioid dependence	LAAM (80 mg) versus low (50 mg) versus high (100 mg) dose methadone	High dose methadone patients had the best rate of retention. Both LAAM and high dose methadone groups had better global drug use outcomes than the low dose methadone group ($P < 0.005$).
Dose (Strain *et al.* 1999)	$n = 95$–97 patients with opioid dependence	Moderate (4–50 mg) versus high (80–100 mg) dose methadone	Both groups decreased illicit opioid use; high dose had significantly greater reductions in opioid use ($p = 0.01$).
Psychosocial services (Woody *et al.* 1995)	$n = 6231$ patients receiving methadone for opiate dependence	Drug counselling versus drug counselling + psychotherapy with comparable contact hours	Opiate use comparable at 6 months, but cocaine-positive urines less frequent in therapy condition (22% of weeks versus 36%, $P < 0.02$).
Psychosocial services (McLellan *et al.* 1993)	$n = 32$–35 patients with opiate dependence	Methadone prescription only vs. with standard psychosocial services vs. with enhanced psychosocial services	All interventions decreased illicit drug use. Increases in services led to a greater percentage of patients showing heroin abstinence ($P < 0.01$). The enhanced service group had better employment, alcohol use, and legal outcomes ($P < 0.05$).
Cost-effectiveness (Barnett 1999)	N/A	Methadone maintenance treatment versus standard care	Methadone maintenance has an incremental cost-effectiveness ratio of <US$6000/quality-adjusted life year. This is substantially more cost-effective than the usual standard of US$50 000/quality adjusted life year for health care interventions.

Source: this chart is an expansion of one that originally appeared in QUERI Substance Abuse Module Executive Committee (2001).

interventions of indefinite length produce outcomes superior to standardized, demarcated lengths (even a 6-month limit is too short). Supplementing the medication with extensive psychosocial services enhances outcome, and OST is quite cost-effective relative to other health care interventions.

In addition to reducing heroin use, OST increases the odds of gaining employment, reduces criminal behaviour by as much as 60% (Amato *et al.* 2005), and lowers the risk of transmitting infectious diseases. Consistent with these findings, risk of death, particularly from drug overdose, for patients on methadone is less than 25% of that for untreated heroin users (Amato *et al.* 2005; Barnett 1999; Gunne and Grönbladh 1981). Many of these benefits radiate beyond the patient: less crime by drug users produces fewer crime victims, less unemployment decreases demand on public assistance, and less infectious disease among drug users lowers disease risk for the rest of the population. Methadone maintenance also reduces use of illicit drugs other than opiates. This may be because receiving an opiate from a clinic rather than through a street dealer helps move the users away from social networks in which use of a range of drugs is common.

Buprenorphine is a newer OST medication, which can be formulated with **naloxone** to reduce misuse and overdose potential. In some countries (e.g. France, Sweden) buprenorphine is more widely prescribed than methadone. Studies of high dose buprenorphine show impressive reductions in heroin and cocaine use (for example, see Johnson *et al.* 2000; Kakko *et al.* 2003). Comparisons of research on methadone and buprenorphine have varied somewhat in their conclusions over the years, but the latest review (Connock *et al.* 2007) concludes that methadone is slightly more effective and less costly than buprenorphine.

In addition to being orally administered, as in the above studies, OST has sometimes been provided in injected form. Beginning in the early 20th century some British physicians prescribed injectable opiates in a way that would today be called OST. Prescribing morphine or heroin was a legal, well-accepted medical practice for doctors, and consequently came to be known as the 'British system', in which patients were allowed to

Box 9.1 Maintenance as an alternative to detoxification

A randomized, placebo-controlled trial study by Kakko *et al.* (2003) is particularly noteworthy because it found significant effects despite weak statistical power (it enrolled only 40 subjects). Individuals on buprenorphine had a 1-year retention rate of 75%, versus 0% for those on placebo, and those retained in treatment provided about 75% negative urines for all illicit drugs (i.e. not just heroin) as well as showing a 90% drop on a measure of criminal behaviour and legal problems. Underscoring the dangerousness of untreated heroin addiction, the controls had a 1-year mortality rate of 20%, versus 0% in the buprenorphine group. Parallel findings were identified with methadone maintenance versus placebo in another clinical trial over 20 years previously (Gunne and Grönbladh 1981), indicating that regardless of the form of OST employed, maintenance produces dramatically better outcomes than brief detoxification regimens.

inject their prescribed morphine or heroin in the context of ongoing medical care (whether for pain relief, terminal illness care, or for treatment of drug dependence). Without systematic evaluation studies, it is not possible to say whether this approach was more or less effective than alternative forms of heroin-based OST (See Box 9.2).

In the early 1990s, clinicians and policymakers in Switzerland decided to introduce heroin maintenance services. The Swiss approach differed from the British model by opening the clinics 7 days per week, 365 days per year, with all injected medication taken under supervision, on site. This was financially costly, but it virtually eliminated the diversion to the black market sometimes found in the British system. The Swiss system also eliminated the challenge for the physician in deciding on the dose of heroin. Instead, patients were provided with whatever dose of heroin they jointly chose to use.

Following the observational studies in Switzerland, several randomized controlled trials investigating the efficacy of medical heroin prescription were conducted in Europe and Canada (Fischer *et al.* 2007; Lintzeris 2009). Box 9.3 provides a summary of these programmes. Participants in these medical heroin prescription trials were chronic and highly problematic heroin users who had not derived lasting therapeutic benefits from other health and social services (including methadone maintenance). That is, the studies examined the effects of heroin prescription as a last resort. Each of the studies illustrated were multisite and offered medical heroin as an on-site intervention only. The studies compared the benefits of heroin prescription with those of the control intervention, high quality methadone maintenance, usually over a study period of 12 months.

Box 9.2 The British system for heroin substitution therapy

For much of the 20th century, the UK was the only country in which physicians were allowed to prescribe injectable opiates in the context of addiction treatment. The most common formulations were injectable morphine up until the 1960s, injectable diamorphine (heroin) in the 1960s and early 1970s, and injectable methadone from the mid-1970s onwards. However, it was not until the 1960s that any significant problem of heroin addiction among young and disadvantaged people was seen outside North America. Hence, by the time the 'British system' of injectable opiate maintenance treatment was put to the test, impressive results with oral methadone maintenance treatment were beginning to be reported. An influential randomized controlled trial in the mid-1970s (Hartnoll *et al.* 1980) reported a mixture of advantages and disadvantages to injectable heroin maintenance versus oral methadone maintenance: oral methadone maintenance was associated with a polarization of outcomes of the patient population, with a greater proportion having reduced or quit their drug use, but also with a greater proportion deteriorating further. Thereafter, oral methadone has been the most commonly prescribed form of OST across the UK, with the proportion of maintenance prescriptions as injectable maintenance having dwindled to about 10% by the mid-1990s (Strang *et al.* 1996) and down to about 2% by 2005 (Strang *et al.* 2007). Heroin prescribing continued to be rare, accounting for less than 1% of prescriptions.

Box 9.3 Randomized studies of heroin maintenance in The Netherlands, Germany, and Canada

Since the late 1990s, clinical trials of heroin maintenance have been conducted with heroin-dependent individuals who derived no lasting benefit from methadone maintenance and other widely available forms of OST. The Dutch study (van den Brink *et al.* 2003) included the two experimental interventions of inhalable and injectable medical heroin provision. Effectiveness was measured by a combination of health status, illicit drug use, and crime. Co-prescribed heroin (with methadone) was significantly more effective than methadone maintenance alone in both the inhalable heroin trial (response rate: 49.7% versus 26.9%) and the injectable heroin trial (55.5% versus 31.2%). Importantly, the discontinuation of the co-prescribed heroin resulted in a rapid deterioration in 82% (94/115) of those who responded to the co-prescribed heroin (van den Brink *et al.* 2003). In the German study, retention was higher in the patient group receiving heroin (67.2%) than in the methadone group (40.0%). Furthermore, the heroin group showed a reduction in illicit drug use and significantly more improvement on a measure of physical/mental health status (Haasen *et al.* 2007). Similarly, the Canadian ('NAOMI') study (NAOMI Study Team 2008) demonstrated that participants randomized to heroin prescription had higher retention (87.8% versus 54.1%) than those given methadone maintenance. They also had better outcomes (relative to the control group) on a combined measure of reduced illicit drug use and criminal behaviour (67.0% versus 47.7%).

A 2005 **Cochrane review** stated that no definitive conclusions could be drawn about the overall effectiveness of heroin-based OST, but also noted that the studies seeming to support the value of this intervention have come from countries where methadone maintenance is widely available (Ferri *et al.* 2005). Presumably, this is because heroin-based OST has been used in these countries primarily to help hard-core heroin users who have not responded to orally administered methadone maintenance. As mentioned, the role of heroin maintenance in the health service system of these countries is to provide another option when first-line OST has not been effective.

Opiate antagonist therapies

An opiate antagonist reduces the effect, and hence the reinforcing power, of opiates in the brain. Oral naltrexone is the most widely used opiate antagonist. Although a few studies have shown that oral naltrexone reduces heroin use and incarceration rates, a Cochrane review (Minozzi *et al.* 2006) noted that, as a whole, oral naltrexone studies are of poor methodological quality and do not support any strong conclusions about the medication's practical effectiveness. Medications are effective only if drug users comply with the prescription regime, and only 10–15% of heroin-dependent people want to take a medication that eliminates the possibility of getting high. A long-acting depot formulation has recently been developed, and may produce higher rates of compliance than does the daily oral dose form.

9.2.2 Interventions targeting the health risks of drug use

OST affects many areas of health and well-being in addition to heroin use, for example, by reducing risk of overdose and HIV infection. A different class of intervention targets these risks directly, without making the assumption that cessation of drug use needs to be a main therapeutic goal. The health and social services described in this section are primarily accessed by heroin users, but most of them can also be offered to individuals who inject other drugs, such as cocaine.

Needle and syringe exchange schemes

The advent of HIV epidemics has led some policymakers and health workers to focus on the modification of drug users' injecting behaviour. Of the estimated 42 million people currently living with HIV/AIDS (with about 5 million becoming newly infected each year), it is estimated that injecting drug use probably accounts directly for 10% of all infections (UNAIDS 2006; WHO 2006). Because this is largely a result of sharing needles and syringes, any intervention that reduces injecting drug use or leads to less hazardous injecting techniques has the potential to reduce the spread of HIV/AIDS. Syringe exchange programmes are also intended to reduce transmission of HCV, which in approximately half of cases ultimately leads to chronic liver disease, including cirrhosis and hepatocellular carcinoma (primary liver cancer). However, there is no firm evidence that syringe exchange programmes significantly reduce hepatitis C prevalence, based on the continued high prevalence of hepatitis C among IDUs in many countries (50–90%), the reality that most needles returned to needle exchange are shared by multiple drug users (Shrestha *et al.* 2006), and the relatively easy transmissibility of HCV (Pollack 2001). The summary of evidence to follow should therefore be assumed to apply to HIV/AIDS only.

Since the 1980s, needle and syringe exchange schemes have become common in Australia and in most European countries, but elsewhere they have been introduced only recently, minimally, or not at all. There are a large number of descriptive reports and a smaller number of more carefully designed prospective studies of needle and syringe exchange programmes that focus on risk of infection and transmission of HIV. Some researchers have used statistical procedures to model the circulation time of needles and syringes, arguing that needle exchange programmes reduce the likelihood of using infected needles and syringes (Kaplan and Heimer 1994). The lack of any randomized study of needle exchange is a notable weakness of the science in this area.

The most widely cited evidence for needle exchange is a review of 214 uncontrolled studies conducted in 81 cities with over 300 000 drug users (Hurley *et al.* 1997). The seroprevalence of HIV in the user population increased by 5.9% annually in cities without needle exchange programmes, and decreased by 5.8% in cities with such programmes. However, Amundsen (2006) notes that the incidence of HIV infection peaked in many cities during the time of Hurley's analysis, and the establishment of needle exchange programmes was more common late rather than early in the epidemic. For example, HIV seroprevalence had dropped for two full years before needle exchange programmes were established in Glasgow, Scotland (Hurley *et al.* 1997). Amundsen argues that HIV testing became available around the same time, and may also have contributed to the changes attributed solely to needle exchange programmes. Admunsen's questioning of the evidence supporting needle exchange drew a passionate response (Wodak 2007). The other contentious issue concerning needle exchange is whether such programmes 'send the wrong message' and encourage people to become IDUs. Though there is no scientific study proving this claim, it is nonetheless made repeatedly in the policy world. Emotional debates surrounding needle exchange programmes are likely to continue given that such programmes are politically controversial and have never been subjected to a rigorous, randomized clinical trial.

Taking needles off prescription

Another approach to expanding syringe access is to repeal regulations requiring a prescription in order to buy needles from pharmacies. Groseclose and colleagues (1995) found that when the state of Connecticut (part of the USA) implemented this policy, the proportion of IDUs who reported purchasing syringes from pharmacies increased fourfold, and the proportion reporting street purchases of syringes declined by more than 50%. The Connecticut policy was implemented simultaneously with the repeal of a law against possession of needles, which probably aided its impact.

More recent evaluations (e.g. Bluthenthal *et al.* 2004) have not replicated these early findings. This may reflect the reality that needles are much more widely available today in most developed countries. For example, 46 out of 50 US states offer needles without prescription, and needle exchange programmes operate in many cities. Even where needles remain illegal to possess, it is possible that police officers confiscate needles less often than they did prior to the AIDS epidemic, in which case legalization of syringe possession may not show an effect because what has become *de jure* already existed *de facto*.

Increasing the availability of naloxone for heroin overdoses

An opiate antagonist that blocks the ability of heroin to occupy receptor sites, naloxone reduces the acute effects of heroin overdose, most notably the depressed respiration that can lead to brain damage and death. Two strategies have been proposed to expand access to this potentially life-saving medication.

The first approach is for all ambulances to carry naloxone. This is done in some countries, allowing ambulance personnel to administer naloxone when responding to an overdose emergency. However, many drug users (as well as friends and family who might discover their loved one in overdose) will not place such a call for fear of arrest of the drug user. Baca and Grant (2005) argue that to maximize the benefits of naloxone in ambulances, health care and law enforcement professionals should make an agreement—announced the to the drug user community—that emergency calls during overdose will not lead to arrest.

The second, non-competing approach is to distribute naloxone to drug users in the community, along with information on how to use it (Darke and Hall 1997). Because overdose-related deaths sometimes occur when a user is alone, or in the presence of people who are severely intoxicated themselves, there are natural limits on how many lethal overdoses could be prevented in this fashion. But programmes in Spain, Germany, Italy, the UK, and the USA have documented cases of successful resuscitation through distributed naloxone.

No definitive research exists on the effects of these two strategies, either alone or in combination. But what evidence is available is encouraging (Baca and Grant 2005).

Supervised drug consumption rooms

Supervised drug consumption rooms are a recent development in services for drug users. In these sites, drug users can take drugs in a clean, supervised environment that includes staff who can assist in the event of an overdose. They may also be considered beneficial by some members of the public who are upset at the sight of drug users injecting in stairwells, parks, and other public places.

Supervised drug consumption services exist in at least 12 countries on three continents (Kimber *et al.* 2003). Some policymakers have argued that these programmes fail to prevent drug-related problems, and may even encourage injection drug use. At present no research is available that speaks definitively to this charge one way or the other. Observational research with no control groups has reported that such services tend to be accessed by high risk drug users, some of whom go on to seek further services, including programmes designed to reduce drug use (Wood *et al.* 2006).

9.3 **Psychosocial interventions provided for a range of drug problems**

In contrast to the interventions reviewed in Section 9.2, which are primarily designed for heroin users, a variety of psychosocial interventions exist for users of a wide range of substances, including heroin, cocaine, methamphetamine, marijuana, hallucinogens, benzodiazepines, and club drugs. The lack of specificity of these interventions stems largely from the lack of effective, tailored medications to treat drug dependence other than for opiates, despite a substantial investment in medication research. The interventions we discuss here are thus entirely psychosocial in nature, and attempt to address a broad band of drug use and related problems by changing behaviour, cognitions, and social factors. The general therapeutic philosophies underlying these interventions are described in Box 9.4.

Purely psychosocial services are harder to specify than are medication-based interventions. Doses and blood concentrations of medication are easier to measure than are 'productive' counselling sessions and 'strong' therapeutic alliances. Further, real-world programmes typically blend elements of multiple approaches. The developers of the Matrix Model of therapy for stimulant abuse, for example, drew on elements from cognitive-behavioural, 12-step, and family/social network approaches (Rawson *et al.* 2004) which may help explain why major meta-analyses of the literature have failed to find that any one particular psychosocial treatment approach is superior to the others (Prendergast *et al.* 2002). For these reasons the research on psychosocial interventions permits less scientific precision than research on medication-based therapies, but the evidence is no less valuable for the planning of health and social services.

9.3.1 **Comparing services with no services**

Randomized trials comparing one or more intervention with an untreated control group are difficult to conduct for ethical as well as practical reasons, but in some cases a wait-list control group is acceptable. In such research some participants receive the intervention immediately whereas others are asked to wait several months, thereby permitting a short-term comparison of the outcomes of those who received the intervention with

Box 9.4 Philosophies of drug treatment and some representative treatment approaches

Brain disease. Addiction is a medical disorder resulting from prolonged exposure of the brain to psychoactive substances. Changes in the brain may be severe enough to require the indefinite administration of medications in addition to psychosocial services. As a disease, the problem of addiction is not the fault of the drug addict and cannot be resolved by willpower.

Psychodynamic. Though lacking an empirical base, the concept that addiction is merely a symptom of an underlying problem continues to be an influential philosophy of drug treatment. This framework usually does not focus on the drug use itself and pays attention instead to the underlying psychodynamic conflicts and emotional issues that are hypothesized to cause the person to use drugs. As drug users gain insight into their 'issues', drug use is presumed to cease.

Moral/religious. Drug use results from moral inadequacy and alienation from God. Involvement in altruistic activity (of a religious or non-religious nature) as well as engagement in religious activities is believed to result in removal of the addiction by spiritual grace or enlightenment. In some cultures, religious punishment, such as flogging by a holy man, is part of the cure.

Twelve-step. Many treatment professionals have adopted the 12-step philosophy originally developed by members of self-help groups who had alcohol and drug problems. Twelve-step philosophy holds that addiction is an emotional, physical, and spiritual problem that can be arrested but never cured. Spiritual re-awakening and affiliation with mutual help groups such as Narcotics Anonymous (NA) are core features of this approach. Lifetime abstinence is the goal of treatment. The famous Hazelden treatment centre in the USA combined 12-step ideas with psychological theories into what became known as the 'Minnesota Model', which has been disseminated internationally (Mäkelä *et al.* 1996). 'Twelve-step treatment' is often used to describe such eclectic and professionalized approaches, and should be distinguished from '12-step groups' such as NA.

Cognitive-behavioural. Drug use is a learned behaviour, and can therefore be unlearned through the acquisition of alternative behavioural and cognitive skills. This approach also promotes environmental changes such as tangible incentives for non-use (as in contingency management programmes) and changes in the immediate social environment (as in family–couples–social network therapies).

Therapeutic community. Drug use is a part of a disordered, antisocial lifestyle comprising deviant behaviours and attitudes. A highly structured environment is required to re-socialize the drug addict into a mature, responsible person.

Brief intervention. The term brief intervention refers to any time-limited effort (e.g. one to two conversations or meetings) to provide information or advice, increase motivation to avoid substance use, or to teach behaviour change skills

Box 9.4 Philosophies of drug treatment and some representative treatment approaches *(continued)*

that will reduce substance use as well as the chances of negative consequences. Brief interventions are typically delivered to those individuals at low to moderate risk. Among the most cost-effective and time-efficient interventions are brief motivational conversations between a health care professional and a substance user. These motivational interventions are designed to increase commitment to the change process, and to enhance confidence that change is achievable.

those who did not. Trials by Stephens *et al.* (2000) and Copeland *et al.* (2001) show that counselling interventions reduce marijuana use more than does no intervention. These studies also show that no single psychosocial intervention seems clearly superior to another, and that reduced marijuana use is a more common outcome than total abstinence. The largest trial of cannabis dependence treatment (Marijuana Treatment Project Research Group 2004) compared groups receiving either two sessions of counselling, nine sessions of counselling, or no counselling (wait-list control group). As illustrated in Figure 9.1, the reduction in days of use was largest in the nine-session counselling group (59%), followed by the two-session group (36%). The wait-list control group changed the least (16%). Although there was no evidence that counselling improved psychological functioning, medical problems, or alcohol use, it did seem to reduce marijuana-related problems.

Prison-based studies offer another source of controlled research (Simpson *et al.* 1999). The typical design of such studies starts with a group of prisoners who volunteer

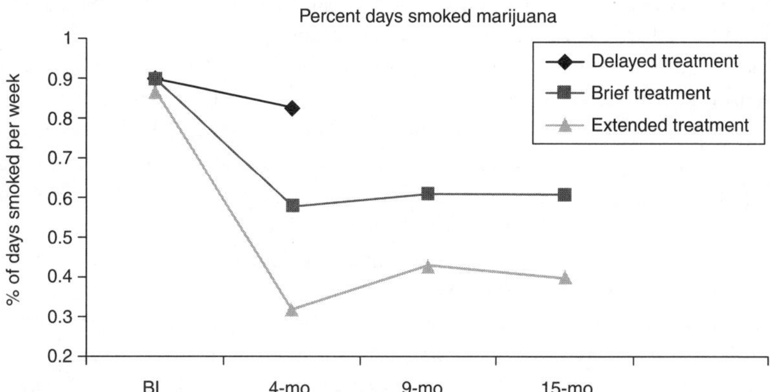

Fig. 9.1 Percentage of days marijuana was smoked before and after 207 chronic marijuana users were randomly assigned to either a wait-list control group (delayed treatment), two sessions of motivational counselling (brief treatment), or nine sessions of psychosocial counselling (extended treatment).
Source: adapted from Marijuana Treatment Project Research Group (2004).

to participate in a therapeutic community. Although the members of this group cannot always be assigned completely at random, it is possible for participation in the therapeutic community to be allotted by external administrative factors, such as availability of space at the time of the prisoner's release. Because the prisoner does not fully control whether he or she ends up in a therapeutic community, more confidence can be placed in the idea that any outcome differences are due to the intervention rather than the prisoners. These studies thus have credible, if imperfect, no-intervention comparison groups, and allow causal inferences to be drawn.

The results show that therapeutic communities significantly increase average time to re-incarceration (e.g. 289 versus 189 days for non-participants, according to Wexler *et al.* 1999), and to drug use relapse (e.g. 28.8 months versus 13.2 months for non-participants, according to Butzin *et al.* 2005). Services received in the period immediately following release from prison seem particularly important. Individuals who receive some therapeutic community treatment in prison but no aftercare do not show better long-term outcomes than individuals receiving no services at all.

A third area of clinical effectiveness research is the study of brief interventions. These studies focus on drug users who are typically not seriously dependent on psychoactive substances, and who are identified through screening in general medical settings and emergency departments. Brief intervention refers to any time-limited effort (e.g. 1–2 conversations or meetings) to provide information or advice, to increase motivation to avoid substance use, or to teach behaviour change skills that will reduce substance use as well as the risk of negative consequences. Bernstein *et al.* (2005) screened over 20 000 patients in a group of hospital clinics and found that 1175 were using drugs and willing to participate in a trial of brief intervention. Those who received a motivational interviewing session and a follow-up telephone call 10 days later had somewhat lower cocaine and heroin use 6 months later than did individuals who only received a pamphlet of information of available services for drug problems. From a policy perspective, it should be noted that the number of screens required to produce this effect was substantial, and no doubt costly.

Baker *et al.* (2005) found that both the provision of a self-help booklet and a single session of motivational interviewing were associated with reduced amphetamine consumption among regular users. Two studies (Bashir *et al.* 1994; Cormack *et al.* 1994) found that general practitioners can reduce excessive benzodiazepine use in their patients using brief interventions such as letters or consultations. The largest brief intervention study of drug users (Humeniuk *et al.* 2008) was conducted by the **World Health Organization** (WHO) in primary health care settings in four countries (Australia, Brazil, India, and the USA). Drug users scoring within the moderate risk range on a WHO screening test for cannabis, cocaine, amphetamine-type stimulants, or opioids were assigned to either a wait-list control group or an intervention condition where they received brief motivational counselling for the drug receiving the highest risk score. Compared with control participants, those receiving the brief intervention reported significantly reduced drug involvement 3 months later. In contrast to these promising results, several investigators have reported negative findings from brief interventions with drug users (Baker *et al.* 2002; Marsden *et al.* 2005). An important question that requires further research is the extent to which brief interventions can be made more effective when combined with strategies that increase the intensity of the intervention for patients who do not respond initially.

9.3.2 Studies without a comparison group

As noted in Chapter 7, randomized controlled trials that compare a no intervention group with one receiving an intervention are the preferred standard in clinical science, but they are often ethically and practically unfeasible. Alternative research designs include **quasi-experiments**, **observational studies**, and randomized trials that compare two active treatments. There are caveats to bear in mind when assessing such studies.

Studies that do not include untreated controls may credit interventions with improvements that would have occurred without intervention, through either **regression to the mean** or **natural recovery**. As the observed level of improvement in a study increases, one becomes progressively more confident that the intervention is responsible for at least some of the change, but experts do not agree on the location of that point for different outcomes. For example, would a 30% reduction in heroin use exceed the natural recovery rate, or is a 60% reduction more defensible?

9.3.3 Meta-analysis of particular approaches

A meta-analysis draws conclusions based on statistical anlaysis of pooled data obtained from a wide range of studies. One such analysis of a range of drug treatments (Prendergast *et al.* 2002) found them comparable in their positive effects on drug use and related problems. Individuals receiving treatment were 36% more likely to have a good drug use outcome than were individuals not receiving the treatment. The effects for positive outcomes on criminal behaviour were about half this size, but still statistically significant. Note that for methodological reasons, only eight of the 78 studies examined in this meta-analysis were OST, so the conclusions above apply to psychosocial interventions.

Two recent meta-analyses examined **contingency management** approaches, one form of behavioural treatment for drug dependence. One meta-analysis (Lussier *et al.* 2006) found that providing gift vouchers for abstinence was about as effective as the services examined in Prendergast and colleagues' 2002 review. Larger value vouchers have a greater influence on patients than those that were small (e.g. less than US$5), although even these smaller value vouchers have a positive influence. Another meta-analysis of contingency management approaches, including but not limited to vouchers, found slightly higher average benefits (Prendergast *et al.* 2006). The authors noted, however, that soon after the contingency management ends, benefits drop significantly. The apparently larger effect may therefore simply be due to most contingency management studies lacking long-term follow-ups.

Stanton and Shadish (1997) conducted a major meta-analysis of interventions targeting the drug user's social network members, such as spouses and parents. Such programmes are designed to change interactional patterns such that they reinforce reductions of drug use and related problems, and support efforts to improve social and coping skills. Programmes designed to change interactional patterns within social networks have better outcomes on a range of measures than do services for the drug user or family interventions that only provide education. The size of the identified benefit was comparable with those identified in the meta-analysis of contingency management approaches described above.

9.3.4 National observational studies of diverse treatment options

Several countries have conducted large observational studies to assess the effectiveness of services for large samples of drug users. These studies are not randomized and do not have no-intervention control groups. Rather, patients are assessed as they arrive seeking help, and are assessed again at subsequent time points. A subset of such studies includes the Australian Treatment Outcome Study, the US Drug Abuse Treatment Outcome Study, and the UK National Treatment Outcome Research Study. These studies typically find that drug patients receiving currently available services show substantial decreases over time in drug use, crime, and related problems (Gossop *et al.* 1998; Etheridge *et al.* 1999; Ross *et al.* 2004). No psychosocial intervention seems to be better than others across all drugs and outcomes. Twelve-step treatments in the USA seem to produce slightly better rates of complete abstinence, an effect that may be in part attributable to the self-help groups that many patients attend for extended periods, as described below.

9.4 Peer-led self-help organizations

Peer-led mutual help organizations are voluntary associations of former heavy drug users who now attempt to help each other to cease drug use and improve their coping skills, prosocial behaviour, and family life. They are typically operated by volunteers, charge no fees to participants, and allow indefinite involvement. Most are self-supporting, though some organizations do accept government and foundation grants (Humphreys 2004). We discuss three examples below.

9.4.1 Pui Hong Self-Help Association

This organization, which has perhaps 3000 members, grew out of the patient alumni club of opiate addiction treatment programmes in Hong Kong. The association provides peer support for abstinence from opiates and also engages in extensive community service projects (Ch'ien 1980; Poshyachinda *et al.* 1982). In the association's only outcome study, a random sample of 100 new members had a 57% 2-year abstinence rate compared with the 9% rate of 100 treatment graduates who were invited to join but declined (Ch'ien 1980). The 1-year readmission rate of about one-third for members is also low relative to that found in most outcome studies (Ch'ien 1980).

9.4.2 Oxford House

Oxford House members manage, reside in, and contribute to the upkeep of a house in which substance use and violence are forbidden. There are about 10 000 Oxford House residents in North America and Australia. Uncontrolled studies document decreases in Oxford House residents' substance use and criminal behaviour (see Humphreys 2004, for a review), and a randomized trial of 157 individuals found that Oxford House residents had, over a 2-year period, half the substance abuse rate, one-third the incarceration rate, and double the monthly income of individuals assigned to usual care (Jason *et al.* 2006).

9.4.3 Narcotics Anonymous

Established in the USA, Narcotics Anonymous (NA) is based on the well-known '12-step model' (see Box 9.4). Despite its name, NA focuses on a range of illicit drugs and not just narcotics. NA has chapters in over 100 countries, having successfully spread from the USA to societies with other languages and religious traditions (e.g. Egypt, Spain, Russia, and Thailand). NA has at least 250 000 members around the world. Although most of them reside in North America, the fastest growth in new members has been in developing societies such as Brazil and Iran.

A study in the UK (Christo and Sutton 1994; Christo and Franey 1995) found that length of NA membership is positively associated with higher self-esteem, lower anxiety, and longer duration of abstinence from drugs. Subsequent work in the US city of Detroit found that drug-dependent patients who attended NA and other 12-step groups after treatment discharge had greater decreases in drug use, drug-related problems, alcohol use, and medical problems at 1-year follow-up than those patients who did not attend NA (Humphreys *et al.* 1994). Other large, prospective, multiprogramme evaluation studies in the USA have found similar results (Etheridge *et al.* 1999; Fiorentine 1999; Humphreys *et al.* 1999; Weiss *et al.* 2000). The only randomized clinical trial involving NA also reported positive results (Timko *et al.* 2006).

9.5 The quality of health and social services for drug users

In every society where the problem has been studied, poor service quality is an enduring concern (Gossop 1995; McLellan *et al.* 2003). Quality problems take many forms, including insufficient staff, demoralized staff, incompetent staff, ignorance of practice guidelines, deteriorated physical facilities, poor integration with medical services, and bureaucratic disorganization. Poor service quality appears to cause worse outcomes (Kraft *et al.* 1997; Prendergast *et al.* 2002). Performance measures and payment systems are sometimes part of the problem, as they often emphasize the number of patients served rather than the quality of service provided.

Without dismissing these concerns about quality, they should be placed in context. Health and social services are often accorded prestige and resources according to the social standing of their clients. Users of illicit drugs are highly stigmatized in most societies (Room 2005a), and consequently drug-related services often receive minimal resources, and are then held to high performance standards (Reuter 2001). As McLellan and colleagues (2000) argue, expecting services for drug users to turn all or even most users into lifetime abstainers imposes a performance standard far beyond that typically used to judge interventions for chronic health problems (and, one could add, well beyond what is used to justify government's educational, criminal justice, military, and financial policies).

9.6 Conclusion

The Appendix at the end of this book summarizes the evidence reviewed in this and other chapters in terms of effectiveness, amount of evidence, cross-national testing, and other considerations. As mentioned, OST stands apart from other interventions in terms of the strong level of evidence supporting its benefits. Therapeutic communities, counselling for marijuana dependence, and brief interventions for moderate level drug use problems have the next strongest level of evidence. The remainder of interventions vary widely in the strength of their evidence base.

For opiate dependence in particular, psychosocial interventions have *relatively* less evidence of effectiveness than does another policy option, OST, which offers psychosocial services in combination with pharmacotherapy. Psychosocial services without pharmacotherapy might be included in a system to provide care for opiate-dependent patients who do not or cannot take medication, but a system that provides only counselling or other therapy programmes will clearly generate what most observers would consider suboptimal outcomes.

Finally, what is judged effective also depends significantly on the desired goals of the service system and its individual components. A policymaker focused primarily on preventing HIV infection, for example, is likely to see a different set of interventions as 'effective' than does a policymaker focused primarily on reducing illicit drug use. The evidence therefore needs to be interpreted in light of the policy goals set in various countries through voting, negotiating, advocacy and other public policy determination processes.

Chapter 10

Supply control

10.1 Introduction

This chapter is about supply control approaches to drug problems, a set of interventions targeting the production, distribution, and sale of illicit psychoactive substances. We begin by explaining the distinctions between law enforcement and supply control. Because supply control traditionally focuses on enforcement against producers and dealers, the second section presents an analytical framework that links different kinds of enforcement to different layers in the drug distribution chain described in Chapter 5. We then organize the remainder of the chapter by the supply level that is targeted by an intervention: production/refining, international trafficking, high level domestic enforcement, and retail enforcement. The final section presents our assessment of what is currently understood about the effectiveness of the different programmes.

10.2 Supply control versus law enforcement

The terms *supply control* and *law enforcement* are sometimes used interchangeably, but that is incorrect. Law enforcement can ameliorate drug problems in four distinct ways. Reducing supply (i.e. lowering the quantity that producers and distributors are willing to provide at a given price) is just one, albeit the most prominent. The other three are reducing demand, driving a wedge between supply and demand, and reducing the harmfulness of drug use. This chapter focuses on supply control. The next chapter discusses programmes aimed at the user, including how the threat of law enforcement sanction might affect use.

To appreciate these distinctions, it is important to use the proper economic definitions of demand and supply, as these terms are often misused. Demand is the population's willingness to purchase drugs at a given price. (Price in this context means price per unit after adjusting for purity.) Note that demand is not the same as consumption (i.e. the amount of drugs actually consumed). A demand curve describes how much would be consumed at each of a range of different prices; in mathematical terms, it is a function, not just a number. Supply is the relationship between price and the quantity of drugs that producers and distributors are willing to provide at that price. The quantity consumed is driven by both supply and demand, and a market is said to be in equilibrium if the market price incentivizes suppliers to provide the amount that users want to purchase at that price, so there is neither a shortage nor excess stockpiling of the drug.

Law enforcement can drive a wedge between supply and demand by increasing 'search costs' for drug users (i.e. the time and effort required to obtain and consume drugs).

For example, 'buy bust' enforcement in which undercover law enforcement agents pose as users could make dealers reluctant to sell to customers they do not know. This strategy is enormously appealing in theory because it promises to increase the effective cost of acquiring drugs (which should reduce drug use) without increasing the dollar cost paid to sellers and, hence, black market revenues (Moore 1973). However, retail drug distribution is often embedded within social networks, and even though search times in street markets are not inconsequential (Rocheleau and Boyum 1994), the strategy may not be viable for established markets when buyers have multiple alternative sources (Riley *et al.* 1997; Caulkins 1998).

Law enforcement can also reduce the harm associated with a given quantity of drugs being sold and used. Often this is framed as avoiding the creation of additional harms, e.g. by not arresting individuals who have overdosed on heroin or by playing a subsidiary role by helping treatment providers (Spooner *et al.* 2004). However, there is also potential for proactive enforcement to reduce harm (Weatherburn and Lind 1999a,b; Caulkins 2002), most notably by reducing market externalities such as violence and disorder. Such enforcement includes problem-oriented policing, disrupting firearm markets (since they provide the means for more lethal activities in drug markets), and focusing on market violence rather than simply on the sale of drugs (Kennedy 1997; Canty *et al.* 2000; Braga *et al.* 2001; Braga and Pierce 2005).

The prototypical supply control effort involves arresting, prosecuting, and incarcerating drug suppliers. However, just as there are dimensions of drug law enforcement besides supply control, there are dimensions of supply control besides conventional law enforcement. For example, restrictions on **precursor chemicals** can, in some cases, disrupt supply sufficiently to reduce drug-related hospital admissions and arrests (Cunningham and Liu 2003, 2005; Dobkin and Nicosia 2005), and well-run prescription drug monitoring programmes may stanch the diversion of prescription drugs such as **OxyContin** (US General Accounting Office 2002). Likewise, alternative development programmes seek to control supply by wooing peasant farmers into growing crops other than coca or opium.

Authorities may also control illegal supply by promoting competitors that take business away from existing, less desirable drug suppliers. That promotion can be passive, as when Dutch authorities allow coffee shops to sell cannabis. Or the promotion can be direct and active, as when the government supplies heroin through medical clinics, as for example is being done in Switzerland and Germany. In either case the objective is to reduce the quantity supplied through harmful illegal markets by substituting another legal or illegal but less harmful alternative source of supply.

10.3 **Conceptual framework**

It was once widely believed that enforcement reduces drug consumption by physically limiting the capacity of the illicit drug industry to produce and distribute drugs. According to this naïve view, a kilo of drugs seized is a kilo of drugs not consumed; one dealer removed from the drug trade is one less person delivering drugs to users. Indeed, under US law, the annual National Drug Control Strategy must include 'an assessment of the reduction of drug availability against an ascertained baseline, as measured by the quantities of cocaine, heroin, marijuana, methamphetamine, and other drugs available for consumption in the United States.'[1]

This often-cited measure, the volume of a drug 'available for consumption', suggests that the main purpose of source-country control is to reduce the volume of drugs available for shipment to the destination, while the function of interdiction is to prevent shipments from entering the country, thus reducing the amount of drugs available for domestic distribution. In turn, domestic seizures remove additional drug volume from the market, while arrests of traffickers and dealers and confiscation of their assets prevent drugs from reaching users. The one major US study reflecting this perspective concluded that interdiction is very effective because the volume of seizures per enforcement dollar is higher than for domestic enforcement (Godshaw *et al.* 1987).

But the idea that crop eradication, seizures, and arrests directly reduce drug consumption ignores the fact that drugs are bought and sold in markets (see Chapter 5) and that the actors involved respond to economic incentives. Indeed, the economic reality that drugs are bought and sold in markets underlies the separation of programmes into demand reduction and supply reduction. Enforcement operations create risks for those in the drug trade, including arrest, imprisonment, and the loss of drugs, money, and physical assets. Farmers, smugglers, traffickers, and dealers take steps to reduce the impact of these risks, such as growing or shipping more drugs to make up for losses, or switching to smuggling or distribution methods that are less vulnerable to detection. To compensate for the costs of eradication, seizures, and arrests, as well as efforts to avoid enforcement, drug producers and distributors charge higher prices to downstream distributors and dealers. These higher prices are then passed on to consumers, which in turn reduces drug consumption.

How well this works in practice depends on two factors: the extent to which various types of enforcement raise prices, and how much drug consumption responds to price changes. We provide here a brief survey of research on each of these factors and then turn to a more detailed examination of how much supply control can influence the supply curve.

10.3.1 The elasticity of demand

Though it was once believed that drug users could not adjust their consumption to changes in price because drugs were addictive, substantial research now shows that drug users are indeed sensitive to price. In particular, a rich economics literature on cigarette smoking, which involves a substance comparably addictive to heroin, shows that consumption is substantially responsive to changes in prices (see Grossman 2005). A parallel, smaller but still considerable literature has examined the 'elasticity' of demand for illegal drugs. Elasticity of demand refers to how much consumption of a good changes (as a percentage) in response to a 1% increase in price. For example, if a 10% increase in price reduces consumption by 5%, then the elasticity is said to be –0.5. Some confusion arises because economists refer to goods with an elasticity smaller than 1.0, in absolute value, as being demand 'inelastic'. Hence, inelastic demand does

[1] Anti-Drug Abuse Act of 1988, 21 U.S.C. §1705(b)(1)(E)(ii).

not mean consumption is impervious to price changes; it merely means the changes in consumption are smaller, proportionally, than are the changes in price.

The elasticity of demand for psychoactive substances is the sum of two separate components: participation response (the decision to use the substance) and intensity response (the amount a continuing user consumes). The extent to which a drug's elasticity of demand is determined by the participation response component is of particular interest for youth, since that decision precedes the decision about how much to use. Studies using general population surveys sometimes estimate only the participation component of the elasticity of demand for drugs because it is easier to measure. Conversely, studies that focus on current users necessarily overlook the participation component of elasticity. But in general both components are important.

The long-term elasticity of demand (i.e. how much consumption changes over a period of years in response to a permanent price change) may be substantially higher than the short-term elasticity because price-induced reductions in initiation take time to affect the stock of users and because current committed users are likely to take time to make behavioral change. A familiar analogy would be how petrol consumption responds to oil price shocks. In the short run people can drive more slowly and cut out optional trips, but they still drive their old cars to work. In the long run people may choose to live closer to work and the stock of gas-guzzling cars can be replaced by smaller cars that get better mileage. Similarly, in the short run the existing pool of drug users can use less, but in the long run the stock of users can also change both in composition and in behavior.

The estimated elasticity of demand varies by drug, user type, and country but in almost all cases the number of users and/or the quantity consumed declines when prices rise, in some cases substantially. The research primarily covers recent decades in the USA, but there are a few studies from other countries (Australia, Norway, the UK) and other times (e.g. opium in The Netherlands East Indies in the early 20th century). Most studies use general population surveys which, as discussed in earlier chapters, miss a large part of the market for dependence-producing and expensive drugs such as cocaine and heroin. The price data are often of low quality, further weakening the analyses, though imprecision in that variable makes it harder to detect a relationship between price and consumption when it is present. The fact that most studies do find price responsiveness is thus all the more compelling.

Marijuana

Pacula and colleagues (2001) used the US high school senior survey, Monitoring the Future, for the period 1986–1996 to analyse participation effects. They found that among high school seniors the participation elasticity is about –0.30 (i.e. a 10% increase in price would lower the number of high school seniors who used the drug in a given year by ~3%). There is great variability in the estimate (–0.06 to –0.47), depending on the specification of the estimating equation. In contrast, Cameron and Williams (2001) used Australian survey data to find a much larger participation elasticity for a broader adult population (–0.88).

There has been a great deal of interest in how changing the price of one drug affects consumption of other drugs. If constraining the supply of one drug increases consumption of a second drug, that second drug is called a 'substitute', whereas if consumption of both drugs falls they are called 'complements'. To the extent that drugs are good substitutes for each other, supply control may have little effect on total drug use even if it can reduce the supply of one drug. Armchair speculation might suggest that drugs are substitutes in the short run, particularly for dependent polydrug users, but complements in the long run since high rates of consumption of one drug may lead to dependence and, hence, greater use of other drugs in the future.

Empirically estimating the extent to which various pairs of drugs are complements or substitutes is challenging, so research has focused on the relationship between marijuana and some other substance (usually alcohol), since data on marijuana use are generally better than are data on use of other drugs. Unfortunately, even with respect to marijuana the empirical findings yield no clear answer that could inform policy development. Some studies find that alcohol is a substitute for marijuana (e.g. Chaloupka and Laixuthai 1997) whereas others suggest it is a complement (e.g. Pacula 1998). Saffer and Chaloupka (1999a) find complementarity between marijuana and cocaine.

Cocaine

Using data on US high school seniors between 1977 and 1987, DiNardo (1993) found no response to changes in the price of cocaine. More recent studies have found substantial price elasticities. For example, Saffer and Chaloupka (1999a) estimate an elasticity of between –0.30 and –0.57 using data from the US National Household Survey on Drug Abuse over the years 1988–1991. For youth, Chaloupka and colleagues (1999) estimate a past-year participation elasticity of –0.89 and an overall elasticity of –1.28 when including the intensity response, similar to what Grossman and Chaloupka (1998) found using a rational addiction approach (participation elasticities ranging from –0.45 to –1.28). Williams and colleagues (2006), using data on US college students, found estimates as high as –0.57, depending on age and gender.

Heroin

It is unclear whether or not the price elasticity for heroin is as high as it is for cocaine. General population surveys provide little information on the prevalence of heroin use so elasticity estimates based on them would be somewhat suspect. Hence, studies of the elasticity of heroin demand usually use other kinds of samples or indicators, and as a result often cannot estimate participation elasticities. For example, Bretteville-Jensen (2006) used interviews with clients of an Oslo needle exchange from 1993 to 2006, so her elasticity estimates (–0.77 for users compared with –0.33 for user-dealers) are conditional on being an IDU. Likewise, Dave (2006) examined the responsiveness of hospital emergency room visits to heroin and cocaine prices. For heroin he found that the elasticity of emergency room visits was only –0.10. Dave (2008) found short- and long-run elasticities of arrestees testing positive for heroin of –0.10 and –0.18, respectively.

A few studies estimate price responsiveness for heroin and another drug using the same data and methods. Most find greater price responsiveness for cocaine (e.g. Grossman 2005; Dave 2006, 2008). However, Saffer and Chaloupka (1999a) are an exception, and Bretteville-Jensen (2006) found greater elasticity for heroin than amphetamines. Furthermore, elasticity estimates are higher for opium when it was legally regulated and therefore better data on its use were available (Van Ours 1995; Liu *et al.* 1999).

In summary, one can say with some confidence that the demand for cocaine, heroin, and marijuana is responsive to price changes. Most findings show moderate responsiveness, but the reliance on survey data that systematically miss the heaviest users and the 'noisy' quality of the price data limit the authority of the findings. Furthermore, it appears that there can be substantial variation in the elasticity of demand across drugs and types of users.

10.3.2 **Unanticipated supply shocks versus ongoing supply control**

Enforcement can affect supply in two ways: disrupting the market equilibrium via actions unanticipated by drug producers/sellers and shifting the equilibrium via ongoing enforcement activity that suppliers treat as an accepted cost of doing business. The logic models underpinning these two mechanisms are different. Failing to recognize this when comparing analyses or conclusions concerning the two mechanisms can lead to great confusion, as happened when the US National Research Council (Manski *et al.* 1999) compared the results of Crane and colleagues' (1997) disequlibrium analysis with Rydell and Everingham's (1994) modelling of the long-term effects of various interventions. Caulkins and colleagues (2000) provide clarification on this matter.

Unanticipated interventions (e.g. the police breaking the 'French Connection' drug smuggling network) can disrupt the equilibrium of a drug market. Ideally the disruption takes the form of physical shortage, and the market never recovers to the old equilibrium. This has been noted for secondary drugs consumed primarily by polydrug users, as with **charas** (hand-made hashish made from the extract of the cannabis plant) in India during the Second World War (United Nations 1953) and methedrine in the UK (De Alarcon, 1972), but rarely happens with major markets. The breaking of the post-Second World War Japanese amphetamine epidemic (Brill and Hirose 1969) and the recent Australian heroin drought, discussed later, are possible exceptions. Usually suppliers adapt to the intervention by changing tactics, and the market equilibrium is restored, although purity-adjusted prices may spike and use may decline in the interim (Crane *et al.* 1997; Cunningham and Liu 2003, 2005).

Enforcement can also shift, as opposed to disrupt, the long-run equilibrium even if sellers correctly anticipate the risks of seizures and arrests. For example, if smugglers know that a quarter of all shipments will be seized, they will respond both by shipping more drugs and by charging higher prices per kilogram delivered to cover the cost of the seized drugs. As just discussed, higher prices lead to lower consumption. Similar logic applies to other risks enforcement creates for suppliers. If small plane pilots know they have a quarter risk of being incarcerated, they will require greater compensation per trip than if the incarceration risk were lower.

In addition to the risks and costs imposed by the government through enforcement, drug dealers face a second source of risks and costs, those arising from the actions of other criminals, notably other market participants. Like the state, these participants attempt to seize drugs and money and sometimes use violence for that purpose; they may also compete for territories, creating another source of violence. Since the trade operates without many written records and often involves male adolescents, it is perhaps not surprising that violent disputes about individual transactions are also common.

The conventional costs of producing and distributing drugs are very modest, particularly relative to the often very high retail prices that drugs command. Hence, these two bundles of risks: those generated directly or indirectly by enforcement and those generated by other suppliers, usually dominate the suppliers' costs of doing business. The 'risks and prices' framework developed by Reuter and Kleiman (1986) posits that in a long-run market equilibrium, drug sellers' revenues (i.e. quantity sold times price) ought to be high enough to compensate sellers for all their costs, including not only tangible costs (e.g. of scales used to weigh the drugs) but also fair compensation for their risks of imprisonment, injury, and death. Because of this coupling between costs and revenues, one might expect prices would rise, other things being equal, if dealers on average faced higher risks either from the state or from other participants. There have been only a few efforts to assess whether this model can explain the level of prices (Reuter *et al.* 1990; Caulkins and Reuter 1998), because the data demands of the model for empirical purposes are very substantial.

Note that in this framework it is not the risks *per se* that determine prices but the sellers' valuation of those risks in monetary terms. Thus prices might change with a constant level of enforcement. For example, an ageing dealer population with prior convictions and few legitimate labour market opportunities might require a smaller amount of dollar profit to accept the same annual probability of incarceration or serious injury relative to a younger dealer population with no criminal record and a range of other economic opportunities.

The focus of this chapter is on the consequences when the state pursues policies designed to raise the risks to drug suppliers. However, the risks caused by other drug market participants may themselves be a direct or indirect function of state actions. For example, more intense enforcement (such as higher probability of arrest or incarceration) increases the incentive for one participant to inform against others. Fear of informing gives incentives for more disciplinary violence, so that the market may be characterized by higher risk of injury. If tough enforcement is geographically localized (e.g. focused on a few street corners), displaced drug sellers may begin to compete violently with other sellers for drug selling posts in nearby neighborhoods. Finally, tough enforcement may also raise risks by influencing who goes into the drug dealing business; those who require lower compensation for a given risk of incarceration may be more willing to use violence to resolve disputes.

10.4 **Enforcement programmes**

Enforcement is not one activity but rather a set of programmes. The multiple levels of the drug distribution chain are mirrored by programmes that target these specific levels. For example, The Netherlands government targets traffickers from

The Netherlands Antilles that ship cocaine into Europe (UNODC/World Bank 2007), mostly through Amsterdam (by air) and Rotterdam (by sea). Quite separately, it enforces prohibitions against the trafficking of cocaine within The Netherlands itself. The first of these programmes should affect the price that traffickers charge for shipping cocaine out of the producing region (i.e. the difference between the export price of cocaine leaving South America and its price on arrival in The Netherlands). Any influence of the programmes aimed at trafficking within The Netherlands should show up in the difference between the import price and the domestic wholesale price. In each instance the result will be an increase in the retail price of cocaine. Table 10.1 provides a general schematic depiction of this for drugs that are trafficked internationally (not particular to The Netherlands). For drugs produced and consumed in the same country, transit zone interdiction is irrelevant. Programmes targeting production and refining still affect the initial sales price, but it is not then an export price.

10.4.1 Source-country control

Chapter 5 noted that, except for cannabis and diverted **psychopharmaceuticals**, most drug production is highly concentrated in a few countries. The supply sources for cocaine and heroin in particular have never been very diverse. Bolivia, Peru, and Colombia are the exclusive commercial producers of cocaine for the world market. Afghanistan and Burma account for over 90% of world opium production, with another three producers (Colombia, Laos, and Mexico) accounting for most of the remainder (UNODC 2005).

Concentration of production in a few countries is not due to any physical or horticultural constraints; coca bushes, opium poppies, and cannabis are all easy to grow in a range of locations. Perhaps the best explanation of why production is so concentrated is that it is easier to grow large quantities of illegal crops in places where the authority of central governments is weak, and illegal crop production in turn undermines governmental authority. So a positive feedback loop makes it easier to grow illegal crops where they are already commonly grown, but historical accident more than anything else determines where that positive feedback loop is initially established.

Most of the illegal drugs consumed in most countries around the world are produced abroad and imported. Some conclude from this that programmes aimed at

Table 10.1 Enforcement programmes and their targets

Programme	Targeted sector	Price affected
Eradication, alternative development, refinery destruction, precursor chemical control	Production and refining	Export
Interdiction	Smuggling	Import minus export
Investigation	High level domestic trafficking	Wholesale minus import
Street-level enforcement	Retailing	Retail minus wholesale

reducing production or export from the source-countries can affect drug problems in consumer nations. Indeed, international programmes aimed at growers and refiners attract a great deal of political and media attention. Intersections with other foreign policy concerns, including terrorism, have helped make these programmes prominent, particularly in Colombia, where the guerillas challenging the central government are financially dependent on coca growing, and Afghanistan, where opium production has returned to world-leading levels despite a ban enacted by President Hamid Karzai.

Four types of programmes aim to reduce source-country drug production: crop eradication; alternative development; precursor control; and in-country enforcement. Eradication, involving aerial spraying or ground-based operations, aims literally to limit the quantity of the drugs available for export from the current crop and to discourage farmers from growing them again in the future. Alternative development is the less coercive version of crop eradication's second objective; it encourages farmers growing coca or poppies to switch to legitimate crops or to related industries by increasing earnings from these other activities. Strategies include introducing new crops and more productive strains of traditional crops, improving transportation for getting the crops to market, and implementing various marketing and subsidy schemes. Precursor control policies refer to the efforts of those nations that have implemented strict regulations on the sale and distribution of chemicals that are used in the production of heroin or methamphetamine. A final form of source-control control is for drug-consuming countries (e.g. the USA and much of Europe) to push source-countries to pursue traffickers and refiners more vigorously, often providing military equipment and training for these purposes.

None of these programmes receives a large share of global drug control spending (**ONDCP** (1997) budgets show they are a small share even in the USA). This reflects some combination of their limited effectiveness and a 'tragedy of the commons' due to the international character of drug markets: unilateral investment by one consumer country would yield benefits shared by all drug-consuming nations. The only nation that consumes more than a quarter of global production of any one drug is the USA, *vis-à-vis* cocaine. Not surprisingly, it is the only nation that invests substantially in source-country control, spending US$1.1 billion in the 2002 financial year, almost entirely directed at cocaine. Still, that is a tiny proportion of the total US drug control spending across all levels of government, which amounts to approximately US$40 billion (Boyum and Reuter 2005). Total expenditures by European nations (both bilateral and multilateral programmes) are probably very much less. The United Nations is the organization most involved in source-country control, and its Office on Drugs and Crime (**UNODC**) had a total budget for the two years 2006–2007 of only US$283 million.[2]

The vast majority of US money went to the Andean region. Mexico has a large role in supplying drugs to the USA, but as a matter of national sovereignty has been unwilling to allow the operation of US programmes on its territory. Only at the end of

[2] Available at: http://www.unodc.org/unodc/en/donors/index.html (accessed 6 January 2008).

2007 was it announced that Mexico might agree to a programme of financial support from the USA (United States Department of State 2008). Only Colombia and Mexico allow aerial eradication; in other nations eradication is done manually, often by the military. Spraying is feared by some to cause significant environmental damage (e.g. Vargas 2002, but see Solomon *et al.* 2005 for an opposing view). Spraying can also generate political unrest, since the immediate targets, peasant farmers, are among the poorest citizens, even when growing coca or poppies. They are often also indigenous groups (e.g. the Aymara in Bolivia and the Wa in Burma) with long-standing grievances against the central government.

Official estimates of the areas eradicated suggest that the effort is quite intense. For example, the Colombian government estimates that the number of hectares of opium poppies eradicated in 2000 was 2500 out of an estimated total planted of 9000 (Uribe 2004). The 1999–2002 estimates for Bolivia indicated that coca eradication accounted for about 50% of the estimated cultivation total (UNODC 2005).

Despite these considerable efforts, there is almost no evidence that eradication has affected the supply of heroin or cocaine to Europe, the USA, or any other country. A rare success story was the drop in Mexican opium production in the mid-1970s, but the circumstances were unusual. An industry that had operated openly in five northern states with large, unprotected fields was seriously disrupted when the government began drug crop spraying. For about 5 years there was a substantial reduction in heroin availability in the USA, particularly in western regions where Mexican supply dominated heroin markets (Reuter and Ronfeldt 1992). Production subsequently became much more widely dispersed, and growing fields were reduced in size and hidden in remote locations. By the early 1980s, Mexico was supplying as much heroin as before the spraying.

There is even less reason to believe that alternative development is an effective way to control drug use, but it tends to have a broader base of political support in developed countries than does crop eradication, perhaps because it provides services to marginalized farmers. Indeed, a common argument against eradication and enforcement against growers is precisely that it leaves a large number of poor people in even worse economic straits. There is a good deal of discussion of sequencing alternative development and eradication, with the former providing a base for the latter (World Bank and Department for International Development 2008). However, unless farmers believe the government will maintain its commitment over a long period, they will not be willing to incur the costs of shifting crops. In situations of political instability there will understandably be scepticism about the ability of, say, the Bolivian government to ensure a dependable market and a reliable transportation infrastructure for pineapples from the Chapare. Furthermore, for source zone interventions to affect downstream consumption—as opposed merely to outcomes in that particular producing area—they have to strike quickly, before production in other regions can expand. Alternative development for an entire drug-producing region is not easily accomplished within one or two growing seasons. Though there are a few instances of well-executed local crop substitution programmes, they do not appear to have reduced drug production in any *region* of the world, let alone consumption in downstream markets. As described in Box 10.1, Bolivia presents perhaps the most interesting current example of large-scale source-country intervention.

Box 10.1 Bolivia: an example of large-scale source-country intervention

Over the past 15 years, the USA has invested in intensive eradication and alternative development. The Bolivian government, starting in 1997 with the election of General Hugo Banzer, placed a large military force in the Chapare to back the USA's efforts. The result was a rapid and substantial decline in Bolivian coca production, from 255 tons of potential cocaine in 1995 to 43 tons in 2001 (Gamarra 2002). Coca production in Colombia rose during this period, leaving Andean total production almost unchanged (International Narcotics Control Strategy Report 2007). The crack-down also led to rising political tensions as well as violent clashes between the police and military on the one hand and the cocaleros on the other, which contributed to the resignation of President de Loszada. The two sides signed an agreement in October 2004 that allowed each cocaleros household to grow on-sixth of one hectare of coca leaves, ostensibly for the legitimate market; almost certainly all of this production went to the illegal cocaine market. Estimated illegal production also began to rise. However it is also likely that the roughly US$50 million invested annually in development programmes in that region of Bolivia has facilitated the exit of some cocaleros households into the legal sector. The December 2005 election of Evo Morales, former cocaleros leader, as president of Bolivia signalled how much popular hostility there was to the US-induced campaign, since he emphasized his fight against coca eradication in his electoral speeches (Reuter and MacLean-Abaroa 2008).

Source-country control is sometimes seen as synonymous with programmes pertaining to crop production, but source-countries are also the venue of most drug production (including the conversion from crops to chemicals) and the greatest market concentration of traffickers. Hence, the UNODC emphasizes the increase of law enforcement capacity along with alternative development in source countries.[3] Its current programmes range from strengthening Iran's drug interdiction capacities with respect to both imports and exports, training sniffer dogs in Southern Africa, improving information sharing among countries in South East Asia and the Caribbean, and strengthening chemical precursor control in Brazil and Colombia.

The USA also invests in building institutional capacity to deal with the drug trade. Each year the State Department, in its *International Narcotics Control Strategy Report* (INCSR), argues that the central problem of drug control in other countries is a lack of political will and integrity (see, for example, US. Department of State 2003, II-10). Efforts to deal with this issue include training investigators, strengthening the judiciary, and improving extradition procedures. Unfortunately, in both Colombia and Mexico (the dominant sources of foreign drugs to the USA), the corruption

[3] Available at: http://www.unodc.org/unodc/en/drug_supply_reduction.html. (accessed 31 January 2006).

problems have been significant, embedded in a larger system of weak integrity controls. For example, in Mexico, near the end of the 6-year administration of a reformist president, Vicente Fox, the level of drug-related violence and corruption remained so high that in the city of Nuevo Laredo 305 of 765 police officers were dismissed and the new police chief was assassinated within hours of being appointed (Carpenter 2005).

There have been two recent successes in cutting heroin production in major source-countries. In 2001 the Taliban government of Afghanistan reduced opium production by over 90% as compared with the previous year (see Box 10.2). In the period 1998–2003 the Shan United Army, an irredentist group in Myanmar, cut opium production in one major growing region of that country by more than 75% (Transnational Institute 2003). As part of the process, the Shan United Army forcibly moved the mountain tribes that were growing opium to more controlled areas near the border with Thailand. The Myanmar and Afghanistan examples are thus both cases of authoritarian regimes reducing drug crop protection at all costs in response both to internal dynamics and external political pressure.

10.4.2 **Interdiction**

Interdiction is the set of programmes aimed at international drug traffickers at the border and in the so-called 'transit zone' between export and arrival in a final market country. Though the retail sales of illicit drugs in rich nations generate tens of billions of dollars in sales (perhaps US$100–150 billion globally), the physical mass and volumes of drugs being transported are tiny. Including what is seized at the borders and

Box 10.2 The Taliban cut-back

In July 2000, the Taliban regime announced, for the third time, a ban on opium poppy cultivation, rooted in its interpretation of Koranic teachings. Though initially greeted with scepticism (partly because it did not include trafficking or refining) the ban met its goal. Afghanistan's opium acreage declined dramatically, to less than 10% of the 2000 figure. The Taliban used its reputation for tough enforcement of law and the promise of foreign aid to affected farmers to obtain compliance with relatively little punishment of offenders. Total world opium production plummeted from 4690 tons in 2000 to only 1600 tons in 2001, a 65% drop. In 2002, following the overthrow of the Taliban regime, planting resumed at near-record levels.

The response to the ban has not been analysed in much detail. Prices for opium and heroin in Afghanistan and its near neighbours shot up in the 12 months following the ban, but seizures in those countries fell only by 40%, indicating the existence of large inventories of the drug. In 2002 and 2003 there were signs of modest shortages in Western European markets. However, whether the ban could have been maintained for more than 1 year and whether this would have led to substantial reductions in world opiate consumption or to shifts in the location of production remain matters for speculation.

Source: Paoli *et al.* (2009a).

in the interior, global imports are estimated at about 400 tons for heroin and 500 tons for cocaine. (Hence, it would take only six Boeing 747-8s to hold the entire world's annual drug cargo.)

The drugs travel in every conceivable mode of transport. Heroin shipments from Tajikistan to Russia may be hidden in fresh produce; cocaine from Colombia has been shipped to the USA in wooden furniture and in frozen fruit pulp containers. Some is carried internally by 'body-stuffers' who swallow up to 750 grams of cocaine or heroin wrapped in condoms.

Given the enormous volume of legitimate traffic and commerce across international borders, it is not hard to hide a few hundred tons of drugs. Indeed, it is remarkable that authorities seize such a large share of cocaine production, perhaps 40% or more over the whole production, international transport, and domestic distribution system. Heroin seizure rates were traditionally lower, only rising to around the traditional 10% figure that orthodoxy has enshrined as the share generally seized by enforcement agencies after 1995 (UNODC 2005).

Many nations have specialized units for interdiction, generally located within the Customs Service. For example, in the UK, Her Majesty's Customs and Excise Service (since 2005 part of HM Revenue and Customs) reports each year on total seizures, some generated by random search but an increasing number from intelligence-targeted investigations.[4]

The USA is perhaps the most aggressive nation in interdiction, taking a 'defence in depth' approach of interdiction throughout the 'transit zone' through which drugs travel, not just at its borders. The USA, along with the UK and The Netherlands, places naval and air assets near the exporting regions of Latin America and the Caribbean. The USA also has a significant number of Drug Enforcement Administration staff in many embassies throughout the world. Interdiction was the principal federal US enforcement programme in the mid-1980s, accounting for 28% of federal drug control expenditures (ONDCP 1997). Other interdiction efforts are collaborations between law enforcement agencies in consumer, producer, and trans-shipment nations. For example, some believe that the heroin drought in Australia (see Box 10.3) was precipitated in part by activities the Australian Federal Police and Royal Canadian Mounted Police undertook in Thailand and other parts of South East Asia (Hawley 2002; Australian Crime Commission 2003).

The UNODC tracks global seizures of cocaine and heroin in its annual *Global Illicit Drug Trends* report. In recent years the total for opiates (mostly heroin but including morphine and opium) has risen beyond the traditionally believed 10%, in 2000 reaching a record 100 tons of heroin or its equivalent, representing about 20% of world opiate production. Large opiate seizures are made primarily by neighbours of Afghanistan and Burma. Iran, for example, consistently reports the highest seizure figures, including a puzzlingly large quantity of morphine (UNODC 2005).

[4] For a recent statement of HMCE performance and goals with respect to drug interdiction see http://www.hm-treasury.gov.uk/performance/targets/perf_target_90.cfm (accessed 29 January 2006).

Box 10.3 The Australian heroin drought

The Australian heroin 'drought' merits special mention following a discussion of interdiction and high level domestic enforcement for two reasons. First, it stands out as a singularly large market disruption. It is not clear that any sizable illicit drug market in modern times has been disrupted so dramatically (overdoses dropping by ~80%) and in such a sustained fashion. Secondly, although it is very likely that the drought stems from some supply disruption, it is not clear whether the drought was triggered by international events versus high level Australian enforcement (Degenhardt *et al.* 2005b).

As background, Australia has a major heroin problem, as serious in relative terms as that of any other western nation (Hall *et al.* 2000b); the pre-drought estimate of 67 000–92 000 dependent users represented 4 per 1000 population, comparable with the 3 per 1000 figure for the USA (ONDCP 2001b), the UK (Millar *et al.* 2006), and Switzerland (Nordt and Stohler 2006). Heroin addiction principally occurs in the two largest cities, Sydney and Melbourne, which account for almost half of Australia's population. The populations of heroin addicts there are large enough that these cities have efficient and mature markets.

Around Christmas of the year 2000 there was a sudden and unanticipated heroin drought in both cities. Purity plunged and street prices rose in the space of 3 months (see Moore *et al.* (2005) for a detailed analysis of the Melbourne data). Though there was some rebound in purity, during the next 3 years the prices per pure gram remained higher and purity lower than prior to the year 2000. The market had arguably reached a new equilibrium.

It is clear that this change was not caused by any demand side shift, such as a sudden increase in demand or a decreased availability or efficacy of services for drug users. It was a supply side shift. Degenhart and colleagues (2005b), after considering a wide range of possible explanations (e.g. the ban on opium production in Afghanistan, weather in Burma) conclude that the sudden shortage was primarily the result of some intervention or interventions aimed at the connections between the South East Asian heroin-producing areas (the 'Golden Triangle'), the source of Australia's heroin, and Australia.

Explanation by elimination of alternatives is an uncomfortable analytical strategy in general. It is particularly so in this instance because of the lack of clarity about the intervention that might have produced the effect. The Australian Federal Police (AFP) had embarked upon an explicit strategy of removing key traffickers exporting large quantities from South East Asian countries, with a number of noteworthy successes (Hawley 2002). The paucity of very large seizures in more recent years suggests that smuggling has shifted to (perhaps less cost-effective) smaller shipment sizes.

What is important for these purposes is that supply control measures could make a substantial and lasting effect on the supply of drugs to a major market. Prior to this event there was remarkably little positive evidence of enforcement success, particularly enforcement directed at the higher market levels.

For cocaine, the seizure total in recent years has been stable at about 350 tons, representing approximately 45% of estimated production. Colombia and the USA account for the majority of cocaine seized. These figures are crude estimates. The reporting of seizures is erratic and questionable in some nations, particularly those with corrupt enforcement, while the production estimates themselves suffer from considerable technical problems (Walsh 2004). Nonetheless, it seems reasonable to assert that an increasing and substantial share of both heroin and cocaine production is being seized.

Interdiction involves an unending series of adaptations by both smugglers and enforcement agencies. There are large-scale shifts in routes, modes of transportation, and techniques for hiding drugs. For example, in the early 1980s much cocaine entered the USA through Florida, but an early Reagan administration interdiction effort, run by then Vice President George H. W. Bush, pushed traffickers farther out in the Caribbean and into Mexico. Mexico is said to have remained the dominant route in the first decade of this century, but there is some evidence of renewed smuggling through the Caribbean (UNODC 2003b). In Europe, which has higher heroin seizure rates, there is also evidence of frequent shifts in routes of smuggling, some reflecting changes in political stability. The wars generated by the break-up of Yugoslavia and the instability of Albania have increased the centrality of the Balkans route since the Soviet era.

Modes change too. In Central Asia since about 2000 there has been a shift from body packing to use of cargo shipments to conceal heroin smuggled into Russia. In the 1980s, a large share of US cocaine was brought in by private planes, typically carrying 250–500 kg on each trip (Reuter *et al.* 1988). By the early 1990s, smugglers had shifted to intermingling their loads with legitimate commerce, especially in trucks crossing the border between Mexico and the USA, a method thought to have become more common following the North American Free Trade Agreement (NAFTA).

Technological innovations in detection appear from time to time. For example, machines that can scan containers from the outside and identify drugs hidden within were developed and deployed from the mid-1990s. There is no way of determining how such innovations individually affect the drug trade.

The Institute for Defense Analysis produced a study (Crane *et al.* 1997) later extended by Anthony and Fries (2004) suggesting that sudden increases in cocaine interdiction can produce spikes in purity-adjusted retail prices. There are no other studies of disequilibria effects of interdiction, and the original study's methodology was severely criticized by the National Research Council (Manski *et al.* 2001).

Equilibrium effects introduce an important set of observations. Bogotá is approximately 1500 miles from Miami; Miami is roughly 2700 miles from Seattle. Yet the difference between wholesale cocaine prices in Miami and Seattle (<20%, or US$5000 per kg) is very small compared with the tenfold markup (from ~US$1500 to US$15 000) between wholesale prices in Bogotá and Miami. Interdiction clearly imposes high costs on cocaine smuggling, and these costs have a significant effect on the import price of cocaine in the USA. Even across apparently porous borders, the markups are often very large. For example, wholesale heroin prices double between Afghanistan and Quetta, Pakistan (UNODC 2003a).

International borders are locations where the government has unique authority to search and inspect. They are more dangerous for smugglers than any other place. But that fact does not necessarily mean interdiction is a particularly effective policy for reducing drug consumption. The key issue is how changes in the import price affect retail prices. Assume that a kilogram of heroin sells for US$50 000 at import in Bristol and the equivalent of US$250 000 per kg when sold at retail units of 200 mg in Edinburgh. Now imagine that more effective interdiction boosts the import price by 50% to US$75 000. How would this affect the retail price of heroin in Edinburgh?

This question is crucial because the answer determines the ultimate value of the enhanced interdiction efforts. One theory of vertical price relationships, which Caulkins (1990) has termed the 'additive model', argues that the import price is essentially a raw material cost (Reuter and Kleiman 1986). Thus, the wholesaler who previously bought heroin at US$50 000 and now pays US$75 000 has had roughly US$25 000 added to the per-kilo costs. The actual cost increase will be somewhat more than US$25 000 per kilo; due to seizures, thefts, and other losses: wholesalers have to buy more than one kilo of drug for each kilo they sell.

In a competitive market, the wholesaler simply passes these increased costs along to the next stage of the distribution chain. The buyer at this stage will thus face an increase of about US$25 000 in costs, which will be passed along to the next market level. Eventually, the approximately US$25 000 cost increase reaches consumers, and the end result is that the retail price of heroin increases by US$25 per gram (or somewhat more, when all the losses and seizures along the distribution chain are factored in), which is just about 10% of the initial retail price. Doing this exercise for cocaine and imported marijuana in the USA, Reuter and colleagues (1988) projected, based on some assumptions that were reasonable but not empirically tested, that a doubling of the import price results in only a 10 or 20% rise in the retail price. Or, put another way, it would take a quintupling of import prices to effect a doubling of retail prices.

Of the few empirical analyses of interdiction, most have assumed the additive model. And because the replacement cost of seized cocaine and heroin is a small fraction of their final retail price—as little as 1% in source-countries and usually no more than 20% at the point of entry into the final market country—these analyses have concluded that the potential contribution of interdiction to the reduction of drug abuse is small, or at least that it is not cost-effective compared with domestic enforcement and treatment (Rydell and Everingham 1994).

Although the additive model is conceptually compelling, some scholars have noted that it does not fit very well with some historical price data drawn from the lower end of the distribution chain (see Boyum (1992) and Caulkins (1990)). In fact, some historical price data appear to be more consistent with what Caulkins has called the 'multiplicative model' of vertical price relationships, which holds that a change of a certain percentage in price at one stage of production or distribution brings about a similar percentage change at subsequent stages. The idea behind the multiplicative model is that many of the costs of doing business in the drug trade, such as the risk of employees and other dealers stealing drugs, are more strongly related to the value of drugs bought and sold than to the quantity trafficked. Thus, the multiplicative model predicts that if the import price of heroin rises 50%, from US$50 000 to US$75 000, retail prices will also rise 50%, from US$250 000 to US$375 000, providing a much more favourable assessment of interdiction.

Cocaine prices in the 1980s and early 1990s followed a remarkably consistent multiplicative relationship between wholesale and retail prices (Caulkins 1990, 1994). Likewise, Rhodes and colleagues (1994), Crane and colleagues (1997), and DeSimone (1998) argue for a multiplicative model. However, the data that indicated a multiplicative model were far from conclusive (DeSimone 2006). Except during occasional shortages, prices consistently declined during this period, and so it is possible that the factors causing the decline operated at all levels of the market. In other words, it may be that declines in retail prices were not so much caused by the decline in import prices, but rather that both import and retail prices were influenced by other factors. For example, the growth in the cocaine industry internationally, and the development of crack markets domestically, may have created economies of scale that lowered the costs of wholesale and retail operations.

In short, the nature of vertical price relationships in drug markets is an open question. The answer may lie somewhere between the additive and multiplicative models. Indeed, Boyum (1993) and Caulkins (1990) have speculated that the multiplicative model may hold when the drugs' price per unit is very high (e.g. for retail cocaine and heroin transactions in the USA and Europe), but that the additive model may apply when prices are less extreme (e.g. for higher level wholesale transactions). Pietschmann's (2004) analysis of data on heroin prices in the Eastern Hemisphere is consistent with such a mixed model.

Interdiction imposes considerable costs on drug traffickers. Import prices are much higher than they would be if borders were unpoliced. What is uncertain, besides the import–retail price linkage, is whether sizeable increases or decreases in the interdiction budget have more than a negligible effect on import prices. It may be that a 50% reduction in interdiction funding would be inconsequential because the remaining seizure effort would be sufficient to prompt traffickers to take costly avoidance actions. It is also not clear whether the current significant markups at national borders can be sustained in the long run given increasing globalization of commerce (Stares 1996; Storti and De Grauwe 2009).

10.4.3 **High level domestic enforcement**

Every nation emphasizes the importance of arresting and punishing those who make the largest revenues from the drug trade: the major traffickers. This is seen as a matter of both justice (those who benefit most should be punished) and efficiency: such cases are believed to have greater effects on price and availability per dollar spent on enforcement (Caulkins *et al.* 1997). However, since senior traffickers invest heavily in protecting themselves against law enforcement, such investigations are sometimes long and expensive, and not all nations allow or have the capacity for the electronic surveillance and undercover investigations typically needed to reach major traffickers.

High level investigations also impose costs on drug suppliers through the seizure of drugs and other assets. These costs can be thought of as a modest tax on the higher levels of the trade. The UK reported total drug-related seizures of £81 million of assets (under the Proceeds of Crime Act) in 2003, a very small figure relative to the estimated

£5 billion in retail drug sales in the UK (Singleton *et al.* 2004). Even in the USA, with an aggressive, large-scale effort to seize assets, the annual total has been less than US$1 billion, against total estimated sales of about US$60 billion.

It is particularly difficult to assess the effects of high level enforcement because neither inputs nor outcomes can be measured well. For example, no studies estimate how much risk is imposed on high level dealers, and that would indeed be a challenging figure to estimate. The imprisonment risk in the USA is probably lower for retail than for above-retail sellers, but a lower rate applied to much larger numbers still implies that the majority of those imprisoned are not high level dealers (Sevigny and Caulkins 2004). Furthermore, the greater risk among above-retail sellers may be borne by low level, not high level, wholesale dealers. Similar concerns pertain in other countries, including Australia, which has a much lower overall rate of imprisonment for drug-law violators (Green and Purnell 1996).

The share of the retail price of cocaine and heroin accounted for by high level dealers is large relative to production costs but small relative to the value added at the lower retail levels. For example, in the UK, heroin sells for £20 000 per kg when it enters the country and for £32 000 when it reaches the lower wholesale level (~1 oz or 30 g) and £70 000 at the retail level (Matrix Knowledg Group 2007). Whether the wholesale margin can be increased in a cost-effective manner by targeting high level dealers is a matter of impression rather than science. The main reason for believing that incarcerating high level dealers is more cost-effective than enforcement against retail sellers is the ease with which retail sellers can be replaced. Since the taxpayers' costs of arrest and prosecution are modest relative to the cost of a long prison term, it is worth investing more in police investigation if that investment helps focus expensive prison terms on dealers whose imprisonment is more valuable (Caulkins *et al.* 1997).

10.4.4 **Retail enforcement**

In budgetary terms, most enforcement targets retail markets, simply because the pyramidal nature of drug distribution implies that the great majority of participants in the drug trade operate in the retail sector (see Chapter 5). Retail drug selling varies dramatically across drugs, locations, and time in ways that matter crucially for the nature, appeal, and effectiveness of retail enforcement. The first crucial distinction is whether the retail selling is covert or brazen. Covert sellers survive enforcement by being difficult to see, which also limits their visibility to customers and their irritation to neighbours. Brazen sellers are like schools of fish or herds of wildebeest. Predators (enforcement agents) know where to find them, but they are so numerous that each individual's risk is moderate. Brazen selling typically increases drug availability and harm to neighbours more than does covert selling (Kleiman 1988).

Markets can shift from one form to another. One hears most often about flagrant street markets developing where there previously had not been any, but the other direction is possible as well. Some Australian street markets disappeared during the heroin drought. New York City law enforcement efforts drove many retail sellers from the streets and into 'beeper sales' or other covert modes of operation. Other US cities have had similar experiences (Johnson 2003). However, stability of both types of markets is the norm. Robust street markets can seem impervious to even very large numbers of arrests because retail dealers can so easily be replaced (Kleiman 1997a). Likewise, if a market is entirely covert and a single dealer attempts to switch to the brazen strategy, that non-conformist dealer faces speedy arrest.

Hence, when confronted with brazen markets, enforcement can be extraordinarily efficient in terms of process outcomes yet extraordinarily ineffective in terms of final outcomes. A standard policy prescription in such circumstances is to make a conscious choice between one of two strategies. Strategy one (eradication or 'crackdown') applies overwhelming force in an attempt to tip the market back into a covert form. But the market will spring back if the effort is half-hearted. Strategy two (containment) tries to control externalities by focusing enforcement effort on the most destructive dealers and providing an incentive for users to stop or reduce using drugs, with or without the aid of helping professionals (Weatherburn and Lind 1999a, b). For example, police may overlook cannabis distribution in order to focus on dealers of 'hard drugs'.

When confronted with covert selling, law enforcement officials may be tempted to do nothing because finding such dealers is difficult and pressure for arrests from neighbours is usually minimal. A modest level of enforcement may, however, be a wiser long-term investment than doing nothing, particularly when the market is growing, because it is far easier to keep a brazen market from developing than it is to push an existing one back below ground (Kleiman 2009).

Another useful distinction among markets pertains to whether the country has a high level of violence, particularly firearm-related violence. As was noted in Chapter 5, brazen selling in the absence of guns is a nuisance; brazen selling in a country such as Brazil or the USA can unleash waves of homicidal violence, with attendant ripple effects on the economic vitality of surrounding neighbourhoods (e.g. Mingardi 2001). Hence, the willingness to tolerate brazen markets and the specific harm-reducing objectives of a containment strategy might differ in Europe and the USA. In a low violence country facing injection drug use supplied by an open street market, aggressive enforcement might do more harm than good (cf. Maher and Dixon 2001; Kerr *et al.* 2005; Friedman *et al.* 2006). Such relative passivity might be much less appealing where there are violent street markets for crack cocaine.

The strong dependence of retail enforcement on the character of the particular drug market complicates efforts to make summary judgements about its efficacy. A further impediment is the scarcity of empirical research on retail enforcement's effectiveness and its skew toward US-based studies (Scott 2003; Mazerolle *et al.* 2006). However, with some exceptions (e.g. Weatherburn and Lind 1997), the international literature is generally not any more optimistic about the potential of retail drug law enforcement to reduce drug use (cf. Edmunds *et al.* 1996; Best *et al.* 2001b; Wood *et al.* 2004; Kerr *et al.* 2005). Indeed, a recent review of police crackdowns, one of the more popular local drug enforcement tactics, did not even describe reduced drug use as an expected outcome; rather, the objectives were primarily to reduce crime and disorder (Scott 2003).

10.5 **Sentencing**

The emphasis above has been on efforts to apprehend traffickers and dealers and seize their assets and drugs. There remains the question of what is done with offenders once

Table 10.2 Arrest, conviction, and incarceration rates per 100 000 for seven countries, 1999

Country	Arrests	Arrests for trafficking	Convictions	Convictions for trafficking	Sentenced to prison	Average sentence length (months)
France	166	22	40	13	14	15
Germany	226	11	66	7	11	
The Netherlands	73		44		20	13
Sweden	113	19	81		16	15
Switzerland	612	110	111	71	42	11
UK	202	27	93	22	17	29
USA	590	120	125	85	65	30

Source: *European Sourcebook on Crime and Criminal Justice* (2003) and *Uniform Crime Reports* (Federal Bureau of Investigation 1999).

Note: the UK data are for England and Wales only. Although the specific number is not available, most arrests in The Netherlands may be safely assumed to be for trafficking because Dutch police do not make arrests for simple possession of marijuana.

they are apprehended. Table 10.2 presents data from seven developed nations on drug arrests (separately for drug trafficking), convictions (also separated by trafficking), and prison sentences in 1999.[5] The data show large variation in drug arrest rates per capita, even though all seven nations have substantial drug problems. Only in Sweden is marijuana use not normative among recent birth cohorts reaching the age of 21. In Switzerland, the arrest rate per hundred thousand is 612, three times that of neighbouring France and about equal to the US figure (590). Outside of The Netherlands, most arrests in these nations are for drug possession.

Arrest is just the first part of the enforcement process. Greater penalties are associated with convictions and incarceration. A key observation is that drug trafficking is the only drug crime for which an arrest results in a conviction even in a simple majority of cases. Only a minority of drug arrests (other than for trafficking) are followed by a conviction, even in countries such as the USA that have a reputation for tough enforcement. For example, whereas the rate per 100 000 for arrested drug offenders was 612 in Switzerland, the number convicted (i.e. 111) was barely one-sixth as high.

The last two columns of Table 10.2 show the rates at which citizens were sentenced to prison for drug offenses and the mean length of those sentences.[6] Switzerland again

5 Comparable data on sentence length in European nations were not available for any more recent year.

6 Note that time spent incarcerated pre-trial is not necessarily included in these data. Nor do we know what share of the sentence is actually served.

stands out with its relatively high rate of incarceration but relatively low sentence length. The UK has much longer average sentences than any other European country. A very small number of those arrested for drug offences serve time in prison, which is true even when we begin with the numbers arrested for drug trafficking.

The USA has received particular attention because of the size of the population incarcerated for drug offenses, estimated at about 500 000 in 2005 (Caulkins and Chandler 2006), which is more than Western Europe imprisons for all criminal offenses. Each year about 340 000 persons are convicted, and approximately 135 000 receive new prison sentences with an average maximum sentence length of 48 months. The proportion of these sentences actually served varies considerably by state. The low ratio of prison sentences to drug arrests (<10%) is largely explained by the fact that most drug arrests in recent years in the USA have been for simple possession of marijuana.

The high arrest numbers and low prosecution rates in the USA are dominated by low level offenders who are relatively easy to catch and whose incarceration has little impact on the prevalence of crime. From the point of view of objective utility, to respond to a low level crime with a punishment that is highly severe and does little to reduce further crime is hard to justify. But sanction severity is rarely determined only on utilitarian grounds; it is often an expression of the social values of the communities affected by drugs, the members of which often feel moral outrage about drug use and wish that those involved in the trade will be punished. Sometimes this emotional climate can lead to sanction regimes that defeat their own intent. For example, the state of Massachusetts passed a School Zone Statute that imposes a mandatory 2-year sentence on anyone caught dealing within 1000 feet of a school,[7] but most urban areas are within 1000 feet of a school, so the statute does not effectively create graduated sanctions that dissuade selling near schools as opposed to elsewhere. This is one of a number of examples in US drug policy when sentence lengths grew indiscriminately in response to particular crises, whether real or primarily media-driven 'moral panics' (Goode and Ben-Yehuda 1994).

Other nations apply severe sanctions far exceeding those in the USA. Iran may have executed as many as 10 000 drug traffickers in the 1990s (Samii 2003). Human Rights Watch (2004) associates Thailand's 2003 crackdown with 2275 extrajudicial killings over a 3-month period, officially attributed primarily to intergang wars, but at a time when the government was encouraging violence against drug traffickers.

A considerable criminal justice literature seeks to evaluate how imprisoning offenders affects crime generally (Spelman 2000). Arguments have been advanced that long sentences for drug offenders increase non-drug crime (Rasmussen and Benson 1994), for example by displacing more violent criminals from overcrowded prisons. Little is known about the effect that sentence lengths for drug offenders have on drug distribution. Two studies of the possible effects of variations in sentences across jurisdictions in the USA (Bushway *et al.* 2004; Kuziemko and Levitt 2004) failed to find substantial effects of time served on cocaine prices, but that may be explained by weaknesses in

[7] Massachusetts General Laws, C.94C, s.32J.

the data on incarceration length. For example, Kuziemko and Levitt estimate that increasing drug-related incarceration from 82 000 to 376 000 between 1985 and 1996 increased retail cocaine prices by only 5–15% over what they otherwise would have been. Model-based analyses (Rydell and Everingham 1994; Caulkins *et al.* 1997) are somewhat more optimistic but still suggest that reducing use of an established mass-market drug by incarcerating its distributors is expensive, requiring prodigious amounts of incarceration to have a significant impact. Furthermore, those models presume deterrence works more or less the way the economics of crime theories suggest it should. However, the psychological literature on risk perceptions suggests that assumption may be overly optimistic for drug dealers (Caulkins and MacCoun 2005), a population that is particularly prone to value immediate rewards over long-term costs (Bretteville-Jensen 1999; Kirby and Petry 2004).

10.6 **Conclusion and policy implications**

Though developed nations vary considerably in the degree of aggressiveness they bring to supply-oriented enforcement activities, enforcement consumes the largest share of drug-related government spending in many countries (Moore 2005). Even The Netherlands, often stereotyped as being 'soft on drugs', attributes 75% of its total drug policy spending to drug law enforcement (Rigter 2006). It is striking then that so little can be said about how effective such enforcement is in accomplishing its goals.

The Appendix at the end of Chapter 16 summarizes this sparse and spotty literature in a format consistent with that used in the other chapters in this section of the book. However, the reader should be aware that there are essentially no opportunities to study the effects of supply control policies on drug markets with methodological rigour even approaching that of the randomized controlled trial design that is the touchstone of quality for studies of drug treatment and prevention.[8] Furthermore, not only are most conclusions heavily dependent on studies conducted in or from the perspective of the USA, a single supply control intervention may produce inconsistent results within a single country. Results may vary depending on the epidemic stage. For example, supply control may be more effective early, when demand grows rapidly, than it is later, when demand has stabilized and distribution networks have matured (Tragler *et al.* 2001). There is also a dynamic, even competitive component to enforcement against traffickers that can modulate effects. It has been claimed that interdicting the Peruvian air bridge (the route used to fly coca from Peru to processing sites in Colombia) had a noticeable effect on cocaine prices in 1995 (Crane *et al.* 1997), but now that most coca production is within ground or water transport radius of the cocaine production facilities, that same intervention might be much less effective. At a much more local level, idiosyncrasies of the physical, built infrastructure may make a given local policing strategy very effective in one neighbourhood but completely ineffectual in another otherwise similar neighbourhood (Caulkins *et al.* 1993).

[8] For an assessment of the difficulties faced by such studies in policing generally see National Research Council (2005).

Hence, the effectiveness statements in the Appendix pertain to potential for effectiveness, not guarantees of effectiveness.

Finally, it is important to ask: 'Effective at what?' Interventions that reduce drug demand generally reduce not only drug use but also many other measures of drug-related problems (e.g. drug-related crime, morbidity, and mortality). In contrast, there is perennial concern that supply-side interventions might reduce drug use at the cost of raising drug-related consequences per unit of use and perhaps drug-related consequences in total. The classic example used to illustrate the concept is the possibility that driving up price will suppress use somewhat, but less than proportionately (see this chapter's earlier discussion of demand elasticity), leading to increased spending on drugs and, perhaps, increased drug-related crime. For all these reasons, the judgements embodied in this chapter are more tentative and more speculative than are those reflected in the other intervention chapters.

Any discussion of policy implications of the evidence reviewed above depends largely on what types of evidence one requires before reaching a judgement and making a recommendation. Anyone who waits for an evidence base that is rigorous by the usual standards applied in health research would say there are few if any implications of any kind to date, nor should more be expected in the future given the limitations inherent in studying interventions on markets and the lack of research in the area (Reuter 2001).

For those willing to draw tentative conclusions based on an amalgam of evidence and arguments of a more general sort, four observations can be made. First, we should not regard alternative development as a drug use control programme given the lack of even case study evidence suggesting that it has had a noticeable effect on use in a downstream market country. Alternative development can be appealing for humanitarian reasons in those countries where it has been shown to reduce poverty. But promoting alternative development as part of global *drug* control is fundamentally unwarranted; if it has a role in a drug policy portfolio, that role has little to do with reducing drug use.

Secondly, other interventions far up the distribution chain (e.g. crop eradication, interdiction, precursor controls) have apparently in the past produced transient market disruptions sufficient to affect drug use and related health outcomes. But success cannot be replicated consistently because it appears to depend on a fortuitous convergence of circumstances. The scientific literature offers no more than educated guesses for when such interventions are or are not likely to achieve noticeable market disruptions.

Thirdly, the evidence concerning effectiveness is weakest for high level domestic investigations, but it is precisely at that level that such evidence is least relevant. High level dealers operating within a country suffering a substantial drug problem may become enforcement targets out of a sense of what is just, rather than a commitment to efficient public health intervention. However, given that such criminals are apprehended, there remains the question of how severely they should be punished. What little evidence exists suggests that there may be diminishing returns to drug policy goals from extending periods of incarceration, but such beliefs depend as much on deductive economic arguments as on empirical evaluations.

Finally, local or street-level enforcement is probably not a viable strategy for reducing drug use. Rather, its primary effects may be controlling harms associated with drug markets (as discussed in Chapter 5), encouraging dependent users to make contact with service providers, and expressing the moral outrage of some people who live in those communities.

We conclude with one over-riding analytical observation: supply control interventions absorb the bulk of drug control spending in most nations, even nations that have a reputation for tolerating drug use. The evidence base concerning these interventions is distressingly weak. That is in no small part due to inevitable challenges of evaluating interventions for which the market is the unit of analysis. However, it is also due to gross neglect by the funding and research communities. An Expert Committee in the USA bemoaned that 'What we don't know keeps hurting us' (Manski *et al.* 2001) a decade after the journal *Science* observed that we were 'Still flying blind in the war on drugs' (*Science* 1990). In 2010, little has changed. Governments are still flying blind.

Chapter 11

Criminalization and decriminalization of drug use or possession

11.1 Introduction

The previous chapter focused on efforts to reduce drug problems by cutting off the supply of illicit drugs. As noted in that chapter, these efforts focus on the producers or distributors of the drugs, and not on the users, except to the extent that a user is also involved in production or distribution.

At both the international and national level, drug control efforts have also been aimed at the user by criminalizing or otherwise punishing possession or use of illicit drugs. As a practical matter, criminalizing possession can also be used as a tool for enforcing laws against suppliers. (It is easier to catch a dealer in possession of drugs than it is to catch him or her at the moment of making a sale.) Nevertheless, punishing the user is a substantial step beyond prohibiting sale or production of the drug, often involving efforts to police otherwise private behaviour. The federal alcohol Prohibition in the USA from 1919 to 1932, for instance, did not take this step. The focus was on cutting off the trade in alcoholic beverages, and possession or use of alcohol was not criminalized in federal law.

At the international level, the requirement that nations criminalize the possession or use of illicit drugs came relatively late to the drug control system. The 1961 international Convention requires each country, 'subject to its constitutional limitations', to outlaw possession of controlled substances (Article 36). While there have been doubts about whether this required criminalization of use, many countries had criminalized possession or use of controlled substances long before 1988, when the doubt was removed by Article 3, Section 1 of the 1988 Convention, which required possession or purchase of controlled substances to be punished 'as criminal offences under its domestic law'.

Looking globally, the great increase in arrests and criminal processing for possession or use has happened since the 1970s, in parallel with the rapid growth in illicit drug use. The rise in arrests and convictions partly reflected the growth in use, but it is also likely to have reflected the attempts of legislative and administrative bodies at national and subnational levels to deter drug use by enacting or raising criminal penalties for it. Arrests have continued to grow in the last 10 years, which seems to reflect intensified enforcement against cannabis in particular (Room *et al.* 2008).

Starting in the 1970s, a counter-trend to this increased criminalization emerged in a number of countries, including the USA, as rates of use grew. The counter-trend applied primarily to cannabis, but in three countries (Italy, Portugal, and Spain) also to other controlled substances. In the USA, politicians and opinion leaders in a number of states responded in part to the fact that young people of the middle class, often including their own children, were getting swept up in the criminal justice system by the criminal laws on possession of cannabis. This precipitated efforts to mitigate these effects by reducing the penalties for cannabis possession. Since this trend was controversial, a substantial evaluative literature has grown up around the reductions in penalties, which can be seen as offering evidence on the effects of various kinds and degrees of criminalization of drug possession and use. After presenting an analytical framework for how enforcement against users should operate, drawing on the framework used for enforcement against supplies in Chapter 10, this chapter summarizes this evidence.

The existing literature has mostly studied changes in one direction. Studies of the effects of legislation about the penalization of drug use or possession are overwhelmingly concerned with the reduction or elimination of penalties, and most of these studies concern cannabis.[1] Our review of the effects of punishing the user is thus primarily based on studies of what happened when punishments for cannabis use, possession, or growing for one's own use are reduced, changed, or abolished.

11.2 **Analytical framework**

We build on the analysis of Chapter 10 by noting that enforcement can reduce demand via deterrence, incapacitation, and/or rehabilitation.

11.2.1 **Deterrence**

Threatening to arrest, fine, or incarcerate drug users simply for possessing drugs may induce people to cease or reduce drug use by raising the risks of buying drugs. The same mechanism may also lead fewer persons to initiate drug use. This hypothesis reflects a direct effect on demand consistent with a variety of economic analyses (Model 1993; Pacula *et al.* 2001; Farrelly *et al.* 2001; DeSimone and Farrelly 2003; but see Friedman *et al.* 2006) as well as some literature on drink-driving (e.g. Voas *et al.* 1997; Shults *et al.* 2001). For youth, the enforcers and sanctions against users are often outside of the formal criminal justice system: parents revoking car privileges, sports teams barring participation, and schools temporarily suspending students. Even though those enforcers do not prosecute formally, their actions may deter.

Kleiman (2009; see also Harrell *et al.* 2003) has shown that the addition of minor but certain penalties causes substantial decreases in drug use by felony probationers. Specifically, the addition of regular urine screens followed by immediate penalties for

[1] A similar situation exists for the literature on the effects of availability controls for alcohol: most of the studies of the effects of limits on hours and days of sale and on density of outlets, for instance, have studied the effects of removing the restrictions (Room 2002b).

dirty urines to the probation regime (e.g. a trial that same day and a 24-hour jail term beginning that night or the next day) was sufficient incentive for the majority of drug-involved probationers to complete a full year of abstinence. Strikingly, the warning of the new procedure alone was sufficient in many cases to deter drug use. Of those who experienced one sanction, fewer than half earned a second sanction, going through the rest of the year with no dirty urines.

11.2.2 **Incapacitation**

A very small fraction of the user population is in prison for violating drug possession laws, even in the USA (Caulkins and Sevigny 2005), but incapacitation can nonetheless substantially affect demand in countries that have high incarceration rates for drug selling and for other offences (robbery, murder, etc.). Approximately 2.25 million people were incarcerated in the USA in 2005 for all crimes combined. Most of them, including both drug dealers and other offenders, used some illicit drug other than cannabis recently before arrest (NIJ 2003). Approximately one-third—or 750 000—tested positive for cocaine, indicating recent use. A large proportion of those cocaine users were dependent users (NIJ 2004), but few managed to continue use in prison (Feucht and Keyser 1999). The US **ONDCP** (2001b) estimates that about 85% of US cocaine demand is attributable to the approximately 2.7 million chronic users who are not currently incarcerated. If this estimate is correct, it can be inferred that roughly 15–20% (85% × 750 000/(750 000 + 2 700 000)) of all potential cocaine demand in the USA is incapacitated by law enforcement.

Incapacitation probably has a much smaller effect in other countries. We make the comparison in terms of general incarceration rates for Western Europe. The USA incarceration rate was 738 per 100 000 in 2005; the rate for France, Germany, and Italy was only 95 per 100 000. Even though US rates of problematic use are higher than those for Western European countries, the difference is much smaller than the incarceration difference. For example, Germany has a problematic drug use rate of 330 per 100 000 compared with a counterpart rate of about 1000 per 100 000 for the USA. Thus, even if the incarcerated population is just as drug involved as that in the USA, the share of total potential drug consumption that is averted through imprisonment of the users would be much smaller. It should not be assumed without evidence, either, that drug users have no access to drugs while incarcerated.

11.2.3 **Rehabilitation**

The criminal justice system can also reduce drug demand via rehabilitation of convicted drug-involved offenders, either through treatment in prison or by coercing offenders to enter and persist in treatment (e.g. drug courts and drug diversion programmes). For example, the UK saw a doubling of treatment enrolment between 1997/98 and 2005/06, largely reflecting referrals from the criminal justice system (Reuter and Stevens 2007).

The remainder of this chapter deals only with the deterrent effects of enforcement against users. There is no research on any incapacitation effects and little on population-level effects of prison rehabilitation; the latter are discussed in the context of treatment programmes in Chapters 9 and 15.

11.3 The many forms of reducing or removing criminal penalties

A fundamental challenge when designing a deterrence regime is deciding how 'tough' to be and how to be tough. Criminology in general has found that certainty of punishment is more important than severity of penalty (Kleiman 2009; Nagin 1998). But legislators continue to be attracted by the idea that a tough law will be a stronger deterrent. It can be argued that the best solution for a deterrence regime is to appear tough but actually to be soft. Apparent severity is a better deterrent, but after deterrence has failed and someone has been arrested, gentler is better because actually imposing the threatened sanction is costly, both to the offender and to society. The latter consideration becomes particularly salient when the purpose of the deterrence is at least in part to protect the offender from his or her own behaviour. Hence fines for speeding, which directly threatens others as well as the speeder, are typically higher than for driving without a seatbelt or riding a motorcycle without a helmet. However, looking tough but acting soft is always an unstable solution in an open and democratic society: it is easily attacked as hypocritical, and the news about the softness cannot be indefinitely suppressed.

Legislators and enforcers in many places have struggled with this dilemma concerning possession and use of drugs in recent decades. A great variety of approaches have been taken in various places over time. Because the terminology used for these efforts has varied confusingly, it is important to define key terms. *Decriminalization* typically means removal of criminal penalties; *depenalization* typically means reduction in severity of penalties, e.g. elimination of a prison term, yet can still mean a criminal penalty. Thus, decriminalization is a subform of depenalization. There is no commonly accepted term for removing all penalties, criminal or civil, on use or possession. This is often spoken of as 'legalization', but few would describe the situation that existed for alcohol during the US Prohibition, for instance, as 'legalization'. Moreover, legalization suggests a broader policy also eliminating prohibition of supply in some way.

The confusion over language reflects the great variety of efforts that have been taken in one place or another to mitigate what are perceived as harms arising from strict application of laws criminalizing use or possession of one or more controlled substances. These include the following:

- Shifting from conventional criminal penalties to some other form of non-criminal or civil penalty, often in a legal category such as a parking or minor traffic ticket (e.g. cannabis expiation notices since 1987 in South Australia).
- Reducing the level of criminal penalties (e.g. in the 1970s several US states shifted cannabis possession from a felony to a misdemeanour crime, which reduced the possible maximum sentence).
- Abolishing criminal laws on use of drugs (e.g. Spain in 1983, although possession in public was re-criminalized in 1992; an Alaskan court in 2006 freed possession of a small amount of cannabis in the user's home or residence from penalty or sanctions in that US state).

- Various forms of alternative handling for persons picked up by the police for drug use or possession. These include informal handling by the police short of arrest—for instance, 'cautioning' and 'warning' in the UK.
- Other forms of alternative handling, for instance diversion to mandated education or treatment. This can be in lieu of criminal conviction. Portugal's decriminalization of drugs in 2001 provided that cases of possession or use of drugs should be referred to Commissions for the Dissuasion of Drug Addiction. Or it can be subsequent to criminal conviction. California's Proposition 36, passed by referendum in 2000, provides that someone convicted of a non-violent drug offence for the first or second time is put on probation and is referred to a certified drug treatment programme.
- *De facto* legalization of purchase and sale of small amounts, even while possession is kept technically illegal and production is still strictly prohibited. This is the well-known case of The Netherlands system for cannabis, with the primary aim of separating the markets for cannabis and for 'hard drugs'.

In what follows, we consider the available evidence on the effects of changing laws or penalties on personal use or possession. As noted, most of the evidence is from changes in one direction, reducing or eliminating penalties. One exception, discussed below, is the carefully evaluated criminalization of possession and use of a range of illicit drugs in the Czech Republic in 1998. Otherwise, there certainly have been shifts to tougher penalties and to more aggressive enforcement under the same set of penalties. For example, the numbers of arrests for cannabis possession rose from 226 000 in 1991 to 505 000 in 1995 in the USA and to over 700 000 in 2006, while in Switzerland cannabis possession arrests rose from 15 500 in 1997 to 26 000 in 2002. These changes have attracted minimal research. Pacula and colleagues (2004), in one of the few papers examining both increases and decreases, find no evidence that variation in cannabis arrest rates has an effect on the prevalence of cannabis use. However, the underlying methodology is not a strong one, since it cannot disentangle the effects of use on policies.

Beyond the population-level effects of laws and penalties, research on the effects of 'criminalization' of cannabis use also demonstrates a number of personal, social, and economic consequences to the individual drug user. Here the term criminalization refers to the process leading up to and including the finding of guilt for a criminal offence, as well as the consequences following the designation of a criminal label. In one study of 95 'cannabis criminals' in Ontario (Erickson 1980), it was found that there were substantial costs to the individual of being treated as a criminal (effects on first offenders' self-perceptions, family relationships, and on their employment) going well beyond the penalties imposed by the criminal justice system itself.

11.4 **Effects of changes in the kind or degree of criminalization of drug use or possession**

Six interventions or strategies have been aimed at deterring drug use and reducing the societal costs of managing drug users in the criminal justice system.

11.4.1 Shifting from conventional criminal penalties to another form of penalty

The distinction between this category of change and the next, reduction of criminal penalties, is not clear-cut. The boundary between what is a 'crime' and what is something else (an 'infraction', a 'civil penalty', etc.) varies with the legal system and over time. An offence with a maximum penalty of a trivial fine may still be legally a crime, while civil penalties may be very substantial, as for example with day-fines in Scandinavia. However, shifting possession or use out of the category of 'crime' is in itself a reduction in penalty, since there are often legal disabilities entrained by classifying an infraction as a crime, apart from any stigma attached to being a 'criminal'. Thus the shift by Western Australia to 'cannabis expiation notices' in part catered to the wanderlust of young middle-class Australians, who would be denied entry to the USA if they had to report having been convicted of a crime.

In 1973, Oregon changed the status of the offence of possessing less than one ounce of cannabis from a crime to a civil violation, with a maximum penalty of a US$100 fine (Single 1989). A number of US state and local jurisdictions followed suit in reducing the penalties for possession of small amounts of cannabis in the period spanning 1975–1978, though whether a shift out of criminal status was involved in these changes varied among the 'decriminalizing' states (Pacula *et al.* 2004).

The most extensive recent studies of the effects of changes from criminal to other penalties have been the studies of the effects of the shifts in Australia from criminal conviction and penalties to an 'infringement' notice in South Australia in 1987, the Australian Capital Territory (ACT; Canberra and surroundings) in 1992, and in Western Australia in 2004. These schemes also allowed for cultivation of a small number of plants for personal use; that clause is unique to the Australian jurisdictions and there is no discussion of how it might independently affect outcomes. In terms of effects on reported patterns of use, Donnelly and colleagues (1999, 2000) found that adjusted prevalence rates of ever having used cannabis rose from 26 to 36% in South Australia in the 10 years between 1985 and 1995, but that there had also been increases in the same general range in Australian states that maintained criminal laws on possession (26–32% in Victoria, 26–33% in New South Wales, and 21–33% in Tasmania). Specifically for 14- to 29-year-olds, the age group with the highest rates of initiation and regular use, trends in lifetime use and in weekly cannabis use did not significantly differ between South Australia and the rest of Australia. Individual state sample sizes were small, so this was a low-powered test. In surveys of schoolchildren aged 11–16 in South Australia each year from 1986 to 1989, cannabis use levels remained stable (Neill *et al.* 1991; Donnelly *et al.* 1992). A study of the effects on student cannabis use of the similar decriminalization in the ACT, with students in Victoria as a control group, found that lifetime use and frequent use did not vary between 1992, before the change, and 1994 (McGeorge and Aitken 1997).

Cameron and Williams (2001) and Williams (2003) examine the effect of cannabis decriminalization on several waves of the Australian household survey (1988, 1991, 1993, and 1995). Importantly, and unlike other studies, they control for variation in the price of cannabis as well as the change in policy. Cameron and Williams (2001) find that when price is controlled for, living in a state that has decriminalized cannabis use increases the probability of participation. They note, however, that decriminalization was adopted in South Australia before their time period so they could not disentangle the effect of decriminalization from a 'South Australian' effect. Hence, Williams (2003) extended the analysis and incorporated data through 1998, which included new states that had changed policy, again finding a positive and statistically significant effect of cannabis decriminalization on the annual prevalence of cannabis use for specific demographic groups in the population. More specifically, living in a state that has decriminalized has a larger effect on individuals 25 years or older, and, when the policy is evaluated for the population as a whole, the effects disappear as they are offset by statistically insignificant findings for the younger population which are less sensitive to a change in this policy. This is consistent with evidence from the USA that finds a larger impact of penalties on older than younger groups (Saffer and Chaloupka 1999a; Farrelly *et al.* 2001).

In terms of social impacts of civil versus criminal penalties, Lenton and colleagues (1999, 2000b) compared matched pairs of first-time-apprehended cannabis users in South Australia and Western Australia, at a time when there were still criminal penalties in Western Australia. The Western Australian respondents were significantly more likely to report adverse employment consequences (32% versus 2%), further contact with the criminal justice system (32% versus 0%), relationship problems (20% versus 5%), and accommodation difficulties (16% versus 0%) that could be attributed to their apprehension. As compared with the South Australian respondents, the Western Australian respondents also reported being less trusting and more fearful of the police as a result of the apprehension.

An unanticipated consequence of the shift to cannabis expiation notices in South Australia was a substantial shift in police behaviour. The expiation notice was easier to implement than an arrest, and perhaps for this reason the number of notices issued grew by over 250% between 1987/88 and 1993/94. Further, only 45% of those issued notices paid their fines by the due date, with those who were poorer less likely to pay; those who did not pay risked incarceration (Christie and Ali 2000). The South Australian scheme thus resulted in substantial 'net widening', with more rather than fewer cases brought into the criminal justice system. These issues were to some extent addressed in the Western Australian scheme, which allowed a further 2 months after the due date for payment of the fine, under threat of losing one's driver's licence. It is estimated that this brought the compliance rate up to 75%. The extent of net widening from the Western Australian scheme is estimated at only 14%, compared with 250% for the South Australian scheme (Swensen 2007).

All told, there is evidence from the Australian experience that decriminalization and replacement with civil penalties had a beneficial effect in the lives of those apprehended by the police for cannabis possession, though more were apprehended since it became easier for the police to do so. On the other side of the ledger, the Australian evidence shows that effects on patterns of cannabis use are small, particularly for younger users. It is hard to interpret the results in terms of deterrent effect, since larger numbers of individuals received lesser sanctions.

The effects of the changes of the 1970s have been described in a number of North American reports and papers. For instance, a pioneering study of the effect of a municipal cannabis law in Ann Arbor, Michigan, which sought to over-ride state law by which possession was a felony crime and reduced the maximum penalty for cannabis use to a fine of US$5, did not find any impact on cannabis use in high school student surveys, in comparison with three neighbouring communities that did not reduce penalties (Stuart *et al.* 1976). However, the study does not address the issue of what actually happened concerning any concurrent enforcement of the state law. Ten years after California lowered the penalty for possession of small amounts of cannabis to a summons and fine, an analysis of emergency room admissions and street-level arrests concluded on the basis of these two indicators that the change 'did not cause a rise in the use of that drug' (Mandel 1987).

Re-analysing data from four US national drug surveys between 1972 and 1977, Saveland and Bray (1981) found that cannabis use was higher in the 'decriminalizing' states, both before and after the changes in the law, perhaps reflecting changes in enforcement intensity that antedated changes in the formal law. Another reanalysis, of the Monitoring the Future national surveys of high school students (Johnston *et al.* 1981), concluded that decriminalization had no effect either on rates of cannabis use or on attitudes and beliefs about cannabis use. However, Model (1993) analysed emergency room data and found that decriminalization was associated with substantial increases in the number of cases involving cannabis and reductions in mentions for other substances. This is the only study with a positive finding, but the methodology was unusually strong.

These specific studies are representative of a fairly substantial evaluative literature in the first years of the changes, much of which was reviewed by Eric Single (1981, 1989). Single concluded that 'the available evidence indicates that the decriminalization of cannabis possession had little or no impact on rates of use' (Single 1989).

Two important limitations of this early literature are that studies did not generally control for either cannabis prices or for changes in enforcement and legal penalties apart from the formal statutory change. This is problematic because Farrelly and colleagues (2001, p. 51) find 'evidence that both higher fines for cannabis possession and increased probability of arrest decrease the probability that a young adult will use cannabis' and Pacula *et al.* (2003) show that the estimated effects of legal penalties on cannabis use are influenced by the way in which the law is enforced. Pacula and colleagues (2004) deconstruct the dichotomy on 'decriminalization' generally used in these analyses and show how problematic the previous characterization is. Of the 12 'decriminalizing' states, four kept possession as a misdemeanour or felony crime, while by the 1990s seven other 'non-decriminalizing' states did not criminalize a first-time cannabis possession offence. Similarly, the arrest rates in decriminalizing jurisdictions were comparable with those in the others, reflecting the fact that many arrests involve the offence of use in public, which is not typically covered by the decriminalization.

In recent years, the literature on the effects of these US changes has grown considerably, drawing heavily on analyses of the large survey data sets that began to come on line around 1990, comparing respondents in the 'decriminalizing' states and other states. According to one review of the more recent literature (Pacula *et al.* 2004), the evidence examining the effects of decriminalization policy on use rates in the USA is mixed. But these studies are largely cross-sectional econometric analyses. A cross-sectional analysis, however many other variables are controlled for, is very weak evidence concerning causality. For example, while Saffer and colleagues (2001) report that 'Marijuana decriminalization was found to increase the probability of marijuana participation by about 8%', that should not be interpreted as causal evidence. Much more compelling are '**natural experiment**' studies: before-and-after studies, if possible with controls, of effects of the policy change. Those results (e.g. Johnson *et al.* 1981; Model 1993) are conflicting.

A key weakness of most studies in this area, including the older and the more recent research, is that they implicitly assume that the law prior to the change was routinely enforced. Without knowing the extent to which law enforcement officers make cannabis a priority and follow the letter of the law, one cannot conclude that a weakening of *de jure* sanctions has actually resulted in a change in the typical interactions of police officers and cannabis users. One study (Williams 2003) shows that in Australia estimates of the impact of cannabis decriminalization on cannabis use are very sensitive to the inclusion of data on the penalties imposed for use offences (i.e. fines and imprisonment).

A recent paper (MacCoun *et al.* 2008) finds that knowledge of the penalties for cannabis use in the USA is very inaccurate. Dividing states into those that have removed the threat of incarceration and those that have not, MacCoun and colleagues report that in four waves of the National Survey on Drug Use and Health similar proportions of respondents in the two groups of states believe that this offence would be potentially punishable by a jail term. Thus one reason for finding little effect of differences in law in recent years is simply that residents of different states are not well informed.

There has been little analysis of the variation in arrest rates for drug offences across states. As noted above, Farrelly and colleagues (2001) found that higher arrest rates did reduce the probably that a young adult would use cannabis.

11.4.2 Changing the level of criminal penalties

While consumption of cannabis remains prohibited by law in Switzerland, there is considerable variation among the 26 cantons in how and to what extent the law is applied. Using cross-sectional data on Swiss 15-year-olds in the Health Behaviour of School Children study, Schmid (2001) found no evidence that the arrest rate per capita was related to the rate of cannabis use in that age group.

11.4.3 Abolishing or introducing criminal laws on use of drugs

As already noted, the Czech Republic criminalized the possession and use of a range of drugs in 1998, after sharp controversy and over the veto of President Vaclac Havel. In the aftermath the government commissioned a substantial evaluative study by a group of Czech experts, advised by US academics (Moravek 2008). In a descriptive analysis, time trends in Czech data were compared with prior time trends. Several propositions about the effects of the introduction of penalties for the possession of illicit drugs for personal use were tested with quantitative data. The propositions that 'availability of illicit drugs will decrease' and that the 'number of [...] illicit drug users will decrease' or at least stabilize were rejected on the basis of the study, while a number of other hypotheses could not be reliably tested. Qualitative studies filled out the picture of the effects of the legislation, including no evidence of effects on 'drug scenes'. However, the new law provided the police with opportunities to pressure persons of interest for other reasons. One law enforcement informant commented about this, 'I must admit it is not completely legal. In a way, it is a bit of blackmail' (Zabransky *et al.* 2001). While penalties for possession for personal use were only enforced randomly and occasionally in the 2 years after adoption of the legislation, there were substantial costs to the state from the legislation, without any apparent benefit (Zabransky *et al.* 2001).

Italy has had a complex history concerning penalization of drug use or possession. A strict penal regime dating from the 1950s was succeeded by a full decriminalization of use or possession in 1975. Personal drug use was re-criminalized in 1990, and decriminalized again in 1993. Though this seems to offer a wonderful research opportunity to investigate the effects of large-scale changes, the available data are few and little analysis has been done. The available indicators were of drug-related arrests, incarcerations, deaths, AIDS cases, treatment admissions, and police drug seizures (Solivetti 2001), all of which are influenced by changes in response systems as well as in drug-using behaviour. While overdose deaths fell after the 1990 re-criminalization, that also occurred in Germany and Spain. Moreover there was also a decline in the number much later in the 1990s. Treatment numbers rose steadily throughout the period 1984–1997. Solivetti (2001) argues that there is little visible impact of the various changes, but this must remain a tentative conclusion.

MacCoun and Reuter (2001b) examined retrospectively the effects of the introduction of the system of *de facto* legal distribution in The Netherlands. Starting in 1976, the Dutch government allowed a few outlets (including youth clubs and coffee shops) to sell small quantities; this was much more restrictive than the broad distribution system that emerged in the mid-1980s. In comparative analyses involving 28 different studies, MacCoun and Reuter (2001b) concluded that this decriminalization in The Netherlands had little effect on cannabis use. Their further conclusions about the later functioning of the coffee shop system are discussed below.

11.4.4 **Measures involving informal handling by the police short of arrest**

British police have long had a procedure for a formal cautioning of an apprehended person, rather than arresting them, in case of a minor offence. Unlike a warning, a caution requires the admission of the crime, and goes in the police records. With variations from place to place, cautioning rather than arrest had long been used in England and Wales for minor cannabis possession offences. An increasing share of all police apprehensions for cannabis took the form of cautions; whereas in 1985 cautioning accounted for about 12% of all dispositions for drug offences, by 1997 the figure was about 50% (Independent Inquiry into the Misuse of Drugs Act 1971 2000, p. 30). In 2004, the British government reclassified cannabis from a Class B to a Class C drug (lowering the potential penalties) under the national drug control legislation, though a specific clause in that 2004 reclassification allowed the police to make an arrest, which was not the case for any other Class C drug; in 2008, the government decided against professional advice to change the classification back again. There is no full study of the effects of the 2004 reclassification on cannabis use, which reduced the criminal penalties for possession. The British Crime Survey figures show that cannabis use started decreasing around 1998, well before the change. As measured by use in the previous 12 months, it decreased thereafter (Nicholas *et al.* 2007) from about 10.5% for 16- to 59-year-olds in the 5 years before the change to 8.2% in 2006/07, and from 26 to 20.9% among 16- to 24-year-olds. Police contacts for cannabis use increased, from 88 263 in 2004/05 to 130 406 in 2006/07. Nicholas and colleagues (2007) note that this may reflect increased use of warnings for cannabis, rather than real changes in its incidence. Official encouragement of the police to use measures other than arrest seems to have resulted in 'net widening', as in the South Australian experience. It is possible that the police cautioning efforts played a role in pushing down consumption, although the proportion of cannabis users with a police contact concerning drugs within a year remained below 5%.

11.4.5 **Diversion to mandated education or treatment**

Portugal removed the personal possession and use of all controlled drugs from the criminal law in 2001, but maintained their formal illegality as offences. Instead, a system of referral of offenders to Commissions for the Dissuasion of Drug Addiction (CDTs) was set up, with treatment offered to all identified as having a drug use problem. Police refer offenders to the CDT (a three-person panel comprising a medical professional, a social worker, and a legal adviser), with a mandate to appear within 72 hours. Apart from treatment, the CDT can also impose penalties such as fines, community service, and banning the person from designated places (Hughes and Stevens 2007).

From interviews with key informants, Hughes and Stevens (2007) found that there had been difficulties with the operation of the CDTs, and views varied on how the system should be further changed. Presentations for treatment for heroin problems had declined and for cannabis problems had increased. Between 1999 and 2003, there had been a 59% fall in drug deaths, and a 17% reduction in notifications of new drug-related HIV cases. Meanwhile, cannabis use reported among Portuguese 16-year-olds in the ESPAD school survey had increased from 9.4% in 1999 to 15.1% in 2003. However, cannabis use had also increased in the ESPAD surveys in other southern European countries (specifically, Spain and Italy) in this period, in the absence of the Portuguese law change. The extent to which the reform had effects on drug use behaviour is thus unclear. A more recent study by Greenwald (2009), using data through 2006, was consistent with the findings of Hughes and Stevens (2007).

In California, Proposition 36, passed by an initiative referendum in 2000, provided that eligible non-violent drug offenders on their first or second such arrest could avoid incarceration, but rather should receive a probationary sentence conditional on completing a certified drug treatment programme; 30% failed to show up for treatment and many others did not complete treatment but received no penalty for doing so

(Kleiman 2009). The measure is thus a post-conviction diversion measure, with the effect of depenalization for those successfully complying with its requirements. Other states have implemented programmes that are similar in spirit, beginning with Arizona's Proposition 200 in 1996.

The final report of the evaluation programme for the Proposition (Integrated Substance Abuse Programs 2007) reports that in the Proposition's fourth year, 75% of the 48 473 offenders referred under it actually entered treatment, and that 32% of those who had entered the previous year completed treatment. Almost half of those treated had at least 90 days of treatment. Reoffending rates were, as might be expected, less for those who completed treatment than for those who did not. But there were more new arrests for programme participants than for an equivalent cohort before the era of the Proposition, which the report notes is probably due to greater opportunity to offend because of more time in the community. The report attempted to test any impact of the Proposition on trends in the statewide crime rates, and found no significant effects. However, the statistical power available was limited, because of delays in the availability of crime statistics. Another impact of the Proposition, a separate study has suggested, has been some displacement of voluntary clients in the drug treatment system by those mandated under the Proposition (Hser *et al.* 2007).

The cases that enter the system created by Proposition 36 are relatively serious and experienced drug users. California police in practice are not arresting neophytes caught experimenting with cannabis. Methamphetamine is the drug most commonly involved. Cost analyses focusing on outcomes for the offenders themselves (i.e. ignoring potential spillover effects) suggest that Proposition 36 diversion results in significant budgetary savings (estimated at US$2.50 for every US$1 invested), since reduced prison and jail costs offset greater spending on treatment and higher re-arrest rates (Integrated Substance Abuse Programs 2007). Broken down by prior record, the results look best for offenders with shorter criminal histories and much less favourable for those with five or more prior convictions.

11.4.6 **Switching between prohibition and *de facto* full legalization with a controlled market**

Only the Dutch coffee shops offer the opportunity to study the case of switching between a regime prohibiting personal use or possession and a regime where a drug cannot only be used and possessed but also purchased. We have already discussed above the *de facto* removal of all penalties for personal use which is involved in this system. However, the system extends beyond this to a highly regulated retail sale system. The system was cobbled together pragmatically as a compromise between conflicting goals. A primary aim was to separate the market for cannabis from the market for 'hard' drugs. One might say, indeed, that the driving consideration was a Dutch version of the 'stepping-stone' theory. If one could separate cannabis transactions from the market for other controlled drugs, then cannabis use would be less likely to be a stepping stone to other drug use. The general conclusion is that with respect to this goal, the system has been relatively successful. Compared with Amsterdam, where only 15% reported that other drugs were available from the same source that supplied their cannabis, about half of users in Bremen and San Francisco reported that other drugs were available (Borches-Tempel and Kolte 2002). However, the ESPAD survey of 16-year-olds found little difference between German and Dutch 16-year-olds in how easy they perceived it to get various classes of drugs. On the other hand, substantially higher proportions of US teenagers reported it would be easy (Hibell *et al.* 2004, p. 415). Only one analysis has examined whether cannabis users in The Netherlands (Amsterdam) were less likely than those in other countries (San Francisco, USA) to go on to use harder drugs. In this analysis (Reinarman 2009), lifetime use of other drugs by cannabis users was found to be higher in San Francisco than in Amsterdam. There is some suggestion in this that the 'separation of markets' in the Dutch system may affect cannabis users' use of other drugs. The study suffers from the usual problem of cross-sectional comparisons, this time with a sample of just three jurisdictions. Also, the choice of an exceptionally liberal city, San Francisco, to represent the USA limits the persuasiveness of the study's findings.

A conflicting goal was to keep the Dutch system as far as possible within the bounds of the international drug control treaties. Since these treaties do not allow any private entrepreneurs selling to a non-medical market, and require that sales and use be criminalized, there are two major quirks in the Dutch system. None of the actions involved in the coffee shop market is actually legalized. They are simply tolerated, so long as the actors obey a set of quite specific guidelines on conditions of sale and use. And the system has what is known as its 'back door problem'. Once the cannabis is for sale on the counter of the coffee shop, its sale is tolerated (though not technically legal). But there is no official tolerance for how the supplies come in the back door of the coffee shop, i.e. for growing and wholesale distribution. In its present form, the system is thus necessarily criminogenic: someone has to provide that supply, somehow.

MacCoun and Reuter (2001b) argue that, while there was no apparent change in use at the inception of the system, as the system grew and became more commercialized in the 1990s the use of cannabis in The Netherlands increased—in terms of use in the past month, from 8.5 to 18.5% in the period 1984–1996. Though MacCoun and Reuter point out that the increases in prevalence in The Netherlands in the early 1990s were similar to trends that occurred then in Canada, Norway, the USA, and the UK, they argue that the increases before the early 1990s were distinctive to The Netherlands and may be the result of the shift to a more accessible and commercial regime. Other researchers (e.g. Korf 2002) have argued against this interpretation, giving more emphasis to the latter period. It is worth noting that, despite the relatively easy access to cannabis that the Dutch (over the age of 17) have had for two decades now, prevalence of use remains in the middle of the European countries.

11.5 **Conclusion**

As summarized in the Appendix at the end of this book, most interventions aimed at deterring drug use and reducing societal costs of managing drug users in the criminal justice system show modest effectiveness, but the amount of research has been minimal and the evidence base is concentrated in only a few countries.

The evaluative record seems fairly consistent for cannabis. There is no clear-cut case in which a reduction in the form or enforcement of the prohibition on use or possession resulted in a substantial change in consumption of the drug. There are a number of cases where there was no measurable change in consumption from such a policy change. For other drugs, Kleiman (2009) has shown the power of sanctions to reduce hard drug use (mainly amphetamine) in the unusually controlled setting provided by the criminal justice system. In the more open system of societies as a whole, reductions in penalties for hard drugs have never been evaluated in a high quality, convincing study, leaving science agnostic as to their effects.

Of course, the evaluative literature we have been considering is drawn from a narrow range of societies, all of which are relatively affluent and open. In such societies, there are cultural and ideological limits to the central direction and monitoring of personal behaviour. Thus the findings of the evaluation studies might well not apply concerning prohibition and punishment for possession and use in a tight village society, for instance, where young people's behaviour may be closely monitored. Kleiman's (2009) work seems to indicate that even within open societies, there are tightly controlled subsystems, e.g. the probation system, where penalties for drug use can be highly effective.

Neither would the conclusion about cannabis suggested here be likely to apply, for example, to use or possession of opium in China in the 1950s, where opium use could be seen as a product of foreign imperialism, and orders were being given by a government with the enormous moral authority of having won a revolution. In such a circumstance, banning possession and use was apparently highly effective (Yungming 2000). The changed policy toward drugs was part of a much larger societal change.

There are three other limitations of the research that bear noting. First, as mentioned, cannabis is the main drug about which there is a significant body of evidence on the effects of changes in legal regime. Though it is by far the most widely used illicit drug, it is also not considered a major source of social and health harms when compared with cocaine or heroin. Moreover, the patterns of use are very different in many respects. Secondly, the analyses are primarily concerned with relaxations rather than tightenings of the law. Thus one must be careful about generalizing to other drugs and to the effects of substantially toughening law enforcement. Thirdly, reductions in cannabis use penalties by definition occurred after a period of tougher sanctions, which may still be influencing values and behavioural norms after the law has changed.

In developed societies, there certainly are examples of centrally directed changes in personal behaviour, even with respect to psychoactive substances. Examples in our current era are the driving down of rates of drink-driving and of tobacco smoking. Drink-driving is something of a special case, since the effort has been not to outlaw the drinking, but rather to outlaw combining it with behaviour. And one thing to notice about both of these behaviours is that effects of the centrally directed policy changes are quite slow. They tend to be a matter of decades, not weeks, and are reinforced by (and in turn reinforce) shifts in popular sentiment.

A notable feature of psychoactive substances, both legal and illegal, in developed societies is the waves of use over time, as already mentioned in Chapter 3. A particular drug, or a particular form of a drug, comes into fashion in a particular youth cohort. Often, it goes out of style for the next generation of youth, which moves on to something else. Lagging the waves of use are waves of societal reaction to the use. Prohibitions on possession and use are brought in as part of the societal reaction. At least for cannabis, it is not clear that these *post hoc* reactions have been potent enough to overcome the inherent power of these societal waves in use.

It is largely heavy and problematic users who are swept up in diversion schemes such as Portugal's or California's Proposition 36. A clear implication of these findings is that the police are being highly selective in who they arrest. Caulkins and Sevigny (2005) have shown that most of those incarcerated in the USA for possession in fact were involved in drug dealing or other crimes. From this perspective, reducing rates of drug use may not be the main consideration in the application of laws against possession or use of controlled substances.

Chapter 12

Prescription regimes and other measures to control misuse of psychopharmaceuticals

12.1 Introduction

As discussed in Chapter 6, many of the psychoactive substances with which this book is concerned have the capacity to bring therapeutic benefits. Most of these substances are made available legally for medicinal purposes because of their great therapeutic value, even though they are attractive to illicit drug users and can also cause great harm. Prescription regimes are the major control structure through which these substances are made legally available for consumption in the modern world. Thus it is important for policymakers to understand the consequences, positive and negative, of allowing a drug to be manufactured in quantity and then sold on prescription.

The regulated legal substances are often used as substitutes for the wholly illegal; occasionally they are complements. Heroin users may choose to consume many kinds of legal opiates, such as morphine, if these legal opiates become more readily available or heroin less available. If the prescription system becomes too loose, as was the case with prescription opioids (most prominently **OxyContin**) in the USA in the 1990s, there may be an outbreak of drug-related problems in a population that has little or no current therapeutic contact with the medical system. Moreover, what starts out as a surge in prescription drug abuse can turn into a new market for illegally produced or stolen drugs, and can also lead to increased theft. Large numbers of prescription opioid (PO) thefts, including at the pre-pharmacy level, have been documented in the USA (Joranson and Gilson 2005), providing part of the supply for PO misuse. Other means are also used to divert pharmaceuticals from legal sources to the illicit marketplace and/or to unintended individuals (Inciardi *et al.* 2007), including theft or sale to others of medications obtained within the prescription system. Apart from diversion, 'non-medical use' also includes non-adherence, which is the non-directed use of a prescribed medication by the prescribee (Larance 2008), such as stockpiling doses, taking more than is recommended, or use of medication by a non-specified route (e.g. snorting, injection).

In Chapter 3 we presented data on what is known about the prevalence of non-medical use of prescription drugs and in Chapter 6 we reviewed studies of how prescription drugs are diverted from the legal market for illicit use. In certain wealthy countries, notably the USA and Canada, the prevalence estimates of non-medical use of opioids legally available only by prescription are comparable with or exceed those for heroin (Compton and Volkow 2006; Fischer *et al.* 2006). Drugs that are prescribed in rich countries, but subject to less stringent or minimal regulation in poorer nations, may also be an important component of **drug misuse** in some of those nations, but the lack of monitoring capabilities in many developing countries makes it difficult to document this phenomenon.

The purpose of this chapter is to examine how well prescription regimes perform their role of allowing psychoactive substances to be consumed for approved, i.e. medical, purposes while preventing their use for non-approved purposes. The chapter does not evaluate the appropriateness of the approval process leading to the definition of a drug's 'approved purpose', a topic over which nations and experts differ. It does, however, note the trade-off between tight restrictions aimed at reducing the risk of diversion and improper use, on the one hand, and the availability of these drugs for proper medical use, on the other. As mentioned in Chapter 6, in many developing countries the balance has been tipped very far against availability for medical use.

The chapter begins with a description of the prescription system that now operates in developed nations and then lays out the regulatory tools that can influence prescription practices. It focuses on a relatively new set of studies that evaluate these interventions in terms of how they affect drug consumption and patient health. Because the literature specific to psychoactive drugs is not large, the review draws in studies of other kinds of prescribed drugs in order to illuminate how various interventions affect prescribing behaviour and related drug abuse. The data come predominantly from Europe and the Anglo-Saxon world (Australia, Canada, the UK and, most prominently, from the USA), but we believe that the issues and interventions have much more general applicability. In the final parts of the chapter, we consider the control of **psychopharmaceuticals** by mechanisms outside of the prescription regimes, such as efforts to control deceptive marketing and to reduce diversion through law enforcement.

12.2 **The prescription system**

The prescription is a written or otherwise recorded instruction from a licensed physician or other authorized health worker, which is filled by a licensed pharmacist or equivalent. Although prescriptions can be provided under other circumstances, we are primarily concerned here with prescriptions in which the physician's script is mandatory, i.e. where the pharmacist may not dispense the substance independently and the customer/patient may not obtain it without a prescription.

This basic triangle of the physician, the pharmacist, and the customer/patient may be surrounded by further complications, depending upon the particular substance to be prescribed. Generally, in any prescription system these further complications are at their most developed for the substances that are under international control.

The existence of the basic prescription system is taken for granted in the **international drug conventions**. In the 1961 Convention, ratifying states committed themselves to 'require medical prescriptions for the supply or dispensation of drugs to individuals'. While the pharmacist's role is not mentioned in the Convention itself, it is mentioned in a matter-of-fact way in the official commentary (United Nations 1973). The 1971 Convention does include reference to 'pharmacists and other licensed retail distributors'.

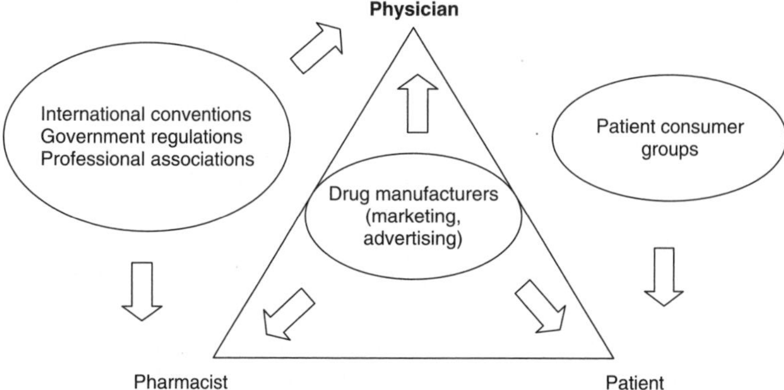

Fig. 12.1 The physician–pharmacist–patient triangle and the groups that influence it.

As illustrated in Figure 12.1, a variety of influential groups surround the triangular transaction of the physician, the pharmacist, and the patient. These include professional associations representing the interests of physicians and pharmacists, and sometimes also groups that act on the consumer's/patient's behalf. As the international conventions make explicit, government is fundamentally involved, setting the basic conditions of the triangle, and often also with a fiscal interest in the cost of the transaction. A further major class of actors is the manufacturers, distributors, and promoters of the prescribed substances, which in recent years has come to include commercial advertising companies engaged in direct-to-consumer marketing.

12.3 The short history of prescription regimes

Though taken for granted in developed societies, the prescription system as we have specified it is less than a century old as a mandatory system or even as a normative mode of practice. In Britain prior to 1913, prescriptions in the modern sense existed, but they were relatively unimportant. Instead there were two largely separate systems of provision of medications. Those who could afford to see a physician received their medicines directly from their doctor (Berridge and Edwards 1981). Meanwhile, the poor purchased medicines from pharmacists or druggists without a doctor's prescription. The National Insurance Act of 1912, with provisions on medical benefits which went into effect in 1913, subsidized the provision of medications to the poor but, as a cost-limiting measure, specified the requirement of a doctor's prescription to be filled by a pharmacist. Within a year, the number of prescriptions filled by pharmacists tripled (Anderson 2006).

In the USA, governance of the health system was long primarily a state matter, and prescription requirements varied from state to state. Although the Harrison Narcotics Act of 1914 introduced a federal requirement of a prescription for opium- or cocaine-based preparations (Crellin 2004), this remained for some years an anomalous exception. A general national prescription regime was an unintended result of regulations adopted by the US Food and Drug Administration to implement the federal Food, Drug, and Cosmetic Act of 1938.

Elsewhere, the triangle of the prescription system is an even more recent legal requirement. Kim and colleagues (2004) describe how South Korea, in line with the traditional system of oriental medicine, allowed both physicians and pharmacists to provide diagnosis and drugs for outpatients until July 2000.

As in the USA, opiates or cocaine were often the original subject for what became modern compulsory prescription systems. In The Netherlands, the 1865 Preparation of Medicines Act took the first step toward a compulsory prescription system by providing that opiates and some other medications could be sold only by pharmacists and physicians (Gerritsen 2000). The first British provision for a prescription-only drug was adopted for cocaine in 1916 as a wartime regulation under the Defense of the Realm Act (DORA, r.40B; Crellin 2004). In the 1905 Opium Proclamation in Australia, the fledgling federal government, with no jurisdiction over health but using its powers over customs and imports, provided that opium could only be imported for 'medicinal use', and only by a medical practitioner, wholesaler, or manufacturing chemist, druggist, or pharmaceutical chemist (Manderson 1987).

12.4 **Alternative controls to a physician prescription system**

Conventionally, medications are categorized as prescription or 'over-the-counter' (OTC). In a majority of developed countries, though not generally in the USA, a third option includes non-prescription drugs that are sold only at pharmacies or by pharmacists and/or are required to be kept 'behind-the-counter' (Crellin 2004; Howley 2005; US General Accounting Office 1995). In 1995, a US report studied the systems in 10 other developed countries, finding 'that little effort has been made to systematically compare systems', and neither were there studies that had 'attempted to link the type of drug distribution system in a country to the frequency of adverse drug reactions or [...] the quality of health care' (US General Accounting Office 1995, pp. 20, 23). In recent years, the USA has begun to move towards a 'behind-the-counter' basis for specific drugs, notably for medications which can be used for the illicit manufacture of methamphetamine (Food and Drug Administration 2006; Dries-Daffner *et al.* 2007).

There is thus considerable modern experience with the pharmacist as the sole gatekeeper for some classes of drugs, including codeine and other opiate preparations. This experience undoubtedly exists in developing societies as well as developed. But research on how well and to what extent pharmacists operate in this function in the course of their daily work is confined to developed countries, and even there the answers to the questions are not well established. On the basis of a review of the literature up to that time and interviews with officials in the countries they visited, the General Accounting Office (GAO) staff were somewhat sceptical about using the pharmacist as counsellor and gatekeeper (US General Accounting Office 1995). According to the GAO report, the officials felt that pharmacists were providing little or no advice about the drugs they sold. Officials gave several possible explanations for this, including time constraints and a lack of counselling skills. On the other hand, it is clear that pharmacists play important professional and gatekeeping roles with respect to controlled substances. In a 2003–2004 survey in the southwest of England, 48% of community pharmacists reported that they provided a supervised methadone consumption service, i.e. they not only dispensed methadone but also supervised its consumption (Britten and Scott 2006). A review of **randomized controlled trials** of care services provided by a pharmacist in the community or an outpatient setting found that in six of nine studies there were significant improvements in medication use (Roughead *et al.* 2005). A Spanish study found that offering counselling without dispensing was negatively associated with long working hours and many customers (Caamaño *et al.* 2006). Clearly, working conditions and the organization of the pharmacy affect whether the pharmacist can act as counsellor and gatekeeper.

Another alternative to the prescription system has been developed around the availability of cannabis as a medication ('medical marijuana'). In The Netherlands, cannabis is available in the regular prescription system, with the cannabis supplied by the government (de Jong *et al.* 2005); in a sample of 200 users, 75% took it in the form of tea, 1-4 times a day (de Jong *et al.* 2005). In Canada a potential medicinal cannabis user must apply to the government with a doctor's signed declaration, essentially a prescription for up to 12 months, with the medical condition specified (Health Canada 2009). In the USA, federal authorities have been strongly opposed to cannabis being made available as a medication through the regular prescription system. Since the federal authorities have the power to remove doctors' prescription powers for opiates and other controlled substances if they prescribe in ways they do not approve, states that make provision for 'medical marijuana' (there are 13 after the elections of November 2008, according to the Marijuana Policy Project (2008)) have been forced to improvise alternative systems. The first and largest of these systems, which has also served as a model for other states, is in California. In that state, a doctor must sign a statement that the patient's health 'would benefit from medical marijuana' as a treatment. In nine states, the patient must also register with the state to be protected from arrest; in these states, 0.17% of the population is registered (Marijuana Policy Project 2008). In California, more than 200 000 persons (i.e. >0.5% of the population) have a medical letter from a doctor entitling them to purchase cannabis (Samuels 2008). The cannabis is not sold through pharmacies (again, federal law would not allow it), but through hundreds of single-purpose dispensaries. An owner of one dispensary estimated that 40% of her clients suffer from serious illnesses such as cancer, AIDS, glaucoma, epilepsy, and multiple sclerosis. The rest have ailments such as anxiety, sleeplessness, attention deficit disorder, and assorted pains (Samuels 2008).

It is clear that the Canadian system, which has been criticized as excessively bureaucratic (Sibbald 2002), serves a narrower range of patients than the California system. But no accounting has been made of the relative benefits and adverse consequences from such a prescription system and from the California doctor's letter system.

12.5 Strategies of drug control through prescription policies

Our focus is on studies that evaluate the effect of regulations and other interventions on the prescription or dispensing of medications. Studies of system changes are valuable because such '**natural experiments**' offer some of the best evidence available on the impact of regulations and interventions, far stronger than cross-sectional comparisons or expert views (see Chapter 7 for a review of research methods). Such studies have focused on a variety of outcomes, consistent with the variety of motivations for such policies. One perspective explores the effect of policy changes on poisonings and adverse drug reactions (ADRs). Other studies target a related but separate outcome: the effect on attempted and completed suicides, since psychoactive drugs are often the means chosen by those intending suicide. A third concern, adverse chronic health effects, has often motivated drugs being withdrawn from the market and other policy changes, but does not seem to be used in policy outcome studies. A fourth and major focus of policy outcome studies has been the effect on costs, both for health insurers (state or private) and for the patient. A final set of outcomes is related specifically to recreational use or **substance use disorders**: the extent or intensity of use *per se*, and indicators of dependence. To the extent the literature allows, we give first priority to the effects of the policy strategy on harms associated with the drug use, and second priority to the effects on use or prescriptions. We also pay attention to policy side effects, both positive and negative.

In the following sections, we discuss prescription drug control strategies that have been evaluated in systematic research. We have organized the research in rough order of ascending intrusiveness of the policy change, in terms of both the patient's freedom of choice and the physician's authority to exercise clinical judgement in the best interests of the patient. Eight strategies are reviewed: (1) changes in costs or reimbursements; (2) restrictions on OTC sales; (3) OTC versus prescription availability; (4) authoritative advice to physicians; (5) enforcement of prescription guidelines; (6) prescription restrictions, prescription registers, and prescription monitoring; (7) restricting the list of prescribers or use to hospitals/clinics; and (8) total withdrawal from prescription availability.

An important limitation of this research base for present purposes is that the effectiveness of a regime or regime change may well be different for different substances, notably whether the drug in question is psychoactive and how pleasurable it is to use. There is a need for caution in extrapolating from studies done concerning just one or a few substances to all substances more generally.

12.5.1 Changes in costs or reimbursement

As governments have assumed increasing responsibility for the provision of medications within national health care systems, the issue of pricing has come to the fore. A burgeoning health economics literature is concerned with the effects of different pricing strategies, from the perspective both of governments seeking to hold costs down and of privately owned pharmaceutical companies seeking to maximize returns. This literature includes some studies of the effects of particular changes in price or reimbursement.

The drug tramadol (Ultram or, when combined with acetaminophen, Ultracet or Tramacet) is an atypical opiate about 10% as potent as morphine. It is a prescription substance used for chronic pain in most countries, but is not 'scheduled' (i.e. subject to special restrictions beyond that). Its marketing material indicates low **abuse potential**, but tramadol clearly has a potential for recreational use. The US authorities approved its non-scheduled status in 1995 on condition that a special programme to monitor potential misuse or diversion from the prescription system be set up (Cicero *et al.* 2005). In July 2002 generic versions of the drug appeared on the market, at a 30–40% reduction in price. The introduction of generic tramadol reduced prescriptions for branded tramadol to only 7% of the market by the second quarter of 2003. The introduction of generic tramadol saw no effect on the rates of misuse (<1 per 100 000 patients) (Cicero *et al.* 2005).

A similar study (Bailey *et al.* 2006) investigated the introduction to the US market in 2004 of a generic competitor to the brand OxyContin, which is the potent opiate oxycodone in controlled-release form. The price of the generic product was about 15% lower than the price of OxyContin. The study found no significant effect on prescription rates either for oxycodone or for other opiates included in the study (hydrocodone, methadone, and morphine).

A study in Sydney, Australia examined the effects of removing government subsidy from prescriptions for the gel form of the benzodiazepine drug temazapam (Degenhardt *et al.* 2008). The gel form of the drug is not intended for injection but is often used for that by IDUs, with consequent injection-related health problems. The change resulted in an immediate drop in prescriptions for the gel form, and a more or less corresponding increase in prescriptions for the tablet form, which was still covered by the government subsidy. However, rates of injection of benzodiazepines in an annual monitoring survey of IDUs did not change.

A **Cochrane review** of reference pricing as a third-party payer strategy for containing drug expenditures found 10 studies, mostly concerning elderly patients in British Columbia (Aaserud *et al.* 2006). Reference pricing, in which the price of one drug in a category becomes the reimbursement standard, produced a shift towards less expensive drugs sharing similar effects. There was no evidence of adverse effects on health and no clear evidence of increased health care utilization.

The general conclusion we might draw from these studies is that doctors pay some attention to price in their choice of drugs to prescribe. The demand for prescription drugs, determined partly by doctors, partly by their patients, and partly by state or other drug benefit schemes, shows some elasticity, though in the absence of substitutes the degree of elasticity is relatively low. On the other hand, a prescription regime appears to dampen the connection between price and the demand for use.

12.5.2 **Restrictions on OTC sales**

Although there has been substantial effort in a number of countries to cut off supplies for illicit methamphetamine manufacture by limiting OTC sales of pseudoephedrine (Sudafed) and other such medications (e.g. Food and Drug Administration 2006), no studies of the effectiveness of these measures had appeared at the time of writing. In fact, only a few studies have investigated the effect of imposing restrictions on OTC sales. The analgesic paracetamol (acetaminophen) was restricted in the UK (Morgan and Majeed 2005; Greene *et al.* 2006) and Canada (Prior *et al.* 2004). The Canadian studies found no effect on poisonings, while the UK studies generally found that restrictions reduced hospital admissions for related poisonings. With conflicting results for the same drug from Canada and the UK, the question of the effectiveness of extra restrictions on the amount of medication sold at once (e.g. through pill strength and number of pills in a package) within the OTC category remains open.

12.5.3 OTC versus prescription availability

A cross-sectional population survey in Santiago, Chile in the early 1990s examined OTC versus prescription use of benzodiazepines. Chile had a very high rate of benzodiazepine use (particularly diazepam). In principle, benzodiazepines were limited to prescription use, but in practice 'most patients go directly to a pharmacy to obtain their medications without getting a physician's prescription' (Busto *et al.* 1996). Of the 471 respondents (31%) who had used benzodiazepines in the last year, 21% used them on the recommendation of family or acquaintances. Of the 32 who obtained their benzodiazepines in a pharmacy, 66% did not always have a prescription. Daily long-term users and those who met diagnostic criteria for dependence on benzodiazepines were no less likely than other users to use by prescription. Thus, in a situation where OTC supplies were readily available, dependence or abuse were no more associated with OTC than with prescription use (Busto *et al.* 1996).

Apart from the Chilean report, the available studies (Lundberg and Isacson 1999; Shih *et al.* 2002; Choudry and Avorn 2005; Trygstad *et al.* 2006; Filion *et al.* 2007) look at drugs that a national regulatory agency had decided were safe enough in use to switch to OTC status. For those drugs, it seems that the switch between OTC and prescription status made little difference in adverse effects. This suggests the agencies had made appropriate judgements in these cases. Indeed, unless zero risk is the criterion of the decision on OTC status, the regulatory process may be unduly conservative in keeping drugs on prescription status. The policy choice between OTC and prescription status is likely to affect use patterns. An important consideration is whether OTC status removes the drug from coverage for reimbursement. If so, the result may be a downward pressure on sales which might counteract the upward pressure from the greater availability and convenience of OTC status. The findings of one UK study (Filion *et al.* 2007) also carry a hint of the symbolic effect of prescription status: the public may come to believe that if the drug is not on prescription, it may not be very powerful or effective.

12.5.4 Authoritative advice to physicians

Evaluation research in Australia (Weekes *et al.* 2005; Mandryk *et al.* 2006) and Ontario (Pimlott *et al.* 2003) suggests that even relatively intensive educational approaches do not easily change doctors' prescribing behaviour. The task for the Australian campaign to get doctors to prescribe antibiotics less often was particularly difficult, since the benefit from the change accrued to the community at large rather than to the individual patient. On the other hand, educational campaigns in the UK (Bateman *et al.* 2003) and the USA (Morrato and Staffa 2007) did produce changes in prescribing behaviour when doctors were warned about a new finding concerning the threat of serious organ damage. However, the main change seems to have been to substitute a different drug. The UK experience with thioridazine (Bateman *et al.* 2003) offers a warning that, in this circumstance, doctors may switch to a drug with an even higher risk of damage.

12.5.5 Enforcement of prescription guidelines

In response to allegations of 'warehousing' of elderly people in nursing homes, including testimony in which some witnesses characterized the practice of using tranquillizer drugs as 'chemical straitjackets' (Ryan *et al.* 2002), the US Congress in 1987 set in motion a series of reforms that led to the development of detailed guidelines on the prescription of psychoactive drugs, including requirements for detailed record-keeping and enforcement by regular inspections (Stoudemire and Smith 1996). Included were a list of behaviours (e.g. fidgeting, impaired memory, and uncooperativeness) for which neuroleptic drugs were declared inappropriate; a timetable for the reduction in doses of neuroleptics and benzodiazepines; a list of maximum dosages for antipsychotics, hypnotics, and benzodiazepines; and rules to discourage prescription of long-acting benzodiazepines or two or more **psychotropics** for the same action. An article reviewing evaluations of the reform (Snowdon and Roy-Byrne 1998) reported that all studies found a reduction in use of antipsychotic medications. This research suggests that the detailed and intense campaign of advice to doctors, backed up with enforcement by regular inspections, produced a substantial change in prescribing behaviour.

12.5.6 Restrictions on prescription, prescription registers, prescription monitoring

Many jurisdictions have a separate class of substances (usually psychoactive drugs) with special requirements for prescription. The physician and/or the pharmacist must often keep a record of each prescription, make the record available to inspectors, and/or send a copy to a central registry. The mention of 'counterfoil books' of prescriptions in the 1961 International Convention is a reference to such a prescription register. Programmes that collect prescription data and send them to a centralized database to detect trends in **diversion** and non-adherence are called prescription monitoring programmes (PMPs).

In the USA, multicopy, serially numbered prescription programmes have been highly unpopular with physicians and pharmaceutical companies, and this coalition has successfully opposed these restrictions in many US states (e.g. Dodd 1993). Some physicians consider such programmes an intrusion into medical practice because they continually remind providers and patients that their prescribing, dispensing, and procuring patterns are being monitored (Simoni-Wastila and Tompkins 2001), while others have been at the forefront of developing the systems that make such monitoring possible (e.g. the national electronic records of the US Department of Veterans Affairs). Nevertheless, by 2006, 32 states had legislation requiring PMPs. Slightly more acceptable have been electronic data transfer (EDT) systems, which typically require pharmacists to submit prescription and dispensing information on an electronic file to a centralized databank. Such systems are clearly less visible to physicians than programmes requiring multiple copies of each prescription. One survey found that 59% of Massachusetts physicians were not aware of the EDT system's existence 6 years after its implementation there, suggesting that there may be little effect on prescribing upon EDT implementation (Simoni-Wastila and Tompkins 2001). However, reductions may occur when the state notifies prescribers that their prescribing is being monitored because of apparent irregularities. For example, when Massachusetts issued an advisory on inappropriate use of glutethimide (Doriden, a sedative–hypnotic with substantial abuse potential) to 100 practitioners who had prescribed it, their average of 50 prescriptions per month fell to four (Simoni-Wastila and Tompkins 2001).

In recent decades, many jurisdictions introduced restrictions on barbiturate prescribing. These restrictions came at a time when doctors, influenced by the same changes in thinking as the regulators, were substituting other drugs, often benzodiazepines, for barbiturates in their prescribing. It is thus not clear whether the restrictions had an independent effect. A Dutch study reports that admissions for barbiturate poisoning dropped sharply due to a more restrictive prescription policy. At the same time, admissions for sedative and hypnotic poisoning also declined, but not for benzodiazepines (van Romunde *et al.* 1992). Similarly, an earlier Australian study reported that restrictions on barbiturate prescriptions (a limit of 25 tablets on a single prescription) led to a 23% decline in drug-related suicide without an increase in suicides by other means (Oliver and Hetzel 1972, 1973).

A number of studies have examined what happens when a drug or class of drugs is added to the 'prescription register' list, which usually involves not only a change in the method of prescription but also prescribing restrictions and potential investigation and enforcement. In 2001, the French drug regulatory agency transferred flunitrazepam (Rohypnol, a benzodiazepene) from regular prescription status to the regulatory regime for dependence-producing drugs, which included more stringent prescribing and dispensing regulations, including prescriptions for no longer than 14 days and dispensing of no more than 7 days' supply at a time. In a follow-up of 738 patients who had been prescribed flunitrazepam, 69% had moved to a prescription for another hypnotic. But nearly half of the patients had stopped using hypnotics altogether during the 8-month follow-up (Victorri-Vigneau *et al.* 2003). A study of the implementation of registration for flunitrazepam prescriptions in Denmark found that consumption of the drug 2 years later had decreased by more than 85% (Hoffmeyer *et al.* 1999).

In January 2003, flunitrazepam was moved up one level in the schedule of controlled substances in Norway. This resulted in a decrease in sales by more than half in 2003 (7.2 to 3.0 defined daily doses (DDDs) per 1000 inhabitants). The decrease was only partly compensated for by an increase in the sales of nitrazepam (from 5.0 to 6.0 DDDs). Meanwhile, between 1999 and 2004 there was a steady increase in sales of benzodiazepine-related hypnotics (zopiclone (Imovane, Lunesta) and zolpidem (Ambien, Stilnox)), which could have taken up some of the slack. In August 2004, one brand of flunitrazepam (Rohypnol) was removed from sale by the manufacturer, leaving another brand (Flunipam) on the market. This had little effect on sales of flunitrazepam (Bramness *et al.* 2006).

In 2003, Swedish authorities introduced restrictions on the prescribing of dextropropoxypene (DXP, Darvon). By the end of 2003, sales were 66% lower than in 1999, though the decrease had already started before the restrictions were in place. Jonasson and Jonasson (2004) suggest the decline would have been temporary without the change in prescription status. Meanwhile, sales of tramadol increased, compensating for much of the DXP decrease. Norway introduced a similar change in prescription policy for DXP in 1982, and Denmark in 1988, both changes preceded by considerable public discussion. A cross-Nordic study of fatal poisoning among drug addicts, conducted before the change in policy in Sweden but after the Danish and Norwegian changes, found that DXP accounted for 20% of the deaths in Sweden and 13% in Finland, but almost none of the deaths in Norway and Denmark, a difference the authors attributed to the difference in prescription regimes (Steentoft *et al.* 2001). However, rates of fatal poisonings among addicts per inhabitant were much higher in Denmark and Norway than in Finland or Sweden, and much more likely to be from heroin or morphine (or methadone in Denmark). It may be that the prescription restrictions on DXP in Denmark and Norway channelled potential suicides towards using opiates, which are more likely to be fatal.

A number of studies have examined the implementation of or changes in state multiple-copy prescription systems in the USA. Several studies have focused on the introduction of a triplicate prescription requirement in New York State for barbiturates in 1981 (Eadie 1993) and for benzodiazepines in January 1989. A study of post-hospitalization prescribing (with New Jersey as the control state) found a sudden reduction of 63.5% in benzodiazepine prescriptions, including a 72.5% reduction for patients who had had heart attacks and a 69.4% reduction for cancer patients. While there were increased prescriptions for substitutes, they did not wholly offset the reductions (Wagner *et al.* 2003). Some striking contrasts have been reported (Weintraub *et al.* 1993) in trends for meprobromate (up 125% in New York, down 9% in the rest of the USA), buspirone (up 116% versus 23%), chloral hydrate (up 136% versus no change), and fluoxetine (up 142% versus 110%). In the view of Weintraub and colleagues (1993), the medications prescribed to replace benzodiazepines can be seen to have major disadvantages. Another study of prescribing patterns in long-term care facilities also found a dramatic drop for benzodiazepines, with 22% of users taken off, but over half of those switched to alternatives including tricyclic antidepressants and antipsychotic drugs. There was no significant change in the risk of falls or hospital admissions for other reasons, although there was a trend toward a reduction in falls (Zullich *et al.* 1992). Studies elsewhere in the USA (Bishop and Vlasty 1993) found declines in overdose mentions or deaths when specific drugs were added to triplicate prescription registers in the 1980s. The switch to triplicate prescriptions also affected prices of the drugs on the illicit market, ranging from a 50% increase for Lorazepam (Ativan) to more than a fivefold increase for Alprazolan (Xanax) (Eadie 1993).

It is clear that prescription registration systems, along with the limitations on dose and duration of a prescription usually associated with them, substantially affect doctors' prescribing behaviour. As a number of studies emphasize, the result can often be not so much a reduction in prescriptions as a substitution of prescriptions for substances that are not so heavily controlled. In the case of barbiturates, the switch that resulted from their inclusion in the prescription registration systems clearly reduced drug-related deaths. It remains an open question whether this benefit happened as completely and as quickly in jurisdictions that did not make the regulatory change. In the case of benzodiazepines, the effect of being included in prescription registration systems is much more questionable in terms of drug-related adverse events, since the switch was often to drugs with a worse record. In the case of opioids, there is some evidence from the USA and Canada that PMPs have unintended effects on physicians' attitudes and practices towards prescribing medications (see Box 12.1), which need to be considered when evaluating the overall effectiveness of these programmes.

Box 12.1 Opioids, prescription monitoring programmes (PMPs), and their unintended consequences

Prescription monitoring programmes (PMPs) have been institutionalized in more than half the US states since the first such programme was established a century ago. PMPs aim to monitor the provision of prescription opioids and enforce rules against providers when violations occur (Fishman *et al.* 2004). PMPs for opioids can have at least three unintended harmful effects.

1. **Less effective pain treatment**
   - PMPs that feature potentially severe punitive consequences for opioid prescribers may compromise the current availability and best practice provision of analgesic treatment for pain patients. Several studies conducted in the 1990s documented that PMPs led physicians to reduce drug doses, to prescribe an alternative drug in a less regulated schedule, or to avoid prescribing opioids for patients with chronic pain 'due to concerns of overzealous regulatory scrutiny' (Fishman *et al.* 2004, p. 317).
2. **Substitution effects among prescribers**
   - As the prescribing of the target drug decreases, prescriptions of alternative (less restrictively monitored) drugs may increase. These alternatives are often therapeutically less optimal, hold a greater chance of toxicity, and carry equal or greater abuse potential (Fishman *et al.* 2004). The introduction of PMP controls for benzodiazepines in New York State in the late 1980s (Hoffman *et al.* 1991) seems to have triggered a substantial shift to non-benzodiazepine sedative–hypnotic prescriptions and concomitant changes in overdoses related to the respective drug categories.
3. **Substitution effects among drug users**
   - An additional issue currently not addressed empirically is whether substitution effects occur among prescription opioid abusers (e.g. street users) when the availability of diverted prescription opioid supplies decreases. Such a situation might, for example, lead to more harmful uses of alternative drugs or create more volatile black markets. There has been some evidence from studies of street opioid user populations that the use of prescription opioids instead of heroin may have public health benefits, such as reduced injecting or infectious disease transmission risks (Fischer *et al.* 2008; Havens *et al.* 2007).
   - PMPs undoubtedly affect the provision, accessibility, and availability of prescription opioids, with both positive and negative consequences for well-being. It is impossible to determine whether or not the gains of PMPs outweigh their substantial 'collateral damage' (Burgess 2006; Simoni-Wastila and Tompkins 2001).

12.5.7 Restricting list of prescribers or use to hospitals/clinics

Another approach to restricting risk of diversion is by restricting the number (and status) of those who can prescribe a drug. This can be seen as a more assertive version of the restriction that a particular medicine needs to be prescribed by a doctor (versus medicines available for purchase over the counter).

Tramadol (Ultram) is an atypical opiate available by prescription in most countries. In 1998 it became the fourth injectable analgesic introduced to the Iranian market. The Iranian Pharmacovigilance Centre (IPC), also established in 1998, collected and analysed ADR reports on tramadol between April 2002 and February 2005. There were 337 such reports, describing 939 adverse reactions, with nausea, vomiting, and vertigo the most common, but also including some severe reactions. Most of the reports (81%) concerned intramuscular injection of tramadol. In August 2003, following assessment of 67 ADRs, the IPC issued a letter to health care professionals with 12 guidelines for reducing adverse effects, covering the speed of injection, the dose, and precautions about patient characteristics such as age and co-existing conditions. Two months later, the Drug Regulatory authority limited distribution of injectable tramadol to hospitals only, and reduced the potency of injectable tramadol by a half (from 100 mg to 50 mg). Analysis of the ADRs by quarter found them to have risen rapidly from eight in winter 2003 to 76 in autumn 2003, and then to have dropped as quickly to 19 in spring 2004, a level they stayed close to in the succeeding three quarters (Gholami *et al.* 2007). The ADR monitoring system and quick regulatory action were therefore considered effective in reducing ADRs from the drug.

Other earlier examples exist, such as the complete ending of a short-lived but florid outbreak of intravenous abuse of methylamphetamine ampoules in London in 1968/69, which were being prescribed (within the legislative framework, but undesirably) by a small number of doctors for dispensing from community pharmacists (Hawks *et al.* 1969). From a virtually zero baseline the preceding year, a small number of private independent doctors began to prescribe massive amounts. In one month of 1968, one single doctor prescribed 24 000 ampoules to 110 individuals (Spear 1975; Power 1994). This outbreak quickly dissolved after coordinated action by the Department of Health, working in collaboration with the pharmaceutical industry/supplier and with pharmacists. The industry applied a self-imposed ban in October 1968 on supply of any pharmaceutical stock to any community pharmacy, thereby preserving supply to hospitals for very limited legitimate medical use, while nevertheless interrupting the supply that was causing concern (Mitcheson *et al.* 1976). A particular advantage of this informal approach was that it could be conceived and implemented much more rapidly than any formal change in the law.

Another example of restricting potential for diversion by limiting the authority to prescribe is the case of heroin prescribing in the UK. In contrast to the rest of the world, the UK has always permitted doctors to prescribe heroin for reasons presumed medically legitimate (such as for severe pain relief, in terminal care, and when treating pain of cardiac origin). However, after 1968, the authority to prescribe heroin for explicit treatment of drug dependence was restricted to a small number of about 100 doctors, almost all being hospital-based addictions specialists. Doctors in the UK still have the authority to prescribe heroin for general medical conditions, but not for treatment of dependence, and they are also able to prescribe other opiate drugs such as methadone for the treatment of dependence. This legislation creates a framework in which the prescribing of heroin is actually controlled by a combination of legislative and professional peer-influence controls. The legislation restricts the authority to prescribe to a small number of doctors with greater experience and expertise, and then professional peer-influence guides the cautious use of this authority. The end result is the very cautious use of this authority to prescribe heroin, with a total of only about 200 patients being treated with heroin (from these 100 specially licensed doctors) for their opioid dependence (for overview of this practice, see Strang and Gossop 2005).

Limiting the number of prescribers may well be an effective way to reduce the number of prescriptions for a drug. Though there is little evidence, it may be expected that physicians no longer able to prescribe the drug may prescribe a substitute. Also, where a substantial demand for a psychoactive substance has been established, the illicit market may take up at least some of the slack.

Restrictions for administering opiate substitution and pain medications

We have already noted one policy change involving an opiate, heroin, which involved restricting the list of prescribers. Restrictions of prescribing to a subset of doctors, or to use in clinics, often combined with other measures, are also common concerning other opiate substitution therapies (OSTs). We deal with these restrictions here, though other control measures are often also involved. One study comparing results from methadone maintenance based in a primary care physician's office and in a clinic found that there was a better compliance and greater patient satisfaction in the office-based treatment (Fiellin *et al.* 2001), without significant differences in functional status or use of other health, legal, or social services.

A review for the **World Health Organization** of 28 national or professional association guidelines on opiate maintenance or antagonist treatment (Uchtenhagen *et al.* 2007) found that 19 of them included legal rules on who could prescribe or who could be taken on as a patient. The provisions included (with the number of guidelines mentioning the provision in parentheses):

- clinics must be licensed (8)
- state-owned clinics only (1)
- health care institutions only (1)
- prescribing doctors must be centrally registered (2)
- prescribing doctors must have a licence for psychiatry (1)
- doctor's licence for prescribing is limited to 6 months (1)
- doctors are allowed to prescribe for a maximum of 20 patients (1)
- patients must be centrally registered (9)
- central register accessible only to treating physician (1)
- patients need individual authorization by health authority or commission (3)

In addition to influencing the behaviour of prescribers, measures restricting access to opiate maintenance are an effort to get patients to adhere to a specified treatment regime.

In the case of methadone, the dose is usually made available daily, often diluted with water or juice, for immediate oral use. Some provision may be allowed for 'take-aways', in which patients can take away one or a few doses at a time. Take-aways involve some risks, including injection of methadone dispensed in a non-injectable form.

Diversion of opiate substitution medications occurs for a variety of reasons, including potential profit from sale, desire to use in a non-therapeutic fashion, and as a potential back-up for when illegally obtained drugs are not available. For this last reason, not all diversion should be considered detrimental. For example, if a regular heroin injector consumes diverted oral methadone to avoid acute withdrawal on a day in which she cannot obtain heroin, both the user and society may benefit. But in most cases, diversion has the potential for serious harm (e.g. overdose by the user or a drug-naïve buyer), a waste of financial resources, and potential for de-legitimizing efforts to provide OST in a community or society.

Multiple strategies can lower the risk of diversion. One approach is to change the formulation of the medication. This can be a physical change, for example by changing it into a form that cannot easily be injected. Thus temazepam capsules were reformulated in the UK to a more solid gelthix capsule (Drake *et al.* 1991) after the previous liquid-filled temazepam capsules came to be widely misused intravenously. However, in the end this was deemed to be an insufficient response and temazepam was put on a more restricted schedule (Fountain *et al.* 1999). Or the change can be pharmaceutical, for example by including **naloxone** in formulations of various opiates, most recently with buprenorphine, to prevent misuse by injection, since naloxone is largely ineffective when swallowed but either prevents any opioid effect or has a highly aversive effect (for those with opioids already present in their system) if injected (Fudula *et al.* 1998). Commonplace strategies that have not been subjected to formal testing include testing urine samples for prescribed opiates as well as illicit use, and directly observing substitution therapy ingestion. Although it would be hard to demonstrate in a research study, most clinical experience indicates that a trusting, respectful relationship between health care staff and patients may reduce diversion as well.

Internationally, there is considerable variability in the regulations around the dispensing of medications such as methadone, and the requirements placed upon clients/patients. Thus, while most countries have systems in place for the supervision of methadone administration (at least during the early stages of treatment), there are some countries or regions in which no such regulatory requirements exist. In Western Australia in the 1970s and early 1980s, methadone was often given as take-home medication, and there was a higher-than-expected problem of opiate overdose deaths. As a result, a new system of supervised methadone consumption was introduced, and the annual opiate overdose figures dropped markedly (Swensen 1988). Denmark had a similar experience with lax controls on the availability of methadone prior to 1996 leading to high overdose rates. Having tightened those controls, Denmark is now the only one of the five Nordic nations to experience a reduction in overdose deaths, although methadone still accounted for 41% of Danish overdose deaths in 2002 (Steentoft *et al.* 2006). More recently, the UK has become aware of the substantial number of overdose deaths in which methadone played a role (Hall *et al.* 2000a). Many of these deaths have occurred in individuals other than the patient to whom the methadone was prescribed (Neeleman and Farrell 1997). Accordingly, from the late 1990s onwards, doctors have been encouraged to stipulate that only one day's dose of methadone be dispensed at a time. The proportion of methadone prescriptions across England for which 'daily dispensing' was stipulated rose from 38% in 1995 to 60% by 2005. Furthermore, new schemes have been introduced for the supervision of methadone administration, such that supervised consumption was a feature of 36% of all methadone prescriptions in England in 2005 compared with 0% 10 years earlier (Strang *et al.* 1996, 2007).

Risk for diversion can also be managed through the decisions a society makes regarding which forms of OST it offers and in what amounts. Basic economic theory teaches that diversion is more likely for substances with a high black market value. Heroin therefore poses a high risk of diversion; buprenorphine combined with an opiate antagonist, much less. A study in the UK found that 37% of heroin-maintained individuals reported diverting some heroin to the black market (cited in MacCoun and Reuter 2001a); as with other self-reports of criminal behaviour, this is likely to be an underestimate. Yet the same text notes that in the closely monitored heroin substitution study of 800 patients in Switzerland, with use required to be on site (described earlier in Chapter 9), illicit market leakage was not a problem.

Ritter and Di Natale (2005) compared methadone take-away guidelines in the six Australian states, and correlated these with methadone injection rates as reported in an annual survey of injecting drug users. The states with the most restrictive take-away policies (Victoria and Western Australia) had the lowest methadone injection rates, although the relationship did not seem 'as straightforward as is sometimes suggested'. The extent of dilution of the methadone as dispensed did not have a simple relationship with the methadone injection rate.

One study (Manchikanti *et al.* 2006b) evaluated the effect of monitoring procedures in a Kentucky pain management centre serving patients on stable doses of opiates as part of their chronic pain management. Patients ($n = 500$) signed an agreement that allowed the centre to contact pharmacies and physicians and to conduct random drug screening and pill counts. The terms of the agreement were regularly reviewed with the patient, and ongoing patient education was provided. While drug abuse (doctor shopping or trafficking) had been found in 17.8% of an earlier cohort of 500 pain management cases, the rate fell to 9% in this cohort. However, 8.6% of the eligible patients refused to participate in the study, raising the possibility that there was little change in the drug abuse rate in the whole cohort of 566.

Even though this type of intervention is under medical jurisdiction, there is surprisingly little evidence on the influence of clinical rules and procedures on adverse events or patient compliance.

12.5.8 **Total withdrawal from prescription availability**

In prescription regimes generally, 'safety withdrawals' of medications are not uncommon. A study of such withdrawals by 31 national authorities or the EU between 1960 and 1999 found such withdrawals more common in the 1980s and 1990s than earlier (Fung *et al.* 2001). Of the 121 withdrawals found from English-language references, 42% were from one or more European market alone, 5% from North America alone, and half from markets on multiple continents. In terms of therapeutic categories, psychoactive substances were fairly common: 31.4% of withdrawals were central nervous system- (CNS) acting agents and 4.1% were CNS stimulants, 7.4% were antidepressants, 4.1% were anorexiants, and 4.1% were barbiturates. In the study's summary of the safety concerns that led to the withdrawals, the emphasis tended to be on toxic reactions and carcinogenicity. Only eight drugs (one of them a steroid) noted concerns such as 'self-poisonings', 'abuse', 'misuse and abuse', 'off-label abuse', or 'CNS stimulation'.

Four of the withdrawals from prescription use were of barbiturates in Norway. One study found that barbiturate overdoses decreased following withdrawal. However, the same study reported that self-poisonings with antidepressants and neuroleptics increased significantly (Ekeberg *et al.* 1987). Following reports of death from zomepirac, a non-steroidal anti-inflammatory drug (NSAID; also described as a non-opioid analgesic), withdrawal of the drug resulted in substitute prescribing not only of other NSAIDs but also of other analgesics, including barbiturates (Ross-Degnan *et al.* 1993). The study stressed the need to weigh apparent gains in patient safety from a withdrawal against the risks of medications likely to be substituted.

In 2004, authorities in the UK withdrew co-proxamol (Darvocet), a widely used prescription combination of dextropropoxyphene (Darvon) and paracetamol (acetaminophen; Tylenol) from the market, after a review (Simkin *et al.* 2005) and consideration of various options. The primary consideration in withdrawing co-praxomol in the UK was the high rate of suicides, accounting for 18% of all suicides using drugs. This was balanced against the uncertain effectiveness of the combination as a painkiller. Despite a trend of reduced prescribing, in 2003 nearly 10% of elderly patients in a sample of 131 general practices were still receiving prescriptions, indicative of the need for policy action, and this was the main difference in a comparison between The Netherlands and the UK of inappropriate prescribing to elderly adults (De Wilde *et al.* 2007).

In 2004, dissatisfied with the results from the withdrawal of government subsidy of gel capsules of temazapam (discussed above), the Australian authorities withdrew the gel capsules from the market altogether. There was a further increase in private (non-subsidized) prescriptions of the tablet form. However, the proportion of IDUs reporting use of benzodiazepines declined sharply, although the overall proportion using benzodiazepines in any form did not change (Degenhardt *et al.* 2008).

There is no doubt that removing a drug from the legal market reduces the number of prescriptions for it. The most frequent physician response to this is to prescribe or recommend something else. These impact studies illustrate that regulators should think ahead to the likely substitutions and assess whether they are better or worse in their risks than the drug in question. If the withdrawal proceeds, it would be wise to try to affect what is substituted.

12.6 **Other interventions to control the supply of and demand for psychopharmaceuticals**

Thus far this chapter has focused on the use of prescription regimes to control diversion of psychopharmaceuticals and prevent non-adherence to their medically appropriate uses. But as suggested in Figure 12.1, there are other types of interventions that have been considered or applied within the context of the triangular relationships among the physician, the patient, and the pharmacist. These approaches include profiling patients to prevent 'doctor shopping' and other abuses, establishing laws directed at patient-consumers and physicians, treating patients with prescription drug dependence, and establishing system controls that monitor and regulate the supply of psychopharmaceuticals.

12.6.1 Profiling patients to prevent 'doctor shopping' and other abuses

Profiles of patients who are likely to misuse psychopharmaceuticals can be used to alert physicians and pharmacists to be more vigilant in their diagnostic, prescribing, and dispensing activities. In the interest of preventing opioid abuse, for example, increasing attention has been given to actual or potential patients 'at risk for addiction', especially in the context of pain treatment, and how they should be appropriately 'managed' (Michna *et al.* 2004; Ziegler 2005; Ives *et al.* 2006; Manchikanti *et al.* 2006b). Such efforts include a large variety of screeners and checklists or symptom indicators for abuse liability, reflecting a predominant spirit of 'universal precautions' or omnipresent risk management as a priority over therapeutic needs in interventions (Gourlay *et al.* 2005). This approach may result in denied, curtailed, or terminated treatment in cases of substantial indications of risk.

In the context of prescription opioids in medical practice, one profiling approach assumes two discrete groups. The first is described as 'with pain, honest and reliable', while the second is 'without pain, dishonest and [diverting and/or abusing] their medication' (Hurwitz 2005, p. 158). In actual clinical practice matters are less clearly delineated. The symptomatologies of both pain and (opioid) dependence markedly overlap or interact in many opioid users. For example, many career trajectories of chronic illicit opioid use involve a history of chronic pain problems, during which tolerance for or dependence on illicit opioids is established by intensive analgesic opioid treatment. Another trajectory begins with the ineffective medical treatment of persistent pain, which leads to illicit opioid use as a form of self-medication (Chabal *et al.* 1997; Khantzian 1997; Rosenblum *et al.* 2003). And there is biological evidence that chronic opioid intake may cause increased pain sensitivity, further influencing the demand for opioids (Streltzer 2005). No research has been conducted to evaluate the effectiveness of patient profiling as a way to prevent doctor shopping.

12.6.2 Laws directed at patient-consumers and physicians

As discussed previously in Chapter 11, a common reaction to drug misuse is to penalize illicit drug users. In the case of prescription medications, some jurisdictions legislate against a wide range of offences intended to deter what is defined as improper patient behaviour. In Florida, for instance, it is illegal to engage in 'doctor shopping', defined as: (1) not telling the doctor that the patient obtained a controlled substance for the same condition in the last 30 days; (2) being in possession of a prescription blank (if not a practitioner or working for one); (3) using misrepresentation, subterfuge, or deception to get a prescription; or (4) possessing a controlled drug without a prescription, or not in the container in which it was dispensed (Palm Beach County Sheriff's Office 2001). There is little literature on the effectiveness of such laws.

The medical community emphasizes the point that physicians' involvement in criminal diversion of prescription opioids is rare. For example, fewer than 0.1% of doctors registered with the US Drug Enforcement Agency were investigated in 2001, with an even smaller proportion having regulatory or punitive action taken against them (Zacny *et al.* 2003). Enforcement authorities suggest that substantial decreases in controlled substance provision following the introduction of PMPs had reduced diversion, and hence are 'the single direct measure of program success' (Fishman *et al.* 2004, p. 317).

12.6.3 System controls that monitor and regulate the supply of psychopharmaceuticals

While there is scant empirical literature on the effectiveness of controls on the production and distribution of psychopharmaceuticals, significant efforts have been devoted to building a supply chain impervious to diversion and counterfeiting of these drugs. At the international level, the three international drug conventions (see Chapter 13) and their implementing bodies have promoted system controls on psychoactive substances and their precursors. Supply control aids are built into the conventions, including provisions for record-keeping, labelling, and notification between sending and receiving countries. While the conventions' provisions were adopted in the era of manual record-keeping, the availability of electronic communication and record-keeping has considerably increased the possibility for surveillance and 'data mining' as an enforcement technique. Currently, a radiofrequency track-and-trace system producing a continuous 'pedigree' of custody of drug lots is in the course of implementation (Laven 2006).

The other side of regulating the supply of psychopharmaceuticals is discouraging the demand for them. For prescription drugs, this includes not only the question of banning or restricting direct advertising or promotion to potential consumers, but also the question of promotion to the prescribers. Sales strategies for psychopharmaceuticals include a variety of procedures designed to influence the prescribing behaviour of physicians, such as free samples, hiring clinical scientists to give lectures, subsidized continuing medical education, and free meals and gifts to doctors. While most physicians believe that they are beyond the influence of marketing, there is growing evidence that these activities affect prescribing behaviour in ways that favour a particular drug as well as the number of prescriptions written (Kassirer 2005; Brennan 2006). Although there are few examples specific to the promotion of psychopharmaceuticals, there is no reason to expect that industry promotional activities differ for this class of drugs. Other writers (Kassirer 2005) have noted a more indirect involvement by industry in the process of evaluating and approving pharmaceuticals. Research suggests that drug companies' extensive contacts with clinical research scientists can affect researchers' objectivity in reporting the results of clinical trials, and patient safety can be compromised when biased research leads to the approval of drugs that are later found to be harmful (Kassirer 2005; Brennan 2006). Three strategies have been devised to minimize the influence of conflicts of interest: disclosure, prohibition, and conflict management (Resnik 2007). Disclosure refers to the practice of informing relevant parties about the physician's or the scientist's financial or other interests in companies that may profit from the use of a particular drug. Prohibition involves preventing or eliminating the conflict. Conflict management refers to policies or procedures that require oversight or review of a conflict situation by an independent third party. There is little evidence to indicate whether these strategies are effective in preventing conflicts of interest and protecting patients from the influence of aggressive marketing practices. As of 2009, the US pharmaceutical industry has agreed to a voluntary moratorium on promotional products such as branded pens and T-shirts promoting prescription of their products (Singer 2008). It will be interesting to see if this limitation on one form of promotion to physicians has measurable effects on prescribing practices.

12.7 Conclusion

There is extraordinary variation among nations in the availability of prescription psychoactive drugs. For example, the ratio between per capita opioid consumption for the USA and Japan was greater than 50:1 in 2002–2004 (INCB 2006b), with Japan's main quantities of opioid consumption actually having decreased substantially since 2000, compared with starkly converse trends in the USA. As noted in Chapter 6, developing countries have extraordinarily low consumption rates of prescribed psychoactive drugs, a topic to which we return in the next chapter. A relevant question is why such highly pronounced discrepancies exist in different countries. Our focus on evidence from a few developed western nations reflects the fact that the problem of misuse of prescription drugs is primarily found in those nations, but it may well spread elsewhere as nations such as Brazil, China, and India become wealthier.

From the point of view of professional autonomy, psychoactive drugs have been perhaps the most poisoned of chalices for both pharmacists and physicians. On the one hand, nothing so well illustrates the power of life and death inherent in the mysteries of each profession than their custody and control over narcotics. On the other hand, narcotics and psychoactive substances have time and again been the territory in which modern states, spurred on sometimes by popular drug scares and sometimes by the international control system, have moved to restrict professional autonomy and to install systems of surveillance, investigation, and prosecution of professionals.

If we look at the results of the policy impact studies on prescription systems from the perspective of public health, what can we conclude? The Appendix at the end of the book summarizes the strategies discussed in this chapter in terms of evidence for effectiveness and amount of research support. Of the 13 strategies considered, seven have evidence of effectiveness, one shows evidence of ineffectiveness, and the rest have not been systematically evaluated. The following points summarize our findings:

- Changes in the cost of medications affect their demand when the medication is freely available to consumers. However, reimbursement programmes for medications affect this relationship. Demand for a medication covered by third-party reimbursement is less price sensitive. Demand for an uncovered medication, where a possible substitute for it is covered, is likely to be particularly price sensitive.

Where prescription is required for a medication, demand is likely to be less affected by its price. Price is potentially a mechanism for channelling demand between two drugs that are substitutes for each other, moving demand from a drug with more adverse consequences to a less risky alternative. However, there is no example of an impact study where this mechanism has been used.

- The evidence on effects of package size and place-of-sale restrictions on OTC sales is mixed. Nor is much evidence available on the effects of restricting OTC sales to 'behind-the-counter' sales or sales by a pharmacist. This is an area worth further investigation, with respect particularly to psychoactive preparations such as codeine cough medicines, where such restrictions are widely in effect. In the context of developing societies, where purchase directly from the pharmacy is often the primary source of medications, it would also be useful to explore extending 'pharmacist-only' purchasing to a wider range of controlled substances.
- At least for medications with limited psychoactivity, whether or not a drug is in OTC or prescription status seems to make surprisingly little difference to the occurrence of adverse effects. The issue of whether the OTC drug is reimbursed by third-party payers probably has more effect on patterns of use than whether a prescription is required.
- Authoritative advice to physicians on prescribing, in the absence of regulatory enforcement, seems to have limited effect unless the advice concerns a new and serious side effect and alternative medicines can be prescribed.
- Prescription guidelines enforced by regular inspections of records and clinical settings can dramatically change patterns of prescribing. The studies supporting this, however, arose from a circumstance of perceived crisis in which a variety of other system changes were being implemented.
- Shifting a prescribed drug onto a special prescription register, in conjunction with guidelines that limit prescriptions, usually causes a substantial drop in prescriptions of that drug. The effect seems to stem partly from the extra trouble involved in a registered prescription and partly from the deterrent effect on the physician of the threat of sanctions. However, a large part of the prescriptions will be replaced by prescriptions for a less controlled substitute drug. If the substitute drugs are less harmful, the result is a clear gain from a public health perspective; if the substitute drugs are more harmful, the shift causes a net loss for public health.
- Restricting prescriptions to a limited group of physicians or to dispensing in hospitals or clinics appears to be an effective way to reduce prescribed use of a drug. As might be expected, withdrawing a drug from the market has an even greater effect on prescribed use. Again, for both of these strategies, the issue that needs investigation on a case-by-case basis is the net public health effect of the substitute prescriptions that will be written, including whether there is a resulting unmet demand for treatment.
- Except for controls on the distribution of opioids in the context of opiate substitution treatment, such as methadone maintenance, there is little evidence that ancillary approaches related to prescription regimes are effective. This is not to say that patient profiling, law enforcement, treatment for those who become dependent on

> prescription drugs, and system controls are ineffective. Rather, it is testimony to the general lack of evaluation research on potentially costly interventions, and to the difficulty in conducting such research.

The debate over interventions to prevent prescription opioid misuse has focused on the controls aimed at the medical providers (e.g. physicians issuing prescriptions), especially the enforcement of rules governing when, how, and to whom these prescriptions are provided. This focus to a substantial degree implies both that legitimate and illegitimate prescription opioid use can be clearly delineated, and that misuse occurs predominantly among people obtaining drugs directly from the system. This ignores the blurred line between use and misuse, as for example in the case of individuals who developed a condition of opioid dependence in the course of pain treatment and are now self-medicating this condition by their own misuse following the termination of medical treatment. Certainly, much of the misuse of opioid analgesics is attributable to recreational and street users, and is supported indirectly via personal, social, or criminal sources rather than directly from the medical system (Joranson and Gilson 2006).

Prescription regimes have become the main way in which psychoactive substances subject to the international conventions are made available for legal consumption. The justification for this is that while the substances are medically useful, they are too attractive or dangerous to be made available for use for other purposes. Recent decades have seen an escalation in the medications covered and the degree of control.

However, the uses to which psychoactive substances are put in the modern world are diverse indeed. These include, for instance, staying awake and alert, improving psychological or physical performance, sleeping better, having better sex, and sensory enhancement. Restricting availability to the prescription regime means that these uses are either medicalized or illegitimized. The result has been a very broad medicalization of activities and conditions of daily life. One outcome of this, given that the state usually pays for prescriptions where there is state-funded health care, is increased pressure on state finances to pay for all prescriptions. The illegitimization of non-prescribed use also, of course, imposes enforcement costs on the state.

Section IV

Drug policy and system issues at the national and international levels

Chapter 13

Drug policy and control at the international level

13.1 Introduction: the great expansion in psychoactive substance use

In its initial stages, the effort to control drugs at an international level was aimed at limiting the reach and effects of colonial empires (Carstairs 2005). Psychoactive substances were a glue of empires in the period of European colonial expansion from about 1500 until the late 19th century (Courtwright 2001; Jankowiak and Bradburd 2003). From the point of view of those seeking to create markets and dependence on trade, psychoactive substances were an obvious choice; once the demand for them has been created, it becomes self-sustaining. Thus psychoactive substances became a favourite commodity from which to extract revenues for the state, either with excise taxes or through a state-run or farmed-out monopoly. In particular, opium monopolies were an important source of revenue for colonial powers in Asia (e.g. Munn 2000).

In the interests of financing their empires, European states had no compunctions about forcing open markets for their psychoactive wares. The most notorious such cases were the Opium Wars that Britain fought with China in the 1840s and 1850s to force the opening of the Chinese market for Indian opium (Courtwright 2001). Particular psychoactive substances often became associated with colonial domination, and rejection of the substances was sometimes a form of insurrection or resistance, as with opium in 20th century China (Yongming 2000).

The globalization brought by the era of European empires and the industrial revolution changed the circumstances of availability of psychoactive substances, as well as the living conditions of many people. Opium in China changed from being eaten, primarily as medicine, to being smoked for pleasure (Edwards 2005). Where production of psychoactive substances had been limited by seasons, available labour, or crop surpluses, now an assortment of such substances was always available to those with cash in the market economy. The availability of such substances increased dramatically as global and imperial trade developed. Habits of heavy use, which previously had often been available only to the wealthy, came within the reach of the poor.

13.2 The inception of international control: limiting colonial and imperial exploitation through drugs

In the latter part of the colonial era, opposition grew to the promotion and provision of psychoactive substances internationally. In part, this reflected the efforts of temperance movements in European metropolitan countries, particularly Britain, and in the USA (see, for instance, Tyrrell 1991). In part, it also reflected indigenous movements among colonized peoples (e.g. Mills 1985; Fahey and Manian 2005). The first expression in international law of the impulse to limit the international trade in psychoactive substances was the Brussels General Act of 1889, which provided that after 1901, for large parts of Africa, distilled spirits would either be prohibited for the 'native population' or would carry a minimum excise tax (Pan 1975). The General Act's provisions were confirmed by the Treaty of St. Germain-en-Laye (1919), one of the treaties concluding the First World War. These international alcohol control treaties were never particularly effective (Bruun *et al.* 1975), and fell gradually into disuse, though as late as the early 1950s there was still some concern among British civil servants about contravening them (Willis 2002).

In the late 19th century, temperance workers seeking to limit the exploitation of indigenous populations through psychoactive substances turned their attention to opium. The main political context of the opium issue was the long struggle between the British and Chinese governments over the marketing of opium in China, with the USA eventually taking an active role against the opium trade. An Opium Conference convened by the USA in Shanghai in 1909 led to the Hague Convention of 1912, which became the foundation document of the present system of international drug controls. Since the Hague Convention required universal ratification, it only came into full effect when Turkey and Germany, defeated in the First World War, were required to accede to it as Article 295 of the Versailles Treaty of 1919 (Bruun *et al.* 1975). The new League of Nations took on responsibility for administration of the Convention. A new International Opium Convention in 1925 extended the range of drugs covered, set up a system of import certifications and export authorizations, and created a Permanent Control Board, a forerunner of today's **International Narcotics Control Board (INCB)** (Donnelly 1992). A further 1931 Convention extended the trade controls and sought to enforce production limits to match estimates of medical and scientific needs. Between 1928 and 1938, recorded world trade in morphine decreased from 6972 kilograms to 1911, and in cocaine from 3230 kilograms to 843 (Donnelly 1992). Whether this change reflected the success of the control regime, the worldwide economic depression, or both, is open to debate.

13.3 The current international drug control treaties

The three main international drug control treaties presently in force (Treaties 2002) build on the foundation of the arrangements in the era of the League of Nations, but are products of three decades after the end of the Second World War. The first, the 1961 Single Convention on Narcotic Drugs (http://www.incb.org/incb/convention_1961.html) as amended in 1972, explicitly collated and extended the pre-war treaties, and covers substances derived from opium, cannabis, and coca leaves, along with cognate synthetics. To the old concerns about controlling colonial exploitation had been added a concern with demand control. Hence the 1961 Convention included criminalization of distribution or sale and punishment and/or treatment of the individual user (Carstairs 2005). The 1961 Convention extended requirements for control within national borders beyond opiates and cocaine to cover also cannabis, a provision adopted under 'heavy international pressure' from the USA, and which 'can be seen as an attempt to globalize the [American] Marijuana Tax Act' (Edwards 2005, p. 153).

The 1971 Convention on Psychotropic Substances (http://www.incb.org/incb/convention_1971.html) considerably extended the scope of the system to cover manufactured and synthetic drugs such as benzodiazepines, amphetamines, LSD, and barbiturates, although with a weaker set of controls than over the plant-based substances covered in the 1961 convention. The third Convention, adopted in 1988 (http://www.incb.org/incb/ convention_1988.html), as Carstairs (2005) argues, represented a further redefinition of the system in terms also of controlling crime, with arguments stressing the danger of drug traffic to national security, the links between the drug trade and corruption, and the role of the drug traffic in undermining economic development. But although the 1988 Convention was primarily concerned with 'illicit traffic', tackled through provisions on money laundering and confiscation of the proceeds of crime, it also included a provision which wrote into international law that 'possession or purchase of any narcotic drug or psychotropic substance' other than for approved medical or scientific purposes, was to be made not just a punishable offence, but specifically a criminal offence under domestic law (Article 3, ¶1(a)(iii)).

Thus, while the inception of the international drug control system was a century ago, and it had immediate effects at that time in the shaping of national drug laws, it was only in the last half-century that it took on much of its present expansive scope and detailed prescription of provisions to be included in domestic law. Despite their scope and intrusiveness, almost all states have ratified and are bound by the three treaties, an unusually large number for such treaties. As of 1 November 2006, there have been 184 ratifications for the 1961 Convention (181 for its 1972 protocol), 179 for the 1972 Convention, and 180 for the 1988 Convention (INCB 2007b). Their application is not quite universal (the INCB's count of nation-states is 203), but it is close.

In characterizing the three drug conventions below, we will offer comparisons with other international treaties in related areas. The main comparisons are with the Framework Convention on Tobacco Control, which was negotiated under the auspices of the **World Health Organization** and entered into force in 2005; the International Convention against Doping in Sport, which was negotiated under the auspices of UNESCO and adopted in 2005, but is not yet in force; and the UN Convention against Transnational Organized Crime (in force since 2003), and its Protocol about firearms (in force since 2005). The last two were negotiated under the auspices of the **UN Office of Drugs and Crime** (**UNODC**), the UN agency also responsible for drugs. While these treaties overlap with the drug treaties in their concerns, there are notable divergences in the approaches taken to international control of markets in hazardous commodities.

13.4 Characterizing the international drug control treaties

13.4.1 Mandated domestic legislation and controls

A prominent feature of the international drug control system is the extensiveness and detail of its concerns with domestic matters in ratifying nations. These may have been international treaties, but they held substantial implications for domestic legislation, and it has been a common experience for national delegations to return from international treaty conferences with the news that amendment of domestic legislation would be required by the new treaty. Thus, the UK Dangerous Drugs Act (1920) was adopted in furtherance of the Hague treaty obligations, and the preamble of the Netherlands Opium Act (1928) stated that it owed 'its existence primarily to considerations relating to international interests' (Gerritsen 2000, p. 132). The Canadian Opium and Drug Act (1911) was adopted in line with the Shanghai Commission's recommendations (Carstairs 2006), and the US Harrison Narcotic Act of 1914 was adopted, according to Musto (1973), in considerable part as an adjunct to foreign policy, to demonstrate sincerity in the wake of the Hague Convention.

The level of control over domestic decisions to which the system aspires exceeds, for instance, the level of ambition of the EU to control national arrangements in the same areas (e.g. concerning Dutch coffee shops), or the level of ambition of national governments in federal states to control state or provincial matters (e.g. concerning supervised drug consumption rooms in Australia). Table 13.1 shows some of the main provisions of the 1961 and 1971 Conventions concerning domestic measures,[1] with the equivalent provisions in the Framework Convention on Tobacco Control for comparison. In the drug conventions, governments are to exert control of their domestic market in drugs through licensing of sellers (or through a government monopoly, in the 1961 Convention) at all levels of the market—producers, traders, and retailers. Detailed records are to be kept of all transactions. At the retail level, medical prescriptions are to be required. The Tobacco Convention includes no requirements on licensing or record-keeping, although it is also much concerned with controlling illicit trade. Its provisions for limits on retail sales are relatively minor and peripheral, for example no free distribution or sales to minors, and bans on vending machine and self-service sales presented as an option.

Advertising and promotion are not restricted in the 1961 Convention, though a requirement of an indication of the generic name is mentioned as desirable; in the 1971 Convention, advertising to the general public is banned where constitutionally permissible (§10.2; reflecting the US limits on advertising of prescription medications at the time of adoption). Counter-promotion efforts are required in the drug conventions only 'if there is a risk that abuse [...] will become widespread'—a provision reflecting worries that counter-advertising might actually have a perverse effect 'by arousing the morbid curiosity of psychologically weak persons' (United Nations 1976, p. 88).

In addition to mandating controls on markets in psychoactive substances, the conventions require criminalization of the drug user, if and when the user is in possession of substances not legally obtained. This is an unusually strong requirement even in the context of national laws on contraband commodities, let alone as a requirement of parties to an international treaty, as noted in Chapter 11; there was no such provision,

[1] The 1961 Convention is as amended in 1972; provisions shown are for Schedule I drugs in the 1961 Convention, and Schedule II drugs in the 1971 Convention.

Table 13.1 Convention requirements of domestic measures to control the market for and use of psychoactive substances

	1961 Convention, e.g. morphine, cocaine	**1971 Convention, e.g. amphetamine**	**2003 Framework Convention for Tobacco Control**
Establishment of national agency	In case of legal cultivation, required (§23, 26, 28); for coordination of 'prevention and repressive action', required where system allows (§35)	Desirable (§6)	—
Limitation of production	For opium, limited to prior estimate of production 'as far as possible' (§21bis); prohibition of opium, coca, cannabis cultivation encouraged (§22)	—	—
Licensing of production, distribution, retailing	Licensing or government monopoly required (§29, 30)	Licensing required (§8); also inspections (§15)	Optional (§15.7)
Record-keeping	Required, to be retained for 2 years, for all involved—government agencies, traders, hospitals, etc. (§34b)	Required for manufacturers, distributors, retailers (§11)	—
Testing, measuring, regulating contents	—	—	Required (§9)
Labelling contents	Required for 'exact drug content', except when dispensed on individual prescription (§30.5); generic name desirable (§30.2)	*(declaration of contents attached to export packages §12.2)*	Required for constituents and emissions (§11.2); and for where to be sold (§15.2.a)
Warnings on or in packaging	Double red band if 'necessary or desirable', but not on exterior wrapping (§30.4)	Required, if deemed 'necessary for the safety of the user' (§10)	Required, detailed (§11)
Taxation	—	—	Urged as 'effective and important' (§6)
Prescription	Required (§30.2.b.i); if 'necessary or desirable', on counterfoil books (§30.2.b.ii)	Required (§9.1)	—
Distribution free or in small quantities	—	—	Prohibited (§16.2&3)

(continued)

Table 13.1 (continued) Convention requirements of domestic measures to control the market for and use of psychoactive substances

	1961 Convention, e.g. morphine, cocaine	**1971 Convention, e.g. amphetamine**	**2003 Framework Convention for Tobacco Control**
Sales in vending machines	*(implicit ban by limitation to prescription use)*	*(implicit ban by limitation to prescription use)*	Optional commitment to prohibit (§16.5)
Self-service sales	*(implicit ban by limitation to prescription use)*	*(implicit ban by limitation to prescription use)*	Optional ban (§16.1.b)
Sales to minors	—	—	Prohibited (§16)
Liability of producers or sellers	*(criminal penalties for illegal trade §36 and confiscation of illicit goods §37)*	*(criminal penalties for illegal trade and confiscation of illicit goods §22)*	Encouraged 'for the purpose of tobacco control' (§19)
Legislation against illicit trade	Required as punishable offence when intentional, subject to constitutional limitations (§36)	Required as punishable offence when intentional, subject to constitutional limitations (§22)	Required (§15.4.b)
Advertising	Indication of generic name desirable (§30.3)	Banned, where constitutional, to the general public (§10.2)	Banned if constitutionally allowed; otherwise restricted (§13)
Other promotion, sponsorship	—	—	Banned if constitutionally allowed; otherwise restricted (§13)
Possession of substance without legal authority	Shall not be permitted (§33); subject to constitutional limitations, shall be a punishable offence (§36a); *(also 1988 Convention as at right)*	*(1988 Convention, §3.2.: possession for personal use to be a criminal offence, subject to constitutional limits)*	—
Limits on times, occasions of use	—	—	Protection required from tobacco smoke in indoor public and workplaces (§8)
Providing and promoting treatment	Encouraged (§38)	Encouraged (§20)	Encouraged (§14.2)

Table 13.1 (continued) Convention requirements of domestic measures to control the market for and use of psychoactive substances

	1961 Convention, e.g. morphine, cocaine	1971 Convention, e.g. amphetamine	2003 Framework Convention for Tobacco Control
Promoting public awareness	Required 'if there is a risk that abuse of drugs will become widespread' (§38)	Required 'if there is a risk that abuse [...] will become widespread' (§20.3)	Required (§12)

Note: the 1961 Convention is as amended in 1972; provisions shown are for Schedule I drugs in the 1961 Convention and Schedule II drugs in the 1971 Convention.

— means that there is no such provision.

for instance, in the US federal alcohol Prohibition laws. The 1961 Convention includes specific provisions that possession of a substance controlled by the Convention without legal authority shall not be permitted, and that, where constitutionally allowed, it shall be a punishable offence. The 1988 Convention adds the requirement that possession of substances controlled under either the 1961 or the 1971 Convention shall be a criminal offence, again subject to constitutional limits.[2] A good deal of energy has been expended in discussions regarding what latitude these provisions leave for national interpretations which would allow **depenalization** or controlled legalization (e.g. Krajewski 1999; Lenton *et al.* 2000a), and, in fact, a number of jurisdictions have moved towards regimes without criminal penalties for use or possession while keeping the criminal offence in principle (see Chapter 11 and Room *et al.* 2008). But it is clear that the Conventions' provisions requiring **criminalization** of use have been a major impediment to efforts at national levels to move away from prohibition towards regulatory drug regimes.

13.4.2 Requirements for cooperation on international control

Table 13.2 shows a few of the main provisions of the 1961 and 1971 Conventions and of the Tobacco Convention concerning requirements for international cooperation by ratifying nations. A system of export and import authorizations is spelled out in considerable detail in the drug conventions. Thus the 1961 Convention specifies that an import authorization is required before a matching export authorization can be issued (§31.4&5). The Tobacco Convention has no such detailed international control regime; the closest it comes is a pledge to consider 'developing a practical tracking and tracing regime'. All three treaties require signatories to adopt legislation on seizure and destruction of contraband equipment and goods.

2 Switzerland and The Netherlands filed a reservation nullifying this provision for them when they ratified the 1988 Convention.

Table 13.2 Convention requirements for cooperation on international control of psychoactive substances

	1961 Convention, e.g. morphine, cocaine	**1971 Convention, e.g. amphetamine**	**2003 Framework Convention for Tobacco Control**
Enacting and strengthening legislation against illicit trade	Required (§35, 36)	Required (§21, 22)	Required (§15.4.b)
Cooperation with other countries and with international organizations	Required (§4.b)	'having due regard to [...] constitutional, legal and administrative systems', required for action against illicit traffic (§21)	Encouraged 'as appropriate' on policies (§5), and 'as mutually agreed' on expertise and assistance (§22)
Requiring and exchanging import and export authorizations	Required; import authorization required before issuing matching export authorization (§31.4&5)	Required; import authorization required before issuing matching export authorization (§12)	To consider 'developing a practical tracking and tracing regime' (§15.2.b)
Support other country's prohibition of specific substance	'not knowingly permit' export to where illegal (§31.1)	Required to ensure no export to that country (§13.2)	—
Sales and imports of tax- and duty-free products	—	—	May prohibit or restrict 'as appropriate' (§6.2.b)
Marking products with destination and origin	*(export authorization including contents with package §31.6)*	*(export declaration including contents with package §15.2.b)*	Required (§15.2)
Monitoring and controlling of goods in transit or bonded	Required (§31); withdrawal from bonded warehouse requires a permit (§31.9)	Required (§12.3.c&f)	Required for products held or moving 'under suspension of taxes or duties' (§15.4.d)
Seizure and confiscation of manufacturing equipment and goods in illicit trade	Required (§37)	Required (§22.3)	Destruction of seized equipment and goods required (§15.4.c)
Confiscation of proceeds derived from illicit trade	*(covered by Article 5 of 1988 Convention)*	*(covered by Article 5 of 1988 Convention)*	To be adopted 'as appropriate'
Elimination of cross-border advertising, promotion, sponsorship	—	—	May ban and penalize such cross-border promotion on basis equal to penalties on domestic promotion (§13.7)

Table 13.2 (continued) Convention requirements for cooperation on international control of psychoactive substances

	1961 Convention, e.g. morphine, cocaine	**1971 Convention, e.g. amphetamine**	**2003 Framework Convention for Tobacco Control**
Assistance to other countries on civil or criminal liability	Extradition for crimes encouraged, required where there is an extradition treaty; but can be refused if 'not sufficiently serious' (§36.2.b) *(also §5 of 1988 Convention as at right)*	*(§5 of 1988 Convention has detailed provisions for collaboration on confiscations)*	Encouraged (§19.3)
Reporting requirements to international bodies	Annual report with text of laws, illicit traffic details, which authorities issue export/import licenses (§§18.1, 20), estimated needs for medical and scientific purpose, amounts for manufacture, stocks held, areas cultivated (§19)	Annual statistical reports; annual report on changes and developments (§16)	Periodic reports, on a schedule to be agreed on, on laws, surveillance, taxation, trade, etc. (§21)

Note: the 1961 Convention is as amended in 1972; provisions shown are for Schedule I drugs in the 1961 Convention and Schedule II drugs in the 1971 Convention.

— means that there is no such provision.

13.4.3 The mixed nature of the drug control conventions

In our era the drug control conventions are conventionally thought of in terms of crime control. Responsibility for them within the UN system is located in the Vienna office, which, as the corridor joke has it, is responsible for 'uncivil society'—not only crime, but also such topics as nuclear weapons control. Crime and drug control are now combined in the same UN agency, the UNODC. The primacy of the crime rubric was set by the 1988 Convention, which focused on 'illicit traffic'. Accordingly, delegations to the occasional ministerial meetings at the Commission on Narcotic Drugs these days are more likely to be headed by interior or justice ministers than by health or welfare ministers (Room 2005c).

The Conventions have a second facet: they are also international agreements concerning hazardous commodities. At the heart of the 1962 and 1971 conventions are lists of commodities evaluated by WHO experts in terms of their '**dependence liability** and **abuse potential**', and in principle distributed between different schedules according to how strongly they have these qualities. Compared with how the world handles other risky commodities, the Conventions represent an unusual degree of international control. The provisions for international control are much weaker, for instance in the 2001 protocol against the Illicit Manufacturing of and Trafficking in Firearms (United Nations 2001).

There is also a third facet to the Conventions: they are a specialized and very unusual form of trade agreement. Along with countering addiction as a 'serious evil', the Preamble of the 1961 Convention refers to a second basis for action: 'the medical use of narcotics continues to be indispensable for the relief of pain and suffering', and 'the availability of narcotic drugs for such purposes' must be assured. In pursuit of this aim, the 1961 Convention sets up a centrally planned economy in opiates and cocaine on a global scale, with the INCB managing the market through a system of national estimates, reports and directives. The 1971 Convention is less ambitious in this regard. Taken together, however, the drug conventions exempt the drugs they control from the common assumptions about the superiority of competition and free movement of goods which have been applied in the era of the World Trade Organization to most other commodities. The drug Conventions are a kind of trade treaty, but with their provisions for designated producing countries and state monopolies they turn the usual assumptions of modern trade treaties upside down.

To think of the Conventions only in terms of crime control, therefore, is a mistake. The evaluation of their effectiveness, accordingly, should be in terms of their multiple purposes. Whether they effectively suppress illicit markets in drugs is a question dealing with only one of their aspects. Whether they indeed are focused on the most hazardous of psychoactive substances, with appropriate rankings on severity of effects, is another important question. And whether they in fact ensure the availability of opiate and other medications to those in pain and need is a third.

13.5 **The implementation of the treaties: the UN drug agencies**

Three specialized international bodies are responsible for the implementation of the treaties (with the WHO also playing a technical role): the Commission on Narcotic Drugs (CND), a political body with states elected as members by the Economic and Social Council of the UN (ECOSOC); the UNODC, the administrative body for the UN's programmes in both the drug area and the crime area; and the INCB (Room and Paglia 1999).

The INCB, with 13 members elected by ECOSOC as experts, supposedly in their personal capacities rather than as representatives of countries, quite self-consciously regards itself as the 'guardian' of the conventions. It defines its responsibilities as 'to promote government compliance with the provisions of the drug control treaties and to assist them in this effort'. This includes both making sure that the licit (medical) market is supplied, and that illicit drug trafficking is suppressed (http://www.incb.org/e/index.htm—'Mandate'). The INCB issues an annual report, in which it regularly scolds governments in diplomatic language for what it views as deficiencies in their actions, and tackles a different special theme each year. For instance, the 2001 report included a discussion of threats to drug control from globalization and the Internet (INCB 2002); the 2006 report focused on the 'unregulated market' in psychoactive medications (INCB 2007b). In addition, its members undertake about 20 missions a year to assist governments in their duties under the conventions (Emafo 2002). The secretariat of the INCB, formally a part of the UNODC, is also involved from time to time in monitoring and admonitory activities which the INCB regards as part of the guardianship. For instance, Herbert Schaepe, the INCB's Secretary, was widely quoted in the Australian press threatening that the INCB would cut off Australia's quota for legal production of opiates if supervised drug consumption rooms were set up (Mann 1999), and engaged in correspondence with an Australian priest on the topic (Schaepe 1999).

As the Australia case shows, for the short list of countries that are licensed to produce opiates, the INCB can threaten action to cut off a legal industry. But otherwise the INCB has no formal powers of enforcement; its powers are limited to persuasion, exposure, and criticism. In recent years, the hard line it has taken in its interpretation of the conventions has encountered increasing criticism, including on the floor of the CND meetings (e.g. International Drug Policy Consortium 2007). The importance of the INCB is therefore somewhat less than its own estimation of it. Perhaps the threat of a scolding from it does affect nations planning to make policy changes, but its specific reports appear not to have affected developed countries such as Australia, Switzerland, and the UK that have been the subject of its criticisms.

The UNODC has altogether about 500 staff, in the Vienna headquarters and scattered across the world. Its operational budget for drugs for 2006 was announced as US$69.1 million (http://www.unis.unvienna.org/unis/pressrels/2007/unisnar988.html). This is a pittance with which to have any impact on global drug use and production, in comparison, for instance, with US expenditures on international 'government assistance' for drugs of US$472.4 million in 2006 (Bureau of International Narcotics and Law Enforcement Affairs 2007). The UNODC must find a specialized niche in support of national governments if it is to make an impact with such a small budget.

The CND consists of representatives of 53 states elected from UN member states in ECOSOC. It meets annually in Vienna for a week or more. Several hundred participants attend Commission meetings, including representatives of states not on the CND and of non-governmental organizations (NGOs) in 'consultative status' with ECOSOC. As the political governing body of the system, the CND each year considers the annual report of the INCB and of the UNODC, and negotiates over and passes resolutions concerning the operation of the system and drug policy issues (see Room 2002a, 2005c).

The WHO plays a technical role under both the 1961 and 1971 Conventions in recommending whether particular substances should be scheduled under either of the conventions, and in which Schedule of the conventions they should be placed. If a substance is scheduled under the 1961 or the 1971 Convention, its production, distribution, and use come under the authority of the international control system. The level of control of a substance is determined by which of the Conventions it is placed under, and by which of several schedules in each Convention it is placed in. The recommendations on scheduling are made by an Expert Committee on Drug Dependence, which is now constituted for a meeting every 2 years.

However, the international control system is increasingly inclined to disregard the scientific advice it receives from the WHO. This is illustrated by the system's lack of action on the rescheduling of dronabinol (Δ-9 tetrahydrocannabinol, THC), the principal psychoactive constituent of cannabis, which is prescribed as a medicine, particularly in the USA. While the plant cannabis and its natural products are included in the 1961 Convention among the substances which are most dangerous and without any therapeutic usefulness (Schedules I and IV), dronabinol was listed under Schedule I of the 1971 Convention (the most restrictive of the schedules for that treaty) at the time of the Convention's adoption. The 1989 WHO Expert Committee on Drug Dependence recommended that that dronabinol be transferred to Schedule II of the 1971 Convention. The CND initially rejected this, but after a reconsideration by the next Expert Committee made the same recommendation, the CND assented in 1991. The 2002 WHO Expert Committee made another critical review, and partly in view of the increased medical use of dronabinol recommended its reclassification to Schedule IV, the least restrictive schedule. The Director of the White House **Office of National Drug Control Policy** (the US 'drug tsar') persuaded the Director-General of WHO not to forward this recommendation, claiming it would 'send a wrong signal and create a tension with the 1961 Convention' (International Drug Policy Consortium 2007). The 2006 WHO Expert Committee reconsidered and updated the review. Hesitating between Schedules III and IV, it finally recommended transfer to Schedule III as a small step forward. In the 2007 CND debate on this, the USA was strongly opposed, and many other countries fell in line. The recommendation was sent back again for reconsideration by the WHO 'in consultation with the INCB' (although the INCB has no formal role in scheduling under the treaties).

One is struck by the contrast between the enormous energy and attention the treaties command in the debating room and their modest impact in daily life in everyday life. Dronabinol was prescribed, primarily in the USA, before, during, and after these heated debates, and its status as a Schedule 3 drug in that country does not seem to be affected by the anticipated change.

13.6 The dominant role of the USA

Ever since the Shanghai Conference, the USA has played a leading role in international drug policy, though during the interwar years its role was hampered by its decision not to join the League of Nations (e.g. Walker 1992; Bewley-Taylor 1999; Room 2005c). At times the driving force has been the internal situation in the USA. For instance, the adoption of the 1971 Convention reflects the rise of the youth counterculture of the late 1960s. At other times, and particularly more recently, the USA's emphasis has been on foreign policy objectives. The rubric of the international war on drugs has often served as a flexible instrument for forwarding general American policy interests, as well as drug concerns (Walker 1992; Nadelmann 1993; Bewley-Taylor 1999). On the other hand, in some circumstances, as for example in Afghanistan since the fall of the Taliban, other US foreign policy interests have over-ridden US drug concerns (Schweich 2008).

The USA plays a self-consciously leading role within the international drug control system. Where the 'ten minutes' assigned to each country in the general debate in the first days of each year's CND meeting is used by most countries to report on developments in their own country, the US contribution is usually a *tour d'horizon* on the world situation.

The weighty US presence is felt in the committee negotiations on the most trivial details of each year's resolutions (Room 2005c).

The activities of the USA in the international drug control system are actually only a small part of its total external efforts on drugs. In 2007 the US Drug Enforcement Administration had 751 staff posted in a total of 59 other countries in 2007 (Office of the Inspector General, Audit Division 2007), considerably outnumbering the total staff of the UNODC. Other agencies, such as the Customs Service and FBI, also had many officers stationed in embassies to help with drug control.

The USA's international effort is pursued through policy statements, diplomacy, bilateral agreements, and unilateral action. Each year, the State Department issues an International Narcotics Control Strategy Report, portrayed on its website as 'the United States Government's country-by-country two volume report that describes the efforts to attack all aspects of the international drug trade, chemical control, money laundering and financial crimes' (http://www.state.gov/p/inl/rls/nrcrpt/).

Under USA legislation, there is also a requirement that the US President produce each year a 'Majors List', which describes major drug transit or illicit drug-producing countries. Separately, the President is required to deny certification to countries which have 'failed demonstrably' to 'adhere to their obligations under international counter-narcotics agreements', a denial which carries serious fiscal and reputational consequences. The President can opt not to deny certification because of 'vital national interest', an option that is often exercised. Twenty countries, none of them high income countries, were on the Majors List in the Presidential Determination of September 2007 (US Department of State, Bureau for International Narcotics and Law Enforcement Affairs 2008, vol. I, pp. 7–12). Burma and Venezuela were the only countries listed for decertification, but the decertification for Venezuela was partially stayed to allow continued US support for programmes there 'to support civil society and other beleaguered democratic institutions', since this was determined to be 'vital to the national interests of the United States'. The global scope of the Determination is indicated by the list of other countries for which the situation was discussed in the Determination: Afghanistan, Bolivia, Canada, Ecuador, Guinea Bissau, India and Nigeria (though Canada and Guinea Bissau were not put on the Majors List).

The US certification/designation programme is a primary and often cited example of external influence on global and local drug policy with serious implications for bilateral and multilateral relations between northern and southern countries (Obot 2004). That the certification programme exists at all is regarded in some circles as insulting (CNN 2001). Beyond this, it has been criticized for being at least as much an instrument of foreign policy as a drug control mechanism (Nadelmann 1993; Ayling 2005; Obot 2004). In 2002 the process of certifying countries was modified so that decertification now has a higher threshold: that the country has 'failed demonstrably [...] to make substantial efforts during the previous 12 months to adhere to counter-narcotics agreements and take certain counter-narcotics measures set forth in U.S. law' (US Department of State, Bureau for International Narcotics and Law Enforcement Affairs 2003, p. I-5). However, now as before, compliance is sought with a big stick and the promise of some carrots:

> If a country is not certified, most foreign assistance is cut off and the United States is required to vote against funding by six multilateral development banks to that country.

> However, assistance may be provided if the President determines at any time after his initial determination that the provision of assistance during the fiscal year is a vital national interest or that the country has made substantial efforts to comply with the standard.
>
> (ONDCP 2006)

The certification/designation process is an important issue in international drug policy because of the implications it has for the development and implementation of national policies. As the experience of Nigeria, the only transit country that occupied a position on the list of decertified countries for several years, has shown, being decertified carries with it many intended and unintended consequences, as countries try to achieve the benchmarks by resorting to extreme measures (Obot 2004).

The involvement of Nigerians in international drug trade dates back to the 1960s, when many young Nigerians were arrested and prosecuted in the UK for trafficking in cannabis (Lambo 1965). Trafficking in cocaine and heroin dates back to the early 1980s, when it came to the attention of law enforcement officials that the country had become a transit point for cocaine and South West Asian heroin meant for the US and European markets (Obot 1990, 1992, 2004). Between 1991 and 2000 the number of arrests for drug offences in the country increased from 293 to 2385; most of the arrests were made at airports and seaports for trafficking in cocaine and heroin. Similar arrests of Nigerians were made in drug-producing countries and at points of entry into major consuming countries in Europe and the USA. By the early 1990s Nigeria and Nigerians had come to be seen as key players in the international drug supply chain. In 1994 the country was put on the decertification list, and for 5 years (1994–1998) was treated as a pariah state by the US government. An analysis of drug policy in Nigeria covering the period from 1994 to 2000 shows that these were very difficult years for the country because of the social and economic losses that resulted from its international status as a country deemed not cooperating enough in the war on drugs (Obot 2004):

> Like drug trafficking, which it was meant to stifle, decertification resulted in significant economic, social, and psychological consequences for Nigeria and Nigerians. The effects of missed economic opportunities, diminished international support for civil society initiatives, the experiences of humiliation at airports around the world are still felt today. More important, because drug control in Nigeria, especially in the second half of the last decade, was focused solely on the achievement of certification benchmarks, a domestic perspective on the solution to drug problems has failed to evolve. Decertification contributed to an existing neglect of demand reduction [and] abuse of human rights, [...] and solidified a war mentality in dealing with the problem [drug use] in the country.
>
> (Obot 2004, p. 25)

The certification/designation statute as an instrument of international drug control and drug diplomacy in general has been widely criticized by experts in the north and south and even within the US policy establishment. One criticism is that efforts to control drug supply 'reflect [...] attempts by western industrialized states to impose their standards and values upon the rest of the world' (McAllister 2000, p. 254). Opposition to the operation of the certification process has been voiced. Some political advocates charge that the decertification process is unfair, ineffective, and leads to human rights abuses (Ayling 2005). A careful scientific evaluation of these charges has not been conducted; what one can observe is that the few countries that have been decertified over the years are typically pariahs to western governments for other reasons, as Nigeria was during the period of military government through the mid-1990s, and as Burma and Syria were then and remain in the 2000s.

13.7 The advent of civil society

The main change in the system in recent years has been the increased attention of 'civil society' to its considerations and meetings. Those involved in the system used to be limited almost entirely to representatives or nominees of governments, but in recent years there has been a substantial increase in representation at CND meetings of non-governmental organizations (NGOs); 81 were represented at the 2007 meeting (International Drug Policy Consortium 2007), and over 300 NGOs took part in an NGO Forum in connection with the 2009 review of the performance of the international drug control system since 1998 (http://www.unodc.org/unodc/en/ngos/beyond2008.html; Vienna NGO Committee 2009). Despite efforts by supporters of the system to counter the trend, many of the NGOs are committed to change of some sort. Along with this has come a growth of critical scholarship on international drug control (e.g. Bewley-Taylor and Trace 2006; TNI 2008).

13.8 The drug control system as an artefact of a particular historical epoch

A century ago, medical concepts of inebriety and addiction commonly linked together opium, alcoholm and tobacco (e.g. Crothers 1902; Towns 1915), with alcohol and opium addicts often treated in the same institutions. The movements to prohibit alcohol which were especially strong in English-speaking and Nordic countries had offshoots which pushed for prohibition of tobacco or of opiates. As we have noted, under the Hague Convention of 1912, opium was actually the second psychoactive substance brought under some kind of international control, preceded by the treaty on alcohol in Africa.

As David Courtwright (2005) has described, drawing primarily on US sources, the 60 years after the Hague Convention were marked by an increasingly radical separation of thinking about alcohol, drugs, and tobacco. The banalization of cigarette smoking after the First World War, and the adoption by a new generation of middle-class youth of cigarette smoking by both genders as a generational symbol (Fass 1977), brought with it the exclusion of nicotine from concepts of inebriety or addiction. In the same era, alcohol Prohibition was implemented and eventually repealed in the USA and elsewhere (Schrad 2007), in part due to rejection by the same generation of middle-class youth (Room 1984). The repeal of prohibition brought in its wake a rethinking of alcohol problems (Roizen 1991), redefining them from problems attributable to the substance to problems located in deficiencies in the person—the 'alcoholic' (Christie and Bruun 1969).

'Narcotics' were thus left as the residual legatees of a conceptualization in terms of inherently dangerous and menacing drugs, a conceptualization transferred from temperance-era conceptualzations of alcohol. Moral panics about drug use (e.g. Kohn 1992; Manderson 1993; Carstairs 2006), with use often associated with derogated racial minorities, had much to do with the demonization of drugs in all English-speaking countries at some time between 1880 and 1940. Though drugs were generally a peripheral political issue before the 1960s, there was thus general support for the restrictive policies pushed forward by the small 'gentlemen's club' (Bruun *et al.* 1975) of the international drug control system, focused until 1971 specifically on substances derived from three plants grown primarily in the developing world.

In recent years, as Courtwright (2005) argues, the divisions have broken down, and alcohol, tobacco, and other psychoactive substances are increasingly seen again in the same conceptual frame. Biological researchers look at the various brain receptors involved in the action of psychoactive drugs very much in a common frame (WHO 2004). Tobacco has been taken back into the addiction concept, now renamed 'dependence'. Alcohol and tobacco are increasingly included in discussions of the dangerousness of drugs, usually ranking considerably higher than many drugs under international control (e.g. Nutt *et al.* 2007), often to considerable political consternation (Room 2006). In the WHO's evaluations of the contribution of risk factors to the global burden of disease (WHO 2002), tobacco and alcohol are indeed each estimated to make five times the contribution to the global burden made by illicit drugs. Drug and alcohol treatment have been reorganized as a single system in many countries (although tobacco treatment is still usually separate), and alcohol, tobacco, and drug education are often combined in schools.

The drug control conventions are an artefact of the historical period when the divisions between different psychoactive substances were at their greatest. The 1961 convention codified and also strengthened the pre-war controls on the three plant-derived substances; the 1971 convention, adopted as a reaction to the rise of youth drug countercultures in western societies, and in the context of the first US political 'war on drugs', extended the 'narcotics' frame to a wider range of substances. Embedded in the conventions are conceptions and categorizations of psychoactive substances which are increasingly at odds with current knowledge.

13.9 The effects of the system

13.9.1 Control of illicit markets and supply

In terms of its most often recognized aim, suppressing the illicit traffic in drugs, in most accountings the international drug control system is pronounced to be a failure. The UNODC's own banner publication, the *World Drug Report* of 1997, noted that ultimately supply reduction strategies 'must be judged by how they affect consumer demand, through the decreased availability of drugs', and that 'in this domain the outcome is undoubtedly less than satisfactory' (UNIDCP 1997).

A decade later, the UNODC's *Annual Report 2007* was no more sanguine: '2006 was a mixed year for international drug control'. The 'good news' of reduction of illicit opium production in the Asian Golden Triangle countries was 'eclipsed by the bad news from Afghanistan, the year's big story [...]. UNODC warned western countries to prepare for a possible increase in drug overdoses as a result of the increased purity of heroin. Rising cocaine consumption in Europe was another cause for concern' (UNODC 2007, p. 11). The 2008 Report has much the same tone: 'In 2007, opium cultivation increased in both Afghanistan and Myanmar: coupled with higher yields, especially in southern Afghanistan, this generated much greater world output. With regard to cocaine, cultivation increased in Bolivia, Peru and especially Colombia, but yields declined, so production remained stable' (UNODC 2008, p. 3).

In these circumstances, the UNODC's best foot forward is often put in terms of accomplishments other than progress towards its main goals. The Executive Director's foreword to the *Annual Report 2007* noted that the UNODC's 'announcement of a record opium harvest in Afghanistan [...] reinforced the Office's reputation for providing the gold standard for drug cultivation data'.

Other voices within the system often agree with the generally pessimistic tone; 'year after year, the situation is worse', as the delegation from Greece put it in the CND general debate in 1994 (Room 1999). Summing up the situation in the 1995 general debate, the Interpol representative noted that

> I am reminded of the film title, *Same Time, Next Year*—as the years go by, there is no real improvement in the situation. There are serious problems in nearly every region [...]. Next year we hope for serious progress, but we can't report it today.
>
> (Room 1999)

Policy analysts who are more at arms length have generally concurred with these conclusions:

> The world today is not any closer to achieving the ten-year targets set by the 1998 UN General Assembly Special Session (UNGASS) on drugs. These goals were 'eliminating or significantly reducing the illicit cultivation of coca bush, the cannabis plant and the opium poppy by the year 2008'. Instead global production of opiates and cocaine has significantly increased over the last ten years. According to the United Nations Office on Drugs and Crime (UNODC) global illicit opium production doubled from 4,346 tons in 1998 to 8,800 tons in 2007.
>
> (TNI 2008)

13.9.2 Ensuring and controlling medicinal supplies

Evaluations of the effects of the system, whether critical or sympathetic, tend to focus only on the effectiveness of the system in eliminating illicit markets and supply. In this context, very little attention is paid to the other aim of the system: making psychoactive medications available for medical and scientific use. On this aim, the system can show some successes. We have already discussed (Chapter 12) the operation of prescription regimes in channelling psychoactive medications into use under medical supervision. As Bruun and colleagues (1975, p. 276) noted some time ago, the system's successes tend to be where 'it has been the conduct of professions and of private enterprise which has been influenced', while the system has had little success where its efforts are 'directly aimed at affecting the individual drug-taker at the behavioural level'. Put in other terms, the successes of the system are in the control of legal markets in psychoactive medications, and exemplify that 'control systems operate most effectively through a license system which restricts sales, provision, or authorization of sales to particular professions or licensees' (Room 2000). Licensed actors in a legitimate market have an interest in supporting and buttressing the system, while if the market is illicit the interests of those active in it are opposed to the system's.

In terms of ensuring adequate supplies of the drugs for medical use, on the face of it the system seems to have operated well except in times of world war. The issue has usually been defined in terms of supplies of opiates for pain medication. In the context of rich developed societies, the INCB in its role as custodian of the world market appears to have made adequate provisions in a timely way for supplies of such medication.

In much of the developing world, however, the picture is very different. The gross imbalance in world consumption of legal opiates, discussed in Chapter 3, is a pointer to severe shortages and indeed the unavailability of effective pain medications in many developing countries. According to a WHO Briefing Note (WHO 2007), 80% of the world's population has either no or inadequate access to treatment for moderate or severe pain, and tens of millions of people suffer from moderate to severe pain each year without treatment. Recognizing this, the INCB's Report for 2006 noted that 'the low levels of consumption of opioid analgesics for treatment of moderate to severe pain in several developing countries continue to be a matter of concern to the Board' (INCB 2007b, p. 12). The problem stems not only from lack of resources to purchase opioids. In countries where law enforcement perspectives dominate drug policymaking, and where prescription systems do not function efficiently, the issue is defined as avoiding the creation of a black market of diverted drugs. The solution seems often to be to cut off the medical supply of opioids.

13.10 **Conclusion**

The self-evaluation of the international drug control system's progress in the decade after the 1998 resolution of the United Nations General Assembly Special Session (UNGASS) duly took place in March 2009. Despite efforts there to put a brave face on the situation, it is clear that the 1998 resolution that the world's drug problems should be substantially reduced 10 years later has not been fulfilled. One may argue whether global drug problems have notably worsened, but it is hardly possible to claim that they have lessened, as is clear from the data presented in other chapters of this book.

The question, then, will be whether there are changes in the international control system that would be likely to improve the situation. There is a good deal of discussion of changes that would involve removing certain of the controls or at least imposing them more flexibly. For example, the INCB might be persuaded to be less disapproving of national experiments such as heroin maintenance in Switzerland and a few other European nations, that add to the world's knowledge about alternative policies and that push the boundaries of the existing system. At present, however, there are no signs that any significant change will be made in the system.

Chapter 14

The variety of national drug policies

14.1 Introduction

Drug policies differ among nations in both appearance and substance. Some nations treat drugs primarily as a problem for law enforcement and give great prominence to efforts to suppress trafficking; others focus their efforts primarily on prevention and education, on helping dependent drug users, and on reducing the adverse consequences of drug use. This variation across nations reflects differences in attitudes toward drug use itself, toward individual rights, and toward the role of government. It also reflects the nature and history of national drug problems, the broader political structure of a country, and the different ways in which drugs affect a nation. For some nations, it is primarily a problem of domestic use, while for others, trafficking to richer nations is the principal way in which illicit drugs damage public health and safety. Policy advice that ignores these differences across nations and assumes that there is a single 'best policy' for all nations is itself likely to be ignored. In this chapter we describe some of the observed policy variation and its sources, so that readers can better understand their own country's choices and how they are framed. This is intended to supplement the descriptions and evaluations of individual programmes that appeared in previous chapters.

The chapter begins by describing the range of drug problems and policies in two very different countries, Mexico and Sweden. These illustrate the interconnections among problems, context, and policies. This is followed by a more parsimonious characterization of the variation in the problems and policies of seven nations: China, India, Mexico, Nigeria, Sweden, the UK, and the USA. All seven have serious drug problems that differ in nature, to which they also have responded in diverse ways. The remainder of the chapter elaborates the nature and consequences of the differences.

The principal focus here is on policy variation across countries, but there is also important variation within a country. Laws are unlikely to differ much across states or municipalities, but they may be implemented in very different ways.

14.2 Mexico

14.2.1 The country

Mexico is the most populous nation between the USA and Brazil, with a total of 110 million inhabitants in 2008. The per capita income in PPP (Purchasing Power Parity) terms was US$10 000 in 2004, making it a middle-income county in terms of the standard UN classification. It has had civilian rule since 1929, with minimal concern about military coups. It was ruled by the Institutional Revolutionary Party (PRI) for 71 years until Vicente Fox of the PAN was elected president in 2000.

14.2.2 Drug problems

Marijuana became the drug of choice in the late 1970s, increasing substantially in the 1990s, but prevalence still remains well below levels in more affluent western nations. In 2002, only 0.6% of the population between 12 and 65 years of age reported use in the last year; this compares with a figure of 11% in the USA. Cocaine use has increased substantially in recent years. Although prevalence remains low in the general population, it has become the dominant drug amongst those seeking treatment. Heroin has been mostly limited to cities on the border with the USA. It has been estimated that 0.4% of the population meets the criteria for substance dependence. Cases of HIV linked to drug injection are low (0.7% of registered cases), mainly due to low rates of injection among cocaine abusers and low rates of heroin abuse. Hepatitis C is highly prevalent among IDUs.

Mexico is the principal country through which drugs flow into the USA. A substantial amount of US-destined cocaine and heroin from Colombia enters through Mexico. In addition, Mexico is the leading producer of heroin for the US market as well as the principal foreign supplier of cannabis and methamphetamine.

The drug industry generates billions of dollars in revenue[1] for Mexican nationals, but this amounts to a small proportion of Mexico's 2006 GDP of US$744 billion. Nevertheless, these earnings are relatively significant in some regions. The bulk of that income is generated by trafficking rather than growing of opium poppies or marijuana. What is more difficult to estimate is the effect of drug trafficking on crime and corruption, as illustrated in Box 14.1.

14.2.3 Politics and law

Political structure and policy

Because the drug problem is considered a matter of national security, drug-related offences (production, possession, etc.) are subject to federal enforcement. Government coordinating councils have been established at the federal, state, and local levels. In the 1990s the National Programme was placed in the Attorney General's Office. Fourteen agencies report to this Office, whose main emphasis is on supply reduction and international cooperation. Crop substitution and alternative development programmes have not been part of the national strategy.

---

[1] Official statements often refer to larger figures but these are probably exaggerated. Working with plausible estimates of total drug expenditures in the USA, US$60 billion in 2000, the most recent year with published estimates (ONDCP 2001b), and taking account of the share of those revenues accruing to producers, exporters, and smugglers and the share of each sector likely to originate in Mexico, the plausible figure is no more than US$5 billion dollars.

Box 14.1 The social and political consequences of drug trafficking in Mexico

For at least two decades the drug trafficking gangs, such as the Gulf Cartel and the Juarez Cartel, have been a source of great violence, leading to many homicides not only of other traffickers but also of police and government officials, and occasionally of journalists. For example, on 17 May 2007 a shoot-out between police and traffickers resulted in 22 deaths in a single day. Over 4000 people were estimated to have been killed in drug-related violence in the first ten months of 2008 (Diaz 2008). In border cities this has occasionally produced extreme levels of disorder; for example, in Nuevo Laredo two police chiefs were killed by drug trafficking groups and the city has had difficulty recruiting a replacement for the job (Freeman 2006). This violence is a prominent part of Mexico's perceived drug problem and in 2006 the newly elected president Calderon made it a major issue for his government, as had the Fox regime in its first year.

Crop eradication and intelligence activities have been prominent in the political discussion since the 1970s when programmes for eradication of illegal opium and cannabis were first implemented. Tension with the USA around drug issues has been a leading concern in the country both officially and in the media as a consequence of the US State Department's annual International Narcotics Control Strategy Report, which passes judgement on whether Mexico's government has 'cooperated fully' with the USA in suppressing drug traffic.

Federal control of domestic drug trafficking was adequate when drug use within the country was limited and the local production of heroin and marijuana, as well as cocaine trafficking, were meant for the US market. Local distribution of drugs became an increasing problem in the late 1980s, but local drug dealers face little risk of apprehension because of the small number of federal police and because local police lack jurisdiction.

Laws

The federal government has the principal role in criminal law. Federal penalties for production, trafficking, and distribution of drugs are harsh by international standards. At the same time, Mexican law considers that drug dependence is a disease and thus should be handed over to health authorities. Possessing drugs for personal use is not considered an offence when the individual is drug dependent. There are in fact very few convictions for personal possession. The law also includes exceptions for first time offenders carrying drugs for their personal use if the offender has not been involved in other offences.

14.2.4 Programmes

Enforcement

Enforcement against illegal production has been a sustained activity since the middle of the 20th century. Major resources are allocated to combat smuggling and trafficking, with many deaths among enforcement personnel. A substantial proportion of arrests are for drug distribution at the local level, but the majority of persons arrested are released because of corruption and the lack of an adequate legal framework to combat drug distribution locally. Yet it is estimated that around two-thirds of persons in prisons have a drug problem.

Efforts to combat corruption and money laundering have been very prominent. However, corruption has been a constant problem, with very senior police and military officials being convicted of close ties to drug trafficking throughout the last 25 years; for example, in 1997 the head of Mexico's drug policy office, a former general, was found to be in the pay of a drug distribution ring (Freeman 2006). The man who succeeded him was arrested on corruption charges as well. Ten years later the set of allegations about federal corruption persist, despite a sustained federal crackdown; the military have been brought more centrally into drug enforcement in part because they are seen as being less corrupt.

Treatment and prevention

A national system oriented to prevention and to the treatment of drug dependence was established in 1969. In 2005 there were 92 centres in Mexico; only three provided treatment on an inpatient basis and only one centre provided methadone maintenance. This system is complemented by a network of local programmes including some supported by non-governmental organizations (NGOs). An important network of self-help groups is also in place, but a substantial proportion of persons with dependence goes untreated. National surveys show that only one-fifth of drug users meeting the criteria for dependence have been in treatment. School-based universal prevention activities have been operating continuously since the 1970s, with little attention given specifically to vulnerable and high risk populations.

14.2.5 Budget

Expenditures on drug control are dominated by supply reduction activities. Even excluding the federal budget for crop destruction and actions to combat organized crime or drug traffic, it is estimated that supply reduction constitutes over 90% of total expenditures. The investment in demand reduction doubled between 1998 and 2002. The dollars spent in prevention are around 30% higher than the budget allocated for treatment.

14.3 Sweden

14.3.1 The country

Sweden is a rich, stable democracy with a population of 9 million. It has been ruled by left of centre governments for most of the last 75 years. The nation has a tradition of paternalistic government that enjoys broad popular support. Perched on the northern edge of Europe, it is away from the major trafficking routes. Municipal governments have substantial powers in some areas, but most political power is concentrated at the national level.

14.3.2 Drug problems

Drug use

Cannabis is the most widely used illicit drug, mostly in the form of hashish. Cannabis use increased during the 1970s, decreased in the 1980s, and has increased again over the past 15 years. Occasional drug use (mainly cannabis) is low by Western European standards; in 2005 past year cannabis prevalence was approximately 2.0% (among 15- to 64-year-olds), compared with 6.9% for Germany and 12% for the UK (EMCDDA 2005).

Most problem drug users take the drugs intravenously, and the estimated number of problem ('heavy') drug users increased from 6000 in 1967 to 15 000 in 1979 and 26 000 in 1998 (1.2, 3.0, and 4.8 per 1000 aged 18–64, respectively). Sweden had a significant problem with widespread misuse of prescription amphetamines in the 1960s, and since that time amphetamines have constituted a large fraction of intravenous drug use in Sweden. However, as the result of a large increase in heroin use, amphetamine and heroin now constitute approximately equal shares of the drugs used among problem drug users. Polydrug use is extensive among problem drug users. In addition to intravenous use of amphetamines and heroin, cannabis, alcohol, and diverted pharmaceuticals (benzodiazepines, flunitrazepam) are popular among problem drug users.

The population of problem drug users has become older; the proportion of users over 30 years of age has increased significantly, as has the length of the drug use career in this group. Women constitute a minority of this group. Problem drug use is concentrated in larger cities, and is more frequently found among the homeless, those with low incomes, and males with immigrant backgrounds.

Consequences

Mortality among problem drug users is high compared with other European countries; the annual mortality rate among heroin users is around 40 per 1000 per annum, and among amphetamine users around 15–20. Since the late 1980s IDUs have constituted around 10% of HIV-positive patients. Rates of HIV among IDUs are around 2–5%, which is lower than in many other European countries. On the other hand, intravenous drug use contributes to the majority of new hepatitis (HCV, HBV) cases, and the majority of IDUs are HCV and/or HBV positive. Problem drug users may cause public nuisance by obtrusive begging and harassment of people in public places. Criminal violence related to drug dealing is not seen as a significant problem.

14.3.3 Politics and law

Drug policy

There is a National Action Plan on Drugs as well as a national drug policy coordinator. The drug policy is seen as an element of social policy aimed at preventing unemployment, segregation, and social distress. The national government is responsible for enforcement of trafficking laws, retailing, and possession laws. Local governments are responsible for most policing and also for administering treatment and prevention programmes, whose financing mostly comes from national grants.

Political rhetoric

Drug policy has been prominent in political discussions for decades. There is broad support for restrictive drug policies, but there is also a strong criticism regarding downsizing of drug treatment. A proposal on a needle exchange programme has been criticized as well on the grounds that it implies an acceptance of drug abuse. In public discourse drug use is considered more of a social problem than a health risk.

Laws

Both minimum and maximum penalties have generally increased over the years. Laws on coerced treatment/care within the social services were introduced in 1982. In 1993 the police were allowed to test for drug use upon suspicion. Medical use of cannabis is not allowed. A national prescription register was established in 2002 in order to monitor all prescriptions of narcotic drugs.

14.3.4 **Programmes**

Enforcement

The number of police officers working on drug-related tasks has increased significantly over the years and is now approximately 12 per 100 000 inhabitants. In 2005, a total of 60 000 drug-related offences were reported, about 10 per 1000 persons (compared with ~7 per 1000 persons in the USA). The vast majority of these (80%) are for possession and/or use of drugs. Another 12% were for drug-driving. In 2003 more than 14 000 persons were prosecuted (around half were fined) for drug offences. The number of correctional inmates serving time for drug offences in 2002 was approximately 2000 (Ramsted 2006), constituting less than 0.3 per 1000 population (compared with the USA figure of ~2.5 per 1000 population). Approximately 5% of imprisoned drug users are sentenced to more than 2 years of prison. Persons convicted for drug crime offences are predominantly male (85%) and over 25 years of age.

Health and social services for problem drug users

Drug treatment, like general health care, is funded by the local government. Treatment services are provided by governmental agencies as well as non-profit organizations under contract to local social service departments. Treatment in residential units constitutes a significant part of the treatment services provided, and the treatment is open for both drug and alcohol abusers. Of dependent users of drugs (excluding dependent users of marijuana), fewer than one-fifth are in treatment at any one time. Sweden differs from the other Nordic countries in its use of coerced treatment. Treatment is also provided in prisons. Almost half of all imprisoned drug users receive drug treatment (this does not included methadone maintenance treatment). Over the past decade funding of drug treatment has decreased whereas the number of problem drug users has increased. Scarcity of services is more prominent with respect to detoxification/abstinence treatment and after-care.

Methadone availability is limited, because of strict selection criteria and low capacity. In 2005 enrolment was less than 800 (Trimbos Institute 2006), no more than 10% of the estimated number of those dependent on heroin. Buprenorphine was introduced in 1999 and had a substantial enrolment of 1300 by 2003 (EMCDDA 2005). Vaccinations for HBV and HIV prevention are provided in prisons, but needle exchange programmes exist only to a very limited extent in one region (and in conflict with the restrictive policy). Disinfectants for syringes are not provided in prisons; there are no specific programmes to counteract overdoses. There are no user/injecting rooms and no heroin prescription programmes.

Prevention

The national government promotes drug prevention through school-based programmes. Prevention of use of alcohol, tobacco, and other drugs is part of the national curriculum. Schools are seen as a major arena for drug preventive measures, and a variety of school-based programmemes have been implemented. The schools have considerable autonomy in choice of programmes. There are also some community coalitions for the prevention of drug use, often also aimed at prevention of alcohol-related harms.

14.3.5 Budget

Total drug policy expenditures in Sweden in 2002 were estimated at around 950 million Euros (range 500 to 1400 million Euros), corresponding to approximately 100 Euros per inhabitant per year (Ramstedt 2006). Most of the expenditure (75%) was for enforcement, 24% for treatment, 1% for prevention, and very little (0.1%) for harm reduction.

14.4 Comparative analysis

These two national vignettes point to the large variation in the nature of drug problems and the responses they generate. The remainder of the chapter draws on the experiences of these two nations and five others (China, India, Nigeria, the UK, and the USA) to illustrate this variation further. We first present a schematic summary of problem differences in Table 14.1. After discussion of the entries in that table, we proceed to discuss differences in policy, summarized in Table 14.2.

14.4.1 Drug problems

In Table 14.1, trafficking refers to trans-shipment to other nations. Violence means the level of violence associated primarily with the drug trade. Crime refers to the contribution of drug users to total crime. HIV refers to the prevalence of HIV or AIDS among problematic drug users. A question mark ('?') indicates that we lack sufficient information to make a judgement. Table 14.1 represents a series of informed judgements but it is still highly approximate. Created with the help of collaborators from these nations, we believe the table is a reasonable portrayal of the drug situation in these seven nations around the year 2005.

Table 14.1 Variation across seven nations in estimated extent of drug use and related problems

	Occasional drug use	Problematic drug use	Trafficking	Violence	Crime	HIV
China	Low	Medium	Medium	low	?	High
India	Low	Low to medium	Low	?	?	?
Mexico	Low	Low	Very high	Very high		Low
Nigeria	Low	Low	High	Modest		?
Sweden	Medium	Medium	Low	Low	Medium	Low
UK	Very high	High	Low	Low?	High	Low
USA	Very high	Very high	Low	High	Very high	Very high

Table 14.2 Variation across seven nations in drug policies

	Enforcement intensity	Treatment availability	Political salience	Principal policy domain
China	High	Medium	Low	Criminal justice
India	Low	Low	Low	?
Mexico	Low	Low	Very High	National security
Nigeria	Modest	Low	High	Foreign relations
Sweden	Medium	High	Moderate	Social policy
UK	High	High	high	?
USA	Very high	Medium	Very high	Criminal justice

14.4.2 Use

Because drug surveys are more difficult to conduct in nations with significant rural populations, it is difficult to provide more than rough indications of differences in prevalence of both occasional drug use and problematic use in these countries. For most of these nations drugs are quite new as mass consumption items and as sources of major social problems, the markets having developed in the last third of the 20th century. China is the major exception. Opium use was extraordinarily prevalent through much of the period of 1850–1950 (see, for example, Newman 1995) and was viewed as one of the nation's major health and social problems. India had traditions of opium use and cannabis consumption but neither was regarded as much of a problem for the nation (Owen 1934).

As described in Chapter 3, occasional drug use is now normative in most western countries. In contrast, illicit drugs are almost unknown in large parts of China. General population surveys in India, Mexico, and Nigeria show lifetime use rates of less than 5%, even when the surveys are confined to large cities, which are more integrated with global cultural trends.

Differences in the prevalence of problematic drug use (involving frequent use of cocaine, heroin, or stimulants) are also substantial. In the USA, the rate of such use is about 20 per 1000 persons over the age of 12.[2] The UK figure is about half of that and Sweden about a quarter (EMCDDA 2006). China provides a sharp contrast. Even making generous adjustment for the official undercount, it would be very unlikely that the figure is as high as 3 per 1000. The other three nations also show perhaps even lower rates.

Although problematic drug use rates appear to be correlated with the prevalence of occasional drug use, there are exceptions. China has a much higher ratio of dependent drug use to occasional drug use than other countries in this sample. Sweden, which has by western standards a low prevalence of drug use in the general population, has a moderately high rate of problematic use.

However, problematic drug use is not evenly distributed within these nations. Opiate dependence in China is highly concentrated in border provinces such as Yunnan, Sichuan, and Xianjing (Tang and Hao 2007). China's emerging stimulant problem is mostly in coastal cities. In India there is a major problem with the misuse of **psychopharmaceuticals** (particularly amphetamine-type substances) in the north-east of the country that is not found elsewhere.

14.4.3 Health consequences

For western nations HIV related to injecting drug use has been the most prominent health consequence of drug use in recent years. Many nations, such as the UK, have managed to prevent high rates of HIV among IDUs through specific programmes. For China, IDUs have been a major vector for transmission, but in other countries, such as India, the rates remain low. High rates of HCV among IDUs appear in almost every nation. Hepatitis B rates vary a great deal. Mortality rates may differ as well, but information is lacking for all but the developed countries.

14.4.4 Crime

The relationship between drug use and crime varies both in form and prominence among nations. In the USA, the most salient adverse consequence of the large populations dependent on cocaine, heroin, and methamphetamine is high rates of both property crime and criminal violence. The rates of drug use among arrestees in the UK are comparably high (Bennett and Holloway 2005). However, with modest violent crime rates generally, the association in the UK is primarily with minor property crimes such as larceny and shoplifting. In Sweden a recent study estimated that approximately 30–40% of all recorded criminality is caused by drug users (National Swedish Police Board 2003). For nations with low levels of drug use, including China, India, Mexico, and Nigeria, crime by drug users is not a major concern.

[2] The figure can be taken from estimates of need for treatment, minus those whose need is based solely on marijuana use. See Boyum and Reuter (2005).

14.4.5 Trafficking and violence

The problems of nations are inter-related. As described above, a large part of the drug-related harm suffered by Mexico is related to its role in trafficking and production for the US market. The same is true for Nigeria, which serves as a trans-shipment point for entry of heroin and perhaps cocaine into the USA. It also suffers, in terms of reputation, from the drug trafficking activities of its diaspora in Europe as well. China, at least until recently, served as an important heroin trafficking route from the Golden Triangle producing area to other markets such as Australia and Canada. With the decline in Myanmar's production since 2000, this may no longer be an important element of the drug-related harm for the country. India suffers from its location between the two major opium-producing nations of the world, Afghanistan and Myanmar, but indications of trafficking on to other nations are slight. Sweden and the UK are almost purely destination countries. The USA, while a net importer of illicit drugs, may export substantial quantities of some synthetic drugs.

Trafficking and production are important sources of revenues, expressed as a percentage of GDP, for only a handful of nations; Afghanistan, Colombia, and Tajikistan are probably joined by a few of the micronations in the Caribbean. However, the income from trafficking can be the source of an important threat to the power of the central government, as in Mexico.

14.4.6 Policies

Table 14.2 presents a set of judgements about differences across the seven nations with respect to drug policies. In the table, enforcement intensity refers to the risk faced by a drug dealer of being sanctioned by the criminal justice system (whether that be arrest or incarceration). Treatment availability is a measure of the probability that a drug user in need of treatment is able to find a service provider. Political salience is an indicator of whether there is much attention paid to drug policy as a public issue in the media. Principal policy domain refers to that aspect of public policy that is most heavily emphasized in drug policy as implemented.

14.4.7 Laws

Differences in formal criminal law are modest. All of these nations are signatories to the **international drug conventions** described in Chapter 13. Consequently the possession, production, and distribution of cannabis, cocaine, heroin, and stimulants are prohibited. Sweden appears to be unique in that it allows for criminal prosecution on the basis of testing for the presence of drugs in the bloodstream or urine of an individual (Brottsförebyggande rådet 2000).

There is some variation in the statutory penalties associated with violations. For example, until 2001 Indian law specified a minimum term of imprisonment of 10 years for possession of more than a quarter gram of heroin. This was lessened in 2001 to allow for sentences of only up to 1 year for less than 5 grams. In the UK, where policies are generally seen as oriented toward harm reduction, the statutory sentences for simple possession of heroin can be as high as 7 years (Reuter and

Stevens 2007). In Sweden, simple possession of small amounts of heroin (up to 50 milligrams) can generate a sentence of up to 6 months (EMCDDA 2003c)

There are, however, large differences in the penalties actually applied. In the USA, approximately 500 000 persons were incarcerated for violations of drug control statutes (principally distribution) on a given day in 2005 (Caulkins and Chandler 2006), i.e. about 2 per 1000 population. Drug incarcerations constituted approximately 22% of all imprisonments around 2005. In Sweden the population rate for drug incarcerations was 0.4 per 1000. Only 5% of Swedish drug offenders had sentences of more than 2 years. In the USA, the median length for drug offenders in state prisons (accounting for 55% of total inmates) was over 3 years and in federal prisons (which account for ~15% of drug incarcerations) the median length was approximately 6 years (Boyum and Reuter 2005). These differences in sentence length reflect, *inter alia*, differences in sentencing generally; US prisoners serve longer sentences for other offences as well.

For the other countries figures are available only for arrests or convictions. China arrested 56 000 persons for drug offences in 2006, representing only 5 per 100 000 persons. This constitutes a tiny fraction of all arrests and is low relative to the estimated 1–2 million problematic drug users. In India the average number of persons prosecuted annually for drug trafficking and selling between 1992 and 2004 was only about 2000 (Narcotics Control Bureau, India 2003, see Table 3), representing a remarkably low level of enforcement per capita or per user.

14.4.8 **Treatment**

There is large variation in the availability of, quality of, and paths into drug treatment. Sweden is estimated to have only about one-fifth of its problematic drug users in treatment at any one time, a number comparable with that for the USA. In contrast, in the UK, after a multiyear campaign aimed at integrating treatment with the criminal justice system, as many as 50% are in treatment at any one time. For India, Mexico, and Nigeria the figures are difficult to estimate.

Sweden allows for coerced treatment. In 2002 about 10% of the treated population was there as the result of a government agency imposing the requirement, sometimes even in the absence of an arrest for criminal violation. In both the UK and the USA the criminal justice system constitutes a major path into treatment. For example, over a quarter of those seeking treatment for crack abuse in the USA were identified as subject to criminal justice pressures (SAMHSA 2006b). For China, treatment has, until about 2005, been fairly close to incarceration itself; few enter except as a consequence of arrest. In India, Mexico, and Nigeria the few who enter treatment do so without coercion.

The nature of treatment available varies, even among the rich nations. As noted previously, fewer than 10% of heroin addicts in Sweden are in a substitution programme, a choice reflecting Swedish views about the appropriateness of substitution therapies. In the USA doctrinal or ideological resistance to methadone has waned in recent years, but financing and regulatory barriers remain. The result is that 30% of the approximately quarter million admissions to treatment for heroin dependence are in substitution treatment, mostly methadone (SAMHSA 2006b). In the UK it is now estimated that over half are receiving methadone. China did not permit methadone until 2004. Even after the central government authorized a large number of experimental sites, the number of patients in methadone maintenance in January 2005 was fewer than 2000, representing local government resistance to substitution therapy (Liu *et al.* 2006). Methadone remains effectively unavailable in India and Nigeria.

14.4.9 **Political salience and policymaking apparatus**

As one might expect, in countries with more severe drug problems there is more press discussion. During the period from 1980 to 1995, the US media provided intense coverage of many aspects of both drug policy and the problem. Though problematic drug use in the USA remains high by international standards, the issue has lost prominence, perhaps because the problem is not seen as growing. Political salience is considered very high as well in Mexico because of the prominence of drug-related violence and corruption. Among the seven nations in this case study analysis, China and India are considered to devote the least media attention to drugs (Table 14.2).

As the drug problem has become more prominent over the last 20 years there has been a tendency toward more centralized drug policy making. The USA may have been the leader in this respect, forming the **Office of National Drug Control Policy (ONDCP)** in 1989, with the director originally having cabinet rank. ONDCP has at times been headed by nationally prominent figures (a former cabinet member and a retired four-star general), at other times by quite obscure figures. In the UK there was a 'drug tsar' in the late 1990s but since 2001 the coordinating function has not been given high status or much power. The Swedish drug coordinator in recent years has been of some prominence. China, Mexico, and Nigeria each have a national coordinating body, but none is very prominent. India does not have such a coordinating body, just a lead ministry in specific policy areas.

In most countries the most powerful agency in drug policy is the equivalent of the Interior Ministry. That may reflect the reality that law enforcement dominates expenditures, even in nations such as the UK and The Netherlands with a strong harm reduction orientation, and that drug problems account for a much higher percentage of the business of the police, courts, and corrections than of doctors and hospitals. In Mexico and Nigeria, the Ministry of Defence and the military have leading roles, suggesting that the drug problem is seen as one of national security (Mexico) and foreign policy (Nigeria).

14.4.10 **The orientation of drug policy**

As summarized in Table 14.1, the drug problems of these seven countries are very different. One might therefore expect that efforts to deal with illegal drugs have different policy orientations, as presented in Table 14.2. For the USA it is clear that drugs have been seen primarily as a source of crime and disorder and that drug policy has been oriented toward criminal justice. It is striking that the annual US *National Drug Control Strategy* makes no mention of AIDS or HIV. In Mexico the Ministry of Defence has a leading role in drug policy, for example being in charge of drug eradication, because the drug issue is defined principally as one of national security. For Nigeria it is more a matter of international relations rather than national security; drug trafficking threatens the respectability of the country.

The differences in drug policy in these countries reflect interplay of politics, culture, and drug use. Sweden is an orderly nation with strong government commitment to helping its citizens. On the one hand it is, by European standards, quite aggressive in law enforcement but at the same time it provides well-funded drug treatment programmes and a considerable variety of social and health services. Mexico's response to domestic drug use has been constrained by the weakness of lower levels of government; the federal government is not well situated either to provide treatment services or to enforce laws against local drug distribution. In the USA the intensity of the enforcement response to drug use is surely conditioned in part by the fact that the cocaine epidemic was thought to be responsible for a rapid upturn in homicide and violent crimes across American cities in the 1980s (e.g. Levitt 2004).

These orientations are not fixed. Nations change over time in how they perceive the drug problem. Until the late 1960s the drug problem in the UK was seen as an issue for physicians, who were charged with the management of a modest number of iatrogenic heroin dependence cases. By the 1990s it had clearly become a major problem for the criminal justice system, which eventually turned to the public health system for help in dealing with it. Changes in Nigeria's drug policy orientation may reflect shifts from civilian to military rule, with the latter favouring criminal justice-oriented policies more than have civilian governments.

14.5 **Conclusion**

This variation across the seven nations does not by any means capture the full range of problems and responses across nations. The USA may be tough in its approach to drug problems but it does not match the severity of some nations in certain respects. For instance, although the UNODC Director-General has now questioned the use of the death penalty for drug trafficking (http://www.unodc.org/unodc/en/about-unodc/speeches/2008-03-10.html), a number of states apply death penalties for drug offences. The city-nation of Singapore, with a population of 5 million, executed 17 persons in 2000 for drug offences; possession of more than 30 grams of heroin is enough to trigger that penalty. Iran, with a population of 70 million, may have executed as many as 1000 per annum in the 1980s. At the other end of the spectrum some nations have a greater commitment to treatment than even the UK; for example, The Netherlands provides methadone, often on a low threshold basis, to any heroin addict who seeks it.

It is clear is that no one set of policies is right for all these nations. What is possible and appropriate in a rich, stable democracy such as Sweden, with a narrowly defined domestic drug problem, may be neither feasible nor desirable for a nation such as Nigeria, whose drug problem is determined largely by market factors outside of its borders. Each nation's policy can be informed by scientific analysis, but the policy choices will not be uniform.

Chapter 15

Health and social services for drug users: systems issues

Drug users receive help from a variety of health and social services that have been specifically developed for them and that were reviewed in Chapter 9. This chapter moves up one level of analysis to consider service programmes in the context of larger systems and their population-level impact. Specifically, this chapter discusses how health and social service programmes interact with each other and with the more generalized types of service programmes that drug users commonly access, for example those that provide vocational training, welfare benefits, and emergency health care. This chapter also discusses how service systems are organized, funded, and managed.

Research on service systems has increased in recent years (Babor *et al.* 2008a), but remains substantially less developed theoretically and methodologically than research on particular interventions. The value of taking a systems perspective is both pragmatic and theoretical: policy choices related to the organization of treatment and social services at the systems level probably have a greater impact on a society's ability to reduce population-level drug problems than do decisions about this or that individual service programme.

15.1 Why do some societies invest in services for problem drug users?

Drug dependence has many 'externalities' that are virtually impossible for societies to ignore, including domestic violence, property crimes, public disorder, infectious disease transmission, and overdose deaths. Even in cases where the drug user sees no reason to change, those in the drug user's immediate social environment are often motivated to take remedial action. Policymakers thus feel substantial need to do *something* about problem drug users, with the most common reaction around the world being to apply some form of punishment. Virtually every society places legal restrictions on some drugs, and applies punishment to at least some drug users, be it in the form of fines, incarceration, or, in extreme cases, execution. Yet a minority of societies also make a substantial investment in health and social services for drug users that are non-punitive in nature. What leads some societies and not others to adopt this policy?

After the Second World War, a number of western societies began to shift from punishment-oriented policy responses to more rehabilitative responses to many social problems, including drug dependence. This phenomenon coincided with the growth of the welfare state and the emergence of social movements desiring to reform addicted people (White 1998). More recently, countries outside the developed western world that historically relied on a punishment approach have introduced a range of medical and psychosocial elements to their response. Sometimes these are parallel to, and at other times integrated with, the criminal justice response (e.g. the recent introduction in several parts of China of methadone maintenance).

One common explanation for why some societies provide services and not just punishment for drug users is that they can afford to. For example, helping professionals across the world most commonly cite lack of fiscal resources as the explanation when services are in short supply (Gossop 1995). Yet this subjective impression may be misleading because providing rehabilitation services to heavy drug users is not necessarily more costly, and in fact may be less costly, than are criminal justice measures.

Simple pragmatism may be a better explanation for the rise of services as a response to problem drug users in some countries. It cannot be overstated that people who do not use drugs can benefit significantly when services are provided to drug users, so policy choices need not be based on whether one wants to help drug users 'versus' society as a whole. Zaric and colleagues (2000), for example, showed that the US methadone maintenance clinic system costs less to maintain than would caring for all the HIV/AIDS cases among non-drug users that the current system prevents. And when the costs of criminal behaviour and the criminal justice response are factored into the calculation, the wider societal benefit from helping drug users becomes even clearer. For example, in the UK, the cost-effectiveness calculations linked to the National Treatment Outcome Study (NTORS) found that, for every pound spent on treatment, there was a reduction of £3 in public costs (Gossop *et al.* 2001; Godfrey *et al.* 2004).

A purely punishment-oriented approach to drug use can be quite costly in itself, particularly as drugs become available to more people and in more countries. Chapter 3 described the extraordinary number of people around the world who use drugs. In the same vein, the UK report on drug misuse from the Royal College of Psychiatrists and Royal College of Physicians (2000) described how observations about the ebb and flow of drug use needed to be understood against the backdrop of the steadily increasing sea level over time as the prevalence of drug use is rising in most societies. As a policy response, incarcerating every drug user contributing to this global pandemic would be extraordinarily costly because of its direct expense and its removal of a significant number of working-age people from economic productivity. Thus some societies have developed service systems not because of any social movement or general change in government, but simply out of practicality. In Iran's case, for example, the sudden legitimization of services for drug users (Vick 2005) was probably driven by fear that the epidemic of heroin use and HIV infection among working-age males could cause complete economic and societal collapse.

15.2 **What is the service system?**

Klingemann and colleagues (1992, p. 4) use the term *system* to refer broadly to those organizations and programmes that provide services to people who have problems related to substance use, and, in a broader sense, to the interconnection of different agencies, programmes, and referral channels that provide supporting services. The term *system* implies coherence and organization, but in fact it is just an analytical convenience (Hunt and Dong Sun 1998). Countries vary in the extent to which system components are integrated, overlapping, or complementary, and meet the needs of their target populations. In most countries, services for substance use disorders are fragmented and heterogeneous, and are financed and managed by multiple agencies that themselves are distributed across different geographic areas and levels and branches of government.

Conceptualizing health and social services for drug users as a system brings numerous questions to light that are not generally apparent in analyses of individual programmes that offer such services. For example, given a fixed amount of financial resources, are there ways of designing service systems that minimize cost while maximizing population impact? If the most costly services (e.g. heroin maintenance) are highly attractive to drug users, will they crowd out other, less costly services, thereby reducing access? How should a system balance the need for high intensity services for the most severely impaired drug users with the desire to be accessible to a broad range of people, including those whose drug problems are less serious? Having focused for decades almost exclusively on the outcomes of individual types of service programmes, such as different kinds of drug counselling, family therapy, needle exchange, or OST, researchers have more recently been giving attention to these types of system-level questions.

Figure 15.1 presents a conceptual model for describing service systems and their effects, adapted from the work of Babor and colleagues (2008a). System policies are the basic decisions made by policymakers about the type, amount, and organization of services. *Siting* refers not only to the physical location of clinics and other facilities, but

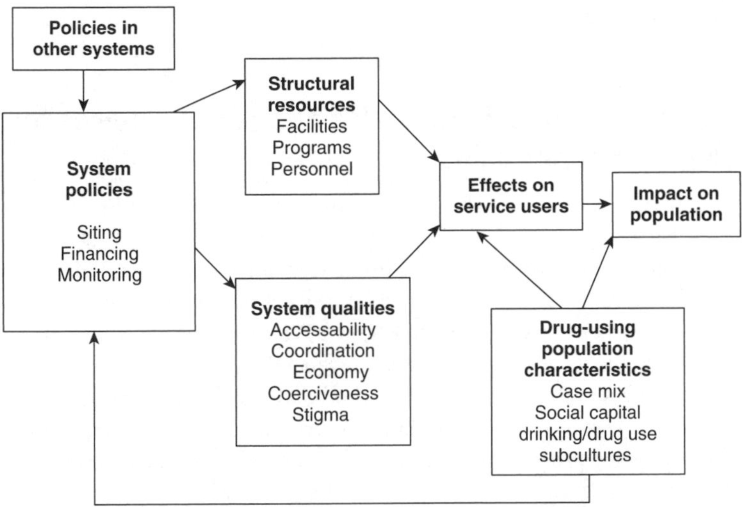

Fig. 15.1 Conceptual model of population impact of service systems.
Source: Babor *et al.* (2008a).

also to where services for drug users are administratively located. For example, in some countries such services are managed by a mental health agency, whereas in others they are linked administratively to law enforcement or social welfare. *Financing* refers to the amount of funds allocated for services, and their source, for example user fees, government budgets, or private sector investment. *Monitoring* refers to whether and how the quality, cost, and outcomes are evaluated and how members of service staff are selected, trained, and supervised.

In making decisions regarding any element described in the conceptual model, policymakers are constrained to some extent by two important factors, namely policy decisions in other systems and the characteristics of the drug-using population. An example of the former are laws specifying what happens to drug users, be it punishment, help, or some combination thereof. An example of the latter is the economic resources of a society's drug users, which will determine in part the extent to which policymakers must rely on public investment to sustain service systems.

As shown in the figure, a service system's policies affect its structural resources and system qualities. The former include the tangible aspects of the system, for example the number and type of facilities (e.g. hospitals, clinics, outreach vans, hotlines), the programmes delivered in those facilities (e.g. brief detoxification, diagnostic assessment, risk reduction counselling, vocational training, psychotherapy), and the characteristics of personnel in those programmes (e.g. certified counsellors, social workers, psychiatrists, recovering persons). System qualities are less tangible, but may be as important as the structural resources of a system. Box 15.1 defines these qualities.

The conceptual model posits that structural resources and system qualities, along with the characteristics of the drug-using population, combine to produce two important outcomes. The first and most obvious outcome is the effect on the service users themselves. The second is the impact on the population, including those who do not have a drug problem. Population impact can come in many domains, including health (e.g. incidence of blood-borne infectious disease), public safety (e.g. amount of property crime), social welfare (e.g. child abuse rates), and finances (e.g. tax burden).

15.3 **Systems research on health and social services for problem substance users**

Systems research has followed three lines of inquiry: historical studies, comparative studies, and analytical studies. Most of the historical research on systems of drug (and alcohol) programmes has been confined to single countries. Some studies have looked at the policies, events, or problem formulations behind major changes in systems, including changes in target groups (Room 1978; Rosenqvist and Stenius 1986; Blomqvist 1998; Stenius 1999; Thom 2000). A general conclusion from these studies is that major changes in the organization, methods, and even the extent of services have been little influenced by scientific findings concerning the effectiveness of a particular model of organizing programmes. Research has, however, been taken into account to a greater extent in nations such as Finland and Sweden, where reforms following the Second World War were inspired by medical science and professionalization. This gradually led in the case of alcohol treatment to increased outpatient care aimed at

Box 15.1 Key qualities of service systems for drug users

- *Accessibility.* Accessibility refers to how easy or difficult it is to enter the service system, and the extent to which necessary services are provided following admission. Services tend to be more accessible in systems that offer many entry points (as might a primary care-based system) versus fewer entry points (as might a system that is based in psychiatric care). Less formal systems, most notably the voluntary sector, may have a further advantage in terms of accessibility because of the low threshold of entry (e.g. no forms to fill out, no bureaucracy to navigate, and little or no financial cost)
- *Coordination.* To the extent that different kinds of services are provided to drug users, coordination refers to whether they are provided in a concerted rather than a haphazard fashion, and whether different programmes in the system work synergistically rather than independently or antagonistically. In general, coordination tends to be better when the services with which a provider wants to coordinate care are offered by the same system in which services for drug users are offered. For example, a drug user system based in primary care may offer easier access to medical services but less access to social services than would a system based in the social welfare system.
- *Economy.* Once the budget is set at the administrative level, the term *economy* refers to whether the services are cost-effective (i.e. given the same total costs, could one achieve better outcomes with a different system?). Economy is often promoted by sharing of fixed costs (e.g. physical space). An example is prison-based treatment services, in which food, shelter, and 24-hour monitoring are already being paid for so the added cost of providing drug services is comparatively small.
- *Coerciveness.* The degree of coercion or pressure placed on drug users to seek services varies across systems. It is highest in the criminal justice system but often present in more subtle ways (e.g. family pressure) in other types of service. Coerciveness increases demand for services and does not appear to reduce effectiveness (Wild 2006), although it can stigmatize drug services and the people who use them and work in them.
- *Stigma.* The extent to which services are subjectively viewed as low status, shameful, and of no value, irrespective of their objective characteristics, is captured by the term *stigma.* Different arrangements may influence whether the use of drug treatment services is considered shameful, and whether providing services is considered a low or high prestige activity. In many societies, medically-based services carry less stigma than free-standing services, prison-based services and mental health-based services.

serving a broader part of the problem drinking population than did inpatient programmes (Rosenqvist and Kurube 1992; Blomqvist 1998. Later developments have resulted in a *de facto* division of the service system into professionalized care for those with better social and economic resources, and a less ambitious type of care for the poor and marginalized population (Kaukonen and Stenius 2005).

Among the best known comparative studies is the **World Health Organization's** survey of services for drug users (WHO 1993), which provides important information on systems arrangements in different regions of the world. Specialized drug treatment services are available in over 80% of countries in the Americas, Europe, and South East Asia. These regions also report that a high proportion of services are located in psychiatric hospitals, teaching hospitals, and general hospitals. In contrast, regions predominantly composed of low and middle income countries (e.g. Africa, Eastern Mediterranean, Western Pacific regions) tend to have high proportions of their drug treatment located in primary care settings. Other countries have located services for drug users in the social welfare service system, in religious and voluntary organizations, and in the criminal justice system. These decisions have been influenced by historical circumstances, legal regimes, funding resources, and professional advocacy (e.g. Klingemann and Hunt 1998; Porter *et al.* 1999). The various components of contemporary health and social systems are described in Box 15.2. Some countries use a combination of components; in other countries only one predominates.

Other international studies have combined historical and comparative perspectives to monitor developments in drug and alcohol service systems during the last quarter of the 20th century (Klingemann *et al.* 1992, 1993). A study of drug treatment services in 23 countries (Gossop 1995) found that helping professionals perceived a scarcity of resources for these kinds of services, and many reported an inadequate level of professional training. However, many of these same countries reported spending significant sums on drug users within the prison system. In countries such as Congo, where there are no specialist services for drug or alcohol problems, native healers provide the majority of care. In many countries the disparity between supply and demand for services is compounded by the highly uneven geographical distribution of services, which tend to be concentrated in large cities. Although 70% of the countries surveyed deliver services primarily in non-residential settings, Ghana, Norway, Nigeria, Spain, and Pakistan were found to favour residential settings (Gossop 1995). In Peru, Japan, Poland, and Germany, problem drug and alcohol users are served in separate programmes. But in most of the other countries they are integrated. In some countries mutual help organizations such as Alcoholics Anonymous (AA) and Croix Bleu are sufficiently well established to provide a substantial contribution to the national system of professionally provided services (Gossop 1995).

Another international comparative study (Rush 1996; Lehto 1998) conducted in 18 countries found that most countries have some specialized treatment services for drug users, but that such services tend to be more fragmented than were general health services in the same country. Many countries with universal health care treat drug poisoning, withdrawal, and dependence in the general medical system. Within countries, variations in availability of services are related to the extent to which services targeted toward drug users are isolated from the rest of the health care system.

Box 15.2 Where services are sited in different countries

1. *Specialized drug and alcohol services.* In many countries, particularly the developed countries, drug treatment services are separately located, managed, and financed. An example would be the hundreds of free-standing methadone maintenance clinics that exist in the USA. Services for drug users are sometimes merged with alcohol services. In many western societies, services for alcohol-dependent people were developed prior to services for drug users. Some governments have always operated under a single 'substance abuse' services model, others have split drug and alcohol services, and still others have switched between one approach and the other. Whatever a society officially designates as its alcohol versus drug services, in most cases the overlap of service users is significant. As shown in Chapter 3, alcohol problems and drug problems are highly correlated at the individual level.
2. *Psychiatric care.* In most regions of the world, services for drug users are located at least partially within the context of psychiatric and mental health services. In many developed countries, drug services developed initially as a subspecialty of psychiatric medicine before growing into an independent system. In other countries, such as Russia, the separation has still not occurred and minimal drug services tend to emphasize medical treatment provided in psychiatric institutions. In recent years, some societies that have distinct drug and mental health systems have begun to merge some services to care for 'dually diagnosed' individuals.
3. *The general medical care system, including primary health care, general hospitals, and teaching hospitals.* This model is most extensively developed in the UK, although it is also applied elsewhere in the developed world (e.g. Australia and New Zealand) and is the only available way to access any services in some developing countries. In the UK, family doctors (GPs, general practitioners) have been encouraged to manage addiction problems, and about a third of all the dependent heroin users who receive treatment do so from a local GP. The nature of the treatment provided is broadly comparable with the treatments provided from hospital-based addiction specialists (Strang *et al.* 1996, 2007).
4. *The criminal justice/prison system.* In many countries (e.g. China, Japan, Russia, and the USA), drug-related services are connected with criminal justice programmes (Porter *et al.* 1999). Large numbers of drug users naturally end up in contact with legal authorities in virtually all countries because the substance they use, the things they do to pay for it, or the actions they undertake while using it (e.g. violence) are illegal. The coordination of criminal justice programmes and drug treatment services takes many forms, including drug courts, prison-based counselling programmes, syringe exchange programmes for incarcerated populations, post-prison discharge therapeutic communities, urine monitoring of parolees and probationers, and indirect coercion (e.g. drug-using individuals voluntarily seeking services in the hopes

Box 15.2 Where services are sited in different countries *(continued)*

that it will lessen the sentence they receive if convicted in an upcoming criminal trial).

5. *The social welfare system/youth services system.* Drug services are embedded in social welfare and/or youth services in some countries, including Sweden, Norway, and Hungary. Such systems may include services related to work training, housing, psychosocial rehabilitation, and family support.
6. *The voluntary sector.* Religious organizations are major providers of services to drug users in many countries. In Ghana and Iraq, for example, there are tribal healers who conduct complex ceremonies intended to drive out psychiatric and addictive problems. In the USA and Mexico, some Christian churches draw all or most of their members from recovered drug users. Religious organizations and programmes are only part of the voluntary sector. Self-help groups, volunteer-staffed drop-in centres, crisis phone lines, and drug user groups that promote safer injection practices are among the services that exist in the non-religious voluntary sector. Poland, Australia, and Peru are diverse examples of societies in which such organizations exist in significant numbers.

Other studies have evaluated the effects of organizational models and service system qualities. In a study of almost 1900 substance abuse clients in social and medical services in Stockholm county in 2000–2004, one half of the county was characterized by more outpatient care and better service integration whereas the other half had more inpatient care and less integration (Stenius *et al.* 2005). The outpatient/integrated system was better at recruiting vulnerable groups into services, and integration and availability were correlated with client satisfaction with services.

In a qualitative study conducted in 12 US states, Gelber and Rinaldo (2005) found that effective collaboration between the lead substance abuse agency and other governmental and community agencies is a key requirement for maintaining effective services. This study also found that organizational placement and positioning of a lead substance abuse agency within state government affects policy authority, agency visibility, funding levels, collaborative ability, and ability to attract and retain talented staff.

Although the research base is modest, it does provide support for the utility of conceptualizing services in a systems perspective. The research also shows that system policy decisions substantially affect (as Figure 15.1 suggests) the structural resources and qualities of the services provided.

15.4 From clinical effectiveness to population effects

From a clinical perspective the benefits of services are thought of in terms of individual patients or clients, but in the public health framework the population impact of intervention systems receives more attention. Health and social services should never be expected to eliminate a nation's drug problem (Reuter and Pollack 2006), but can make a significant contribution to reducing drug-related crime, infectious disease, overdoses, and the quantity of drugs consumed.

Chapter 9 reviewed the research documenting that effective interventions not only reduce service users' drug use, but also result in improved psychiatric, medical, and employment outcomes, as well as reduced risk of overdose, crime, and HIV infection. Beyond these individual effects, service systems can have impacts at the level of communities and populations. Box 15.3 reports three prominent examples of how changes in the service system can have broad effects. Other studies suggesting that such effects are possible have been conducted by UK and US investigators, who have shown that drug users comprise a large share of all cocaine and heroin retailers (Reuter *et al.* 1990; Gossop *et al.* 2003). In the UK National Treatment Outcome Research Study, one-third of imprisoned respondents reported that they had sold drugs in the 3 months prior to treatment (Gossop *et al.* 1999), and the number of drug selling offences after 1 year in treatment was only 13% of the entry level (Gossop *et al.* 2003). If broad service provision significantly reduces the number of drug users engaged in the drug trade, expanding services, could be a more efficient way to reduce drug-related crime than is expanding law enforcement.

The research findings on the effects of service systems for drug users are complemented by more extensive evidence on the population impact of alcohol services, particularly AA groups and professionally provided treatment. In an analysis of data from Ontario, Canada (where the number of alcohol-dependent people receiving services increased 76% between 1976 and 1982), Mann and colleagues (1988) found that increases in the proportion of alcohol-dependent people in treatment were associated with decreases in liver cirrhosis morbidity. In an integrative review of this research, Smart and Mann (2000) concluded that (1) in most studies, increases in AA membership and amount of professionally provided services in a geographic area are associated with decreased rates of alcohol problems; and (2) in some countries such changes may be large enough to have a considerable impact on hospital admissions and death from liver cirrhosis. Although these findings emerged in observational research rather than in randomized studies, they provide a preliminary indication that service systems can affect population health.

15.5 **What is the optimal financial investment in service systems?**

Policy decisions affect not only the resources and quality of the system, but also its impact on the population. Which types and combinations of services are optimal in terms of cost-effectiveness and impact on population health indicators will probably vary across societies, making it difficult to make simple generalizations. This occurs for two reasons. First different societies will weigh different outcomes differently (e.g. whereas one society may consider the added coerciveness of drug courts too high a price to pay for reduced drug problems, another society may not see it as a price at all, but as a public good). Secondly, desirable service system qualities often exist in tension with each other. For example, broad expansion of low intensity services increases accessibility and makes the system more attractive to low severity

Box 15.3 Three service system changes that made a difference

1. *Introduction of large scale opiate substitution services in France and Switzerland.* In the 1990s, France and Switzerland created large systems of opiate substitution services. The number of individuals receiving such services in France increased from close to zero to about 100 000 in the course of a decade; the change in Switzerland was similarly dramatic. Both countries experienced substantial population-level benefits. French data from 1996 to 2003 show an impressive 75% decrease in heroin arrests (Emmanuelli and Desenclos 2005), and drug-related mortality and AIDS cases also declined (Wiessing *et al.* 2009). A downside to this policy was a comparatively small number of overdose deaths from diverted methadone and buprenorphine (17 cases in 1998; see Auriacombe *et al.* 2001). Switzerland also experienced large drops in crime, and the heroin market itself may have been significantly disrupted due to the exit of a large number of heavy users (i.e. former customers), many of whom were also heroin sellers (Killias and Aebi 2000).
2. *Creation of the drug court system in the USA.* Beginning in Miami in 1989, various states and cities in the USA began to create specialized courts that handle only drug cases, and which use judicial power to reward certain behaviours (e.g. entering treatment, providing clean urines) and punish others (e.g. drug use, crime). There are now over 1000 such courts and they exist in all 50 US states. A growing research base, including randomized trials (Gottfredson *et al.* 2003), shows that drug courts reduce crime, promote treatment participation, and are less costly than imprisonment. The other systemic effects of these programmes include greater fusing of the criminal justice and service systems in the USA, which increases the number of individuals who seek services but also may create greater stigma around services than would exist in a purely voluntary system.
3. *Promotion of clinical practice guidelines for opiate substitution in the UK.* Beginning in 1996, the British government began issuing high profile guidelines for improving opiate substitution services and promoted them heavily for a number of years. A 2005 survey (Strang *et al.* 2007) found substantial changes since 1995 in national clinical practices consistent with those endorsed in the guidelines. These included a doubling of the number of opiate substitute prescriptions, an increase in supervised medication use (from zero to 36%), and a rise in average dose provided to bring it closer to the most effective range. Based on the review of evidence in Chapter 12, these system-level changes could be expected to reduce diversion of opiate substitutes, and reduce heroin use by those receiving services.

users, but at the same time may take away from the intensive resources needed by heavy drug users. Having a distinct specialist system for drug users may improve coordination of services within that system, but weaken linkages with other parts of the health care system, such as departments of infectious disease and psychiatry. In many cases, these tensions exist because of resource limitations. It is therefore useful now to consider one of the most basic questions of service systems, namely what amount of resources is appropriate.

There are several ways of estimating the need for services as well as the nature and extent of a drug service system for a society. One common method is to conduct population prevalence surveys of drug problems, and then assume that policymakers should expand services so that every problematic drug user not in contact with services could receive them. This approach generates greatly overstated estimates of service need for four reasons. First, many drug users stop using drugs or reduce their drug-related problems without the aid of health professionals (Klingemann *et al.* 2001). Secondly, many individuals who seek assistance for drug problems do so in the voluntary sector (e.g. from self-help groups) rather than from service professionals. Thirdly, many people with problematic drug use have no desire to change their behaviour, and not everyone who does wish to change would be willing to access services even if they were affordable and available. Fourthly, some drug users who seek services are not helped by those currently available.

Another approach for determining the 'right' service budget is to invest in a system just up to the point that further investment continues to reduce the overall costs of drug use plus services. That is, a service system would theoretically be perfectly efficient if budgets were increased until adding even one more dollar (or pound or yuan) to the budget would return anything less than a dollar in reduced damage from drug use. Meara and Frank (2005) took this approach in the USA, arguing that spending on drug treatment programmes is less than 5% of the amount at which perfect efficiency would be achieved. Although the disparity might not be as large, treatment systems in most developed societies would probably show similar inefficiency. From this standpoint, policymakers in virtually all developed societies would be encouraged to increase spending on services for drug users on the grounds that the costs of services would more than be made up for by reduced costs in other areas (e.g. criminal justice, health care, unemployment benefits).

There are, however, at least two limits to this line of reasoning. First, all helping efforts in a society are in some way an expression of prosocial values. Even if certain intervention efforts, for example counselling provided to mentally ill, HIV-positive drug users in homeless shelters, are cost-inefficient, they may be priceless as an expression of particular individuals' and a society's compassion. Secondly, particularly in societies with a developed bureaucracy, cost offsets rarely go to the agency that paid for the services for drug users. Even if overall costs are reduced, it is difficult to persuade one agency to invest 'its' money in programmes that reduce costs on 'some other department's' balance sheet (Humphreys *et al.* 2009).

A different approach to determining the right budget is to compare service spending not against theoretical perfect efficiency but against other possible policies. One could compare, for example, the cost of achieving a standardized outcome (e.g. eliminating one year of harmful drug use by one person) via prevention, interdiction, and services, and make investments accordingly.

15.6 How can a service system manager promote quality?

Patients, families, politicians, and service professionals agree in the abstract that whatever services society provides for drug users should be high quality. But in concrete instances, most stakeholders do not know how to evaluate quality, so they focus instead on quantity, for example by asking how many programmes have served how many people in how many places. This may partly explain why, as mentioned in Chapter 9, service quality within systems is often uneven. Further, research on ways to improve the quality of services frequently does not find its way into everyday practice (Compton *et al.* 2005a), in part because treatment programmes are often plagued by underfunding, over-regulation, and other organizational challenges (McLellan *et al.* 2003). Spending on quality may produce changes less visible to the purchaser than does spending on quantity, but may be a better investment for improving population health. System managers must therefore determine what strategies they will employ to improve quality and how much resources should be devoted to them.

Within a public health framework, efforts to promote quality face a trade-off between level and distribution of quality throughout a society. Many countries, for example, have a national 'centre of excellence' that provides state-of-the-art services to the most severely troubled patients. Touring such centres, one sees engaged staff members and hears stories from satisfied and improving patients and their families, all of which is quite impressive through the individual clinician lens. But from a population perspective, such centres seem less appealing in the many cases in which they consume a disproportionate share of the country's budget for drug-related services, leaving little money for services in other areas and populations (e.g. less severe drug users who may respond to more modest interventions). In the absence of resources for the most advanced services, system managers have employed three approaches to promote quality services: credentialing systems, process performance indicators, and outcome monitoring systems.

Licensing and certification of service providers. Maintaining the skills and education of staff members is a neglected task in many service systems (Uchtenhagen *et al.* 2008). Many drug treatment service systems try to promote quality by requiring particular credentials for those who provide services. Many of these credentials are created and advocated for by professional guilds, and have no evidence of improving the outcome of services. This is also true of various advanced educational degrees. Indeed, Smith and colleagues' (1980) **meta-analysis** of hundreds of studies enrolling tens of thousands of patients found that the effect of training on counselling outcomes was negligible. Although upsetting to professional guilds, there is no scientific evidence that a professional's training and academic credentials have a significant impact on their success at drug counselling.

This does not mean that credentialing systems are entirely a waste of time and money. There are tasks in drug services beyond counselling, some of which require special training, for example measuring blood concentrations of medications, identifying medical co-morbidities, negotiating regulations, and managing finances. Further, credentialing systems have some power to weed out individual clinicians and other service providers who may be incompetent or dangerous, such as individuals with a history of exploitative or criminal behaviour. Credentialing may also serve a de-stigmatizing function in the society and enhance the morale of the staff who earn certifications. Finally, licensing may minimize diversion of dangerous drugs from the legitimate pharmacy system by making it more difficult to become a prescriber. Thus, licensing and credentialing seem to be blunt instruments to affect service quality, functioning primarily to establish a floor for service quality and integrity rather than helping to raise it step by step to a higher level.

Process performance indicators. In many health care systems, the process by which care is provided is monitored and evaluated against some standard, such as typical practice patterns in the field or, where available, the scientific evidence base. Process measures can be gathered while patients are still receiving services and thus are less costly and provide more immediate feedback than do outcome monitoring systems (described below). By tracking process measures and incentivizing them, health care systems can reinforce clinicians for offering high quality services. One example is the US Veterans Health Administration, which rewards its national system of health care facilities financially if drug-dependent patients are retained in treatment over time (Harris *et al.* 2009). The downside of such approaches is that many process of care measures have inconsistent relationships to ultimate outcomes, whether one is considering individual patient outcomes or the average effectiveness of a particular facility (Harris *et al.* 2009).

Outcome monitoring systems. Health care performance management systems monitor what service providers do during the time of service. Outcome monitoring systems, in contrast, typically assess outcome directly (e.g. drug use and drug-related behaviours) at some point after the service is no longer being provided. Some systems request that each individual service programme conduct such monitoring. Service providers tend to resist this because locating drug users after service termination is often difficult and costly. In addition, it is argued that time spent by service providers conducting follow-up evaluations is time not spent providing services. Another reason why outcome monitoring is resisted is the fear that outcome evaluations will show that services are not as effective as professionals claim. As a result, some service systems have designated organizations that do nothing but conduct such outcome evaluations on all or a sample of all serviced individuals, and this approach typically generates higher follow-up rates and more trustworthy data (Tiet *et al.* 2006).

There is no consensus on the optimal length of time after receipt of drug services when outcomes should be evaluated. Setting the time window too far out may miss the bulk of obtained effects, just as it would for even highly intensive medical procedures. Time windows set close to the conclusion of care tend to fall short of the demand of stakeholders, who expect longer-term benefits from services.

McLellan and colleagues (2005) suggested that the outcomes of drug services should be evaluated concurrently with service provision rather than afterwards. This somewhat minimizes the distinction described above between process and outcome monitoring. One advantage of this approach is that clinicians can gather outcome data as services proceed, which is less costly than conducting post-treatment outcome studies and may also improve quality of care by increasing attention to drug users' progress in services. At the same time, this approach would also allow clinicians to 'fudge' data more easily, for example to make themselves or their service programme look more effective than it really is.

The Methadone Treatment Quality Assurance System (Phillips *et al.* 1995) is an intriguing example of an in-treatment outcome monitoring approach in which staff in OST clinics regularly gathered and faxed to a central research site data on patient's drug use, employment, and mental health functioning. The research site then provided feedback to the clinics on their relative performance. OST clinics are particularly well suited to these sorts of systems because of their high retention rates and regular monitoring of desired outcomes (e.g. through frequent urinanalysis). Such a system has not been successfully implemented and evaluated in an outpatient care system that does not offer OST.

Case mix adjustment is essential for outcome monitoring projects, and for performance process measures described earlier. This refers to the well known variability among treatment clients in demographic factors, psychiatric severity, and drug use history. The most accurate, technically sophisticated case mix adjustment is likely to be inscrutable to those who fund programmes, use services, and are supposed to be incentivized by the performance monitoring system. As a result, many systems adopted very simple case mix adjustments (e.g. three critical, simple variables such as presence of serious mental illness, unemployment, and AIDS) to compare programmes, even though such models sacrifice accuracy to some extent.

Summary of quality improvement strategies. Promoting quality services for drug users is a major challenge for systems managers, and some of the most widely employed methods (e.g. credentialing) have limited evidence of effectiveness. Process performance indicators seem the most promising approach, but will not realize their full potential until evaluation science better specifies which proximal outcomes predict long-term changes in drug users' behaviour.

15.7 **Conclusion**

From the point of view of drug policy, what happens at the systems level matters more than the outcomes of different individual patients and service programmes. The scientific literature has focused historically more on the latter issue than the former, but this chapter shows that some of the research on systems is of value in policy deliberations.

Policymakers who focus only on decisions about individual service programmes will usually find that they have limited impact on the outcomes they wish to produce. In contrast, policymakers who think and act at a system level, and do so in light of the emerging evidence base on the nature and impact of systems, have a much greater likelihood of making a significant contribution to ameliorating drug problems at both the individual and the population level.

Section V

Synthesis and conclusions

Chapter 16

Summary and conclusions

16.1 The evidence

At the beginning of this book we asserted that drug policy can be improved by greater attention to scientific evidence, and thereby better serve the public good. To justify that claim, we discussed the complex nature of drug use and drug problems, and systematically evaluated different intervention approaches. We hope that by this point it has become clear that science offers a range of findings that can inform the development of effective drug policy. Nevertheless, the current patchwork of drug policy responses by modern societies and international organizations takes little account of the available research. This concluding chapter explores the implications of this situation for policymakers and practitioners.

Chapters 8–12 reviewed the scientific research evaluating a wide range of different drug policy strategies and interventions. A summary of that review is provided in the Appendix following this chapter. The table demonstrates that a variety of options are available to the policymaker, ranging from universal approaches aimed at the entire population, to targeted approaches aimed at problem drug users. The table also makes clear that fewer than half of the policy options have been proven effective, either because the interventions have not had their intended effect or because the research has not been conducted with sufficient rigour to provide a definitive conclusion. Even that is a generous assessment, in that a large variety of interventions, particularly involving enforcement, are not included in the list because the evaluation literature is so slight that it was not sensible to break down the categories as finely as was done with other policy domains in which scientific evaluations are far more common. Nevertheless, a great deal has been learned about many of these interventions, and within most of the major areas there are several that have been shown to be effective for a particular drug problem or population group. Seventeen of the 43 show some evidence of effectiveness in more than one country, particularly those devoted to providing health and social services to dependent drug users. Tools are available to deal with many types of drug problems, and the cumulative and combined impact of the most effective policies could have a synergistic effect.

We now present some implications of these findings for achieving various policy goals. In doing so, we recognize that policymaking cannot and should not be solely a technocratic endeavour entrusted to scientists. Scientists are experts in measuring the nature of the problem and in estimating the outcomes of policy, but they have no more standing than anyone else in a society to say which specific outcomes a society should care about the most, or whether such outcomes are good, bad, or indifferent

(Mugford 1993). What follows therefore is not a prescription for what any society or policymaker *should* do but rather an analysis of what science indicates will be the likely consequences of exercising particular options. This information becomes meaningful only in light of whatever goals a policymaker or society has chosen to pursue.

16.2 **Does drug policy matter?**

Poring over the many negative or uncertain findings reviewed in this book, and being cognizant that drug problems continue to spread in the world despite vigorous attempts to stanch them, a sceptical reader might wonder whether drug policy is worth the resources devoted to it. The disappointments of drug policy are numerous, but two lines of evidence suggest that the bother is indeed worth the cost and the effort.

Some of the drug policy efforts reviewed in this book have made a positive difference. For example, as discussed in Chapter 15, the dramatic expansion in availability of Opiate Substitution Therapy (OST) in France led to substantial reductions in heroin-related problems. The reduction in methamphetamine-related problems following the 1995 precursor regulation policies in the USA is another example (Cunningham and Liu 2003). Just as importantly, drug policy has mattered even when it has not produced its intended outcomes. In Thailand in 2004, several thousand suspected drug dealers were killed in extrajudicial proceedings. We do not know whether this policy action had any significant impact on drug use and trafficking in Thailand, but it clearly had an effect on the people who were executed, their families, and their communities, and is therefore worthy of serious discussion. Even more potent examples can be drawn from policies that appear to have made a drug problem substantially worse. In the early 1990s Iran incarcerated thousands of drug users and provided no health services for them. The prisons became incubators for needle sharing, HIV infection, and tuberculosis (Farnam 2005; Mokri 2005). Drug policy compels our attention even when it fails because, like any other extension of government authority, it can have unintended consequences.

In asserting the power of drug policy we still acknowledge that drug problems unfortunately will always be with us in some form no matter what policies are put forward. Unlike technical problems that can be 'solved' and then recede into the realm of routine government administration (e.g. how to purify water or build a sturdy bridge), social problems have to be 'solved' again and again by each generation (Sarason 1978). Policy can minimize the damage drugs cause and influence what sort of drug problems exist, but it does not allow a society to choose to be completely free of drug problems (Kleiman 1992).

16.3 **Scientifically grounded conclusions about drug policy**

Although science is unable to forecast confidently the precise effects of many potential policy changes (e.g. decriminalization of all drugs), it can pronounce more authoritatively on other drug policy options. The authors have come to consensus that the evidence reviewed in this book supports the following 10 conclusions.

16.3.1 There is no single drug problem within or across societies; neither is there a magic bullet that will solve 'the drug problem'

Various sections of this book (Chapters 3, 4, and 14) revealed that societies differ substantially in the specific drugs that are problematic, the patterns in which drugs are used, the damage associated with drug distribution and use, and the ways in which various substances are controlled, among myriad other factors. There are significant variations as well within societies, for example between the sexes, across races and age groups, and at different stages of a drug epidemic. There is, as a result, no single, globally homogenous 'drug problem'.

It follows from this realization that there can be no single or universal solution to the drug problem, either within a society or across societies. The desire for a 'magic bullet', be it a new programme of services, a change in the legal regime, a new medication, or the concentration of resources into a 'war on drugs', is understandable. However, to quote H.L. Mencken, '[f]or every complex question there is an answer that is clear, simple and wrong'. We offer this caution about the search for a simple solution to a complex drug problem, including the assumption that the same drug policy will have the same impact in different societies.

16.3.2 Many policies that affect drug problems are not considered drug policy, and many specific drug policies have large effects outside the drug domain

Chapters 2, 3, and 4 have established that drug problems are often intermixed with other social, psychological, and behavioural problems, and that the predictors of young people developing future drug problems are similar to the predictors of developing many other difficulties. As a result, policymakers would be ill-advised to assume that only specific 'drug policies' influence drug problems. Economic policies, for example, will almost certainly have spillover effects into drug problems because changes in a society's economic situation typically impact a range of health behaviours and outcomes (Kiernan *et al.* 1989; Ruhm 2000). The social welfare net a society provides will also influence its drug problems, for example by determining how long drug dependence can continue before a drug user encounters punitive or rehabilitative social control efforts. Policies governing trade (e.g. the amount of travel and contact permitted between individuals in different countries, the extent to which parcels from abroad are subject to inspection, regulation, and taxation) influence international drug trafficking just as they do other businesses (see Chapter 5). Preventive interventions that promote the social development of young people can impact positively on antisocial behaviour, criminal activity, health, and well-being, as well as drug use and misuse (see Chapter 8). This and other evidence indicates that policymakers who want to form a comprehensive drug strategy can usually find effective policies and agencies outside of the remit those officially charged with addressing specific drug problems.

In parallel fashion, societal efforts to combat other social problems (e.g. crime, poverty, child abuse) could be facilitated by looking to those agencies charged with combating drug problems. A clear example can be found in efforts to reduce property crime and public disorder. The evidence suggests that in many societies, the best method to pursue this goal would be to expand OST for opiate-dependent individuals. Yet many policy planning groups convened to reduce street crime include not a single expert in services for drug users. Although more widely appreciated in most societies, the same point holds for a society's efforts to reduce child abuse or infectious diseases, both of which may be substantially enhanced by coordination with existing drug policies.

16.3.3 Efforts by wealthy countries to curtail cultivation of drug-producing plants in poor countries have not reduced aggregate drug supply or use in downstream markets, and probably never will

Several wealthy countries, most notably the USA, have invested billions of dollars in efforts to reduce cultivation of drug-producing plants in poor countries. One such approach described earlier in Chapter 10 is called alternative development, which encourages substitution of drug-producing plants with legal crops. A Congressional inquiry into US efforts of this sort in Afghanistan showed not only that agricultural development programmes were unsuccessful in that country, but that drug production increased the most in those areas receiving such aid (US House of Representatives, Committee on Government Reform 2005). Other evidence reviewed in Chapter 10 supports equally pessimistic conclusions about crop substitution. The evidence on mass defoliation campaigns is similarly clear: sustained and intense campaigns of crop spraying in Colombia and Mexico have not reduced drug production in those countries.

A proponent of such efforts might argue that cultivation curtailment initiatives have simply not been conducted on a sufficient scale to work. The weakness of this argument lies in the fact that it only requires a very small amount of arable land to provide the world's drug supply. Thus, even a large increase in such programmes would only serve to drive production to a new area, perhaps in a new country, rather than reduce global drug cultivation. Further, the basic rationale for these programmes neglects the reality that drugs are traded in a market, often taking the form of a set of small, semi-autonomous social networks (see Chapter 5). When defoliation or crop substitution reduces the amount of drug-producing crops in one area, the value of the remaining product increases, making it more attractive for other individuals to begin or expand cultivation. Particularly with opium poppy crops, which in some regions can be planted multiple times a year, such adaptations can be very rapid indeed. Moreover, inasmuch as crop substitution programmes may merely shift drug production to another nation, these programmes tend to have negative effects on neighbouring countries.

This does not necessarily mean that drug crop substitution and defoliation programmes should be stopped. A society may decide that removing a small number of people from the illegal economy is morally worthy enough, or that reducing the drug supply in producing nations is noble enough to justify the expense (even though these benefits do not return to the wealthy country). But if a wealthy society hopes to ameliorate its own drug problem with such an approach, the most scientifically grounded conclusion is that it will fail even if current efforts are multiplied many times over.

16.3.4 Once a drug is made illegal, there is a point beyond which increases in enforcement and incarceration yield little added benefit

Drug prohibition is regarded by many policymakers and much of the public as essential. It increases the price of drugs, stigmatizes drug use, and prevents large-scale corporate entities from promoting drug sales through modern marketing techniques. After these 'structural consequences of illegality' are attained and maintained through routine levels of enforcement, increased enforcement against drug dealers produces diminishing returns. That is, even if very large numbers of people are incarcerated, drug prices do not rise and availability does not decline much beyond what could be expected from routine enforcement of drug laws. Further, there may be perverse effects if law enforcement resources are diverted to arresting and incarcerating drug dealers when other crimes that would otherwise claim police attention are neglected (Kleiman 1992; Rasmussen and Benson 1994).

16.3.5 Substantial investments in evidence-based services for opiate-dependent individuals usually reduce drug-related problems

Chapter 9 reviewed a number of health and social services that are intended to reduce drug use and related problems (e.g. crime, transmission of infectious disease). Yet, as shown in Chapter 15, most societies invest in these services at a low level, resulting in limited access and inadequate quality. If a society is committed to 'doing something' about its drug problem, a substantial expansion of such services, particularly for people dependent on opiates, is likely to produce the broadest range of benefits. If the expansion is large enough, some change in health and crime indicators may be manifested at the population level (see French example, Emmanuelli and Desenclos 2005). We emphasize services for opiate-dependent individuals because our review found that (1) the services available for this population, especially OST, have the strongest supporting evidence; (2) opiate use poses a high risk of overdose death; and (3) injection drug use has in many societies produced an ensuing epidemic of AIDS and other infectious diseases. Services for opiate users therefore could have a relatively large effect on population indicators of drug-related harm.

Health and social services for users of other drugs, most notably stimulants (e.g. cocaine, methamphetamine), have less scientific support than those for opiate users. Policymakers may therefore weigh the importance of these substances differently in planning service budgets and drug policy. Opiate dependence is a dangerous condition for which highly effective services are available, so most policymakers will find it logical to prioritize services for that population. Prioritizing services for other substances may be less simple in that services for cannabis users have more evidence of effectiveness than do services for stimulant users, but the latter group of drug users does more damage to the public good. There is no scientific answer to the question of whether it is better for a policy to have a large effect on a less serious problem or a small effect on a more serious one. This is a question that policymakers and society must answer for themselves.

Another important conclusion is that many of the drug-related problems about which policymakers worry are caused by a relatively small group of individuals who use drugs heavily. The programmes and services reviewed in Chapters 9 and 15, despite their limitations, can have a significant impact on population-level drug problem indicators precisely because they are accessed primarily by those individuals who use drugs most heavily and with the most severe consequences. We would emphasize also that the scientific evidence strongly supports the proposition that such services benefit both the drug user and the broader society. Families whose houses might be robbed have as much interest in expanded services for drug users as do the opiate users who commit burglaries to support their drug habits.

16.3.6 School, family, and community prevention programmes have a collectively modest impact, the value of which will be appraised differently by different stakeholders

There are only a small number of high quality studies from the USA that support particular family-based or classroom management programmes in terms of preventing drug use. Interestingly, these programmes do not focus exclusively or specifically on drug use but rather on improving behaviour and social skills more generally, within a family or a classroom environment, and they also show evidence of wider effect beyond drug use and misuse. Prevention programmes that are delivered to younger people before they initiate drug use, that are based on social, psychological, and developmental theories, and that target a broad set of mental, emotional, and behavioural disorders as well as drug use, have emerged over the last 20 years to be the most promising of this kind of intervention (National Research Council and Institute of Medicine 2009). In contrast, purely didactic prevention programmes, whether delivered through the mass media, in the community, or in the classroom, have no evidence of effectiveness.

Whether the modest impact observed in some studies is still worth the costs of school- or family-based prevention programmes is a political judgement each society must make for itself. Caulkins and colleagues (2002) argue that the pay-off of even slightly lower rates of initiation is so large over the lifespan of a drug user that prevention programmes are cost-effective even when they are only modestly effective, suggesting that the proverbial ounce of prevention is worth a pound of cure. Whether this argument is compelling will be likely to depend on the time horizon a policymaker or society uses to assess the return on investment in a prevention programmne.

16.3.7 The drug policy debate is dominated in many countries by four false dichotomies that can mislead policymakers about the range of legitimate options and their expected impacts

Under conditions of conflict and high emotion, human beings are prone to perceive sharper distinctions than are empirically accurate (Weick 1984). This is true in many drug policy debates, and it creates at least four false choices. First, as this book makes clear, the allegedly distinct approaches of law enforcement and health services (sometimes shorthanded as 'cops versus docs') each make significant contributions to the others' allegedly exclusive mission. For example, the illegality of drugs raises prices, which lowers drug use, and OST reduces street crime. Thus, law enforcement can promote public health, and health services can increase compliance with the law.

Secondly, the contrast between policies that support services targeting drug use *per se* versus those that target the damage caused by drug use is less distinct than is often supposed. A society that offers 'harm reduction' services will find that at least some service users become abstainers, and a society that offers only abstinence-oriented services will discover that some service users attain non-abstinence outcomes that reduce harm.

Thirdly, the distinction often drawn between 'good drugs' (meaning those that are legally available or prescribed medically) and 'bad drugs' (meaning those that are neither) is overly simplistic. As reviewed in Chapters 6 and 12, an increasing amount of illegal drug use derives from medications diverted from the legal market. And as noted in Chapter 2, tobacco, a legal substance, causes far more health damage than any of the illegal substances.

Fourthly, the putative trade-off between the interests of heavy drug users and those of the rest of society are also often overstated. To take one example mentioned earlier in the book, service systems established for the benefit of drug-dependent people at taxpayer expense may prevent more HIV infections among non-users than they do among drug users.

16.3.8 **Perverse impacts of drug policy are prevalent**

The iron law of unintended consequences is a commonly cited principle in political science and public discourse. Perhaps all policy analysts in all fields would make the same observation, but in the drug policy field this law seems unusually apt. The examples mentioned in the book include heroin and methadone prescription regimes that led to diversion and overdose deaths in the UK, US decertification threats that led to brutal government actions in low and middle income countries, and stigma-promoting prevention programmes that discourage drug-dependent individuals from admitting that they have a problem.

Drug policies should be judged not just on their intended effects, but also on their potential unintended consequences. For example, a new **contingency management** programme that pays patients US$50 per week for abstinence should be evaluated not just in terms of its effect on patients, but also on whether such a programme would lower drug users' interest in other, less costly, health services, thereby reducing the number of individuals who could receive services each year within budgetary limits. To take a law enforcement example, efforts to break up one well-established drug market should consider where drug dealing is likely to move next, and how its character may change as a result. In offering this stricture we are simply bringing drug policy into the mainstream of policy analysis. Cost–benefit analysis, a standard tool in many fields of policymaking, requires assessment of all the consequences of a policy choice, not just the intended ones (Gramlich 1990).

The law of unintended consequences also implies that it may be possible to improve drug policies by doing less rather than more. Many reform-minded policymakers assume that adding a new policy, programme, or regulation to the current system will improve matters substantially. Given the law of unintended effects, that policymaker would be wise to survey current policies in light of the historical record and make a full appraisal of whether any of them have unintended negative effects in excess of whatever positive benefits they are likely to produce. In many countries, a policymaker's goals might be better served by repealing existing policies or abolishing certain programmes and agencies, rather than attempting new approaches.

16.3.9 **The legal pharmaceutical system can affect the shape of a country's drug problem and its range of available drug policy options**

As noted in Chapters 3 and 6, the misuse of psychopharmaceuticals has been growing rapidly and is likely to accelerate. In our review of various societies and their drug problems and services, a recurrent theme is the influence of the pharmacy system. When a country has no pharmacy system, or a weak one, policymakers often face sharp trade-offs because admitting a drug for medicinal purposes immediately allows its widespread misuse. The alternative, a law enforcement approach in which the drug is outlawed for all purposes, may deprive ill individuals of quality medical care (e.g. adequate pain control for cancer). Even in societies with well-managed pharmacy systems, diversion of prescription drugs is a serious problem that has been increasing in its dimensions. Nonetheless, the existence of strong pharmacy systems creates other policy options, such as implementing widespread buprenorphine maintenance or asking prescribers to replace dependence-producing medications with less dangerous alternatives. Building up the legal pharmacy system in countries where it is lacking could be the first foothold in developing an effective policy for illicit drugs.

16.3.10 **There is virtually no scientific research to guide the improvement of supply control and law enforcement efforts**

The lack of research into strategies for enforcement, interdiction, incarceration, and related measures represents a major failure. Independent of how strongly a policymaker values law enforcement and supply control as policy tools, it is difficult to understand why policymakers would not want their policies to be based on good quality evidence. The lack of careful study thus continues to pose a major barrier to applying these policies effectively.

16.4 **Conclusion**

The conclusions above are fewer in number and less confident in tone than some policymakers and many political activists would prefer. This situation reflects the fact that drug policy research has a modest, if growing, evidence base and that we are hewing closely to that evidence base, striving not to advance our personal opinions about how societies should make democratic and culturally appropriate decisions regarding drugs. Yet even within the limits of present science, there is no doubt that many drug policies that are known to be ineffective continue to exist, and many that are known to be effective suffer from disuse.

More than a decade has elapsed since the international community established a set of ambitious goals at the 1998 United Nations Special Session of the General Assembly (UNGASS). The primary aim of UNGASS was to mobilize enough international cooperation to reduce global drug supply and demand significantly by 2008. A review of that effort (Reuter and Trautmann 2009) found no evidence that the global drug problem has been reduced, a conclusion that is consistent with the findings presented in this book. Whether the systematic application of evidence-informed policies could have resulted in a better outcome merits consideration. Scientific evidence alone is not sufficient to stem the rising worldwide tide of drug problems, but it could be a powerful ally of leaders who have the courage, creativity, and conviction to create more effective drug policy.

Appendix

Summary of policy strategies and interventions reviewed in Chapters 8–12

Intervention	Effectiveness[a]	Amount of research support and cross-national testing[b]	Comments
Chapter 8: School, family, and community programmes			*Target group*: non-users of drugs, casual users, parents, and the general public.
Family/parenting programmes	Some studies show effectiveness in reducing the onset of drug use.	A few studies conducted in the USA only.	Positive findings for the universal Strengthening Families Programmeme for 10-to 14 year-olds, including longer term follow-ups and cost-effectiveness analysis. Replication studies are needed. Other family/parenting programmes have not been evaluated as positively.
Environmental/classroom management programmes	Some evidence supporting the Good Behavior Game.	A few studies conducted in the USA only.	In one study the Good Behavior Game reduced lifetime drug abuse by up to 50% in males 14 years after exposure to the programme, with even stronger effects with boys identified at age 6 as highly aggressive and disruptive. A second study did not find the same level and range of impacts over the longer term. Subsequent research has not provided strong replication.
Social or life skills	Most evaluations have not examined effectiveness beyond immediate and short-term follow-up, where the evidence is equivocal. Some evidence of positive impact over the medium to longer term.	Several high quality studies conducted in USA only.	A small number of evaluations have shown positive intervention effects from a small set of prevention programmes for cannabis use and also for use of other drugs.
Multicomponent community	No evidence of effectiveness.	Only a few small US studies.	Studies have typically combined school and non-school approaches. Effect sizes tend to be small or negligible.

Affective education	No evidence of effectiveness.	Several school-based US studies.	This approach was popular in the 1970s and 1980s.
Information/knowledge only	No evidence of effectiveness.	A few school-based US studies.	There have been few well-controlled studies but many uncontrolled evaluations.
Mass media	No evidence of effectiveness.	Research limited to a few studies in the USA.	Few high quality scientific evaluations. The use of mass media alone, particularly in the presence of prodrug music, drug-using role models, and exposure to images of drug use does not prevent or reduce substance use, although media campaigns can raise awareness of the negative consequences.
Social marketing/norms	Insufficient evidence to determine effectiveness.	Only one US study.	One social marketing intervention showed lower cannabis initiation rates.
DARE	No evidence of effectiveness.	Several well-controlled studies and numerous uncontrolled evaluations.	Despite DARE's widespread adoption, meta-analyses of outcome evaluations showed that the programme is ineffective.
Drug testing in schools	No evidence of effectiveness.	No well-controlled studies available.	Drug testing programmes could have negative effects, such as reduced trust between pupils and staff.
Chapter 9: Services to change behaviour			*Target group*: drug users diagnosed with substance use disorders and/or under legal pressure to obtain treatment. Also, injection drug users.
Methadone maintenance*	Good evidence for reduced heroin use, other drug use, crime, HIV infection, and hepatitis.	Numerous studies in high income countries, some in LAMI countries.	Dosage level is important, as are the populations treated. Overdose risk increases in some populations, but in general methadone reduces overall drug-related mortality. Combination with psychosocial services enhances outcome. Cost-effectiveness is high relative to other treatment interventions.

Intervention	Effectiveness[a]	Amount of research support and cross-national testing[b]	Comments
Buprenorphine maintenance*	Good evidence for reducing heroin use, other drug use, crime, HIV infection, and hepatitis.	Tested in several countries but less in LAMI countries.	May reduce overall drug-related mortality if implemented on a wide scale.
Heroin substitution*	Recent limited evidence for effectiveness as a way to reduce crime and infection among those who have had poor outcomes in other forms of opiate substitution therapy.	Demonstration programmes evaluated in Switzerland, The Netherlands, Germany, Canada, and the UK.	Qualitative and quasi-experimental treatment evaluations as well as randomised trials show positive results and none shows a negative result. This is the most costly form of opiate substitution therapy.
Opiate antagonists (e.g. naltrexone, naloxone)	Some evidence for reduced opiate use but medication compliance is a major limitation.	Few studies outside of the USA.	Studies of oral naltrexone (the most popular opiate antagonist) are of poor methodological quality and do not support the medication's practical effectiveness. Depot formulations may have promise.
Needle exchange programmes (NEP)*	NEPs may reduce drug-related HIV infections and facilitate treatment engagement.	Most research conducted in Canada, the UK, Australia, and the USA.	NEPs may prevent HIV infections but have no evidence of reducing hepatitis C infections. The fear that NEPs will increase intravenous drug use initiation has no research basis. NEPs have never been subjected to a randomized clinical trial.
Psychosocial treatment*	Good evidence for reducing drug use, drug-related problems, and criminal activity.	Numerous studies in many countries, including LAMI countries.	Often combined with other treatment modalities such as methadone maintenance. Typically delivered in both outpatient and residential settings in either group or individual formats. Effective for opiates, cannabis, cocaine, methamphetamine, and other substances.

Peer self-help organizations*	Good evidence for reducing drug use, crime, and infections.	Evidence available from several countries including the USA, the UK, and China.	A very cost-effective way to manage chronic drug users.
Naloxone distribution	Minimal good quality evidence available, but some programmes have documented cases of successful resuscitation.	Only a few studies in a few countries (e.g., the USA and the UK.)	This type of intervention applies primarily to opiate users in subcultures where there is a high risk of overdose. It may have limited applicability in countries and cities where resources are limited.
Brief interventions in general medical settings	Good evidence for reducing drug use by at-risk drug users.	Evidence available from a variety of countries, including the UK, the USA, India, Australia, and Brazil.	Evidence available for a variety of substances.
Chapter 10: Supply control interventions			*Target group*: either producers or illicit market forces.
Alternative development	No known instance of a correlation with reduced drug use.	Programmes have been evaluated qualitatively in several LAMI countries.	Certain types of drug use are related to increasing affluence (see Chapter 3), so alternative development may be counter-productive. Once drug markets have become established it is difficult to change them. Cost is extremely high.
Crop eradication	Can sometimes create a noticeable but temporary market disruption.	Programmes have been evaluated qualitatively in several LAMI countries.	Availability of other growing regions often results in a shift in production and a recovery of the market. Cost is extremely high.
Precursor chemical control*	Good evidence for temporary disruption in drug market.	Several studies in the USA and Canada.	Low cost to implement through legal statutes but enforcement can be costly. Despite market disruptions, there is often a transition to alternative production materials or producers re-locate to other countries.

Intervention	Effectiveness[a]	Amount of research support and cross-national testing[b]	Comments
Interdiction*	May disrupt drug market and supply chain, and thus increase cost to drug user.	Several studies in the USA and LAMI countries.	Price markups over relevant market layers suggest important benefits of modest investments but limited evidence of a dose–response effect. Cost to implement and sustain interdiction programmes is extremely high.
High level enforcement through criminal investigations	Price mark-ups suggest important benefits of modest investments but limited evidence of a dose–response effect.	Only a few studies have been conducted.	Incarcerating high level dealers may be more cost-effective than enforcement against retail sellers because of the ease with which retail sellers can be replaced. This is a matter of impression rather than science.
Street-level enforcement	Stronger evidence of ability to modify markets and market harms than of ability to reduce drug availability.	Only a few studies outside the USA.	Cost to implement and sustain on a local level can be high to achieve maximum impact.
Imprisonment	Some evidence that there may be diminishing returns to expansion of imprisonment beyond certain levels.	Only a few investigations outside the USA and UK.	High cost to manage prison system and community re-engagement services.
Chapter 11: Criminalization and decriminalization			*Target group*: drug users, especially cannabis users.
Shifting between conventional criminal penalties and some other form of penalty*	Modest or no effect on cannabis use, while reducing adverse consequences for the user.	Several Australian and US studies	Some benefits to criminal justice system and to users, with debatable impact on cannabis use and related problems. Net-widening is an issue.
Changing the level of criminal penalties	Moderate or no effects on cannabis use.	A contested literature from the USA, The Netherlands, and Switzerland.	Some benefits to criminal justice system without necessarily increasing cannabis use.

Abolishing or introducing criminal laws on use of drugs	Very little study.	Limited. There is a Czech study of recriminalizing.	Czech recriminalization added state costs without apparent benefit; availability of drugs and number of users did not decrease.
Measures involving informal handling by the police, short of arrest	Little evidence that police cautions are more effective than alternative sanctions.	There are no well-controlled studies.	Changes in criminal processing are difficult to evaluate.
Diversion to mandated education or treatment	Little effect on cannabis-related problems.	Several Portuguese and Californian studies.	Diversion saved money in California.
Switching between prohibition and de facto legalization of use with a controlled market	Circumstantial evidence that Dutch system may be effective in separating cannabis from other drug markets.	Several evaluation studies in The Netherlands, but no well-controlled research.	Effects on consumption levels are contested, though Dutch use rates are relatively low compared with other European countries.
Chapter 12: Regulatory interventions			*Target group* or behaviours: medically inadvisable use of the drug, or prescribing behaviour of doctors, or selling by the pharmacist. The main criteria of effectiveness are reductions in overdoses or other adverse consequences of the drug use, or reduction in sales of the drug.
Change cost or reimbursement*	Some evidence for an effect on prescribing behaviour.	Most published studies are from North America.	Some evidence on drugs for relief of pain, particularly where there are alternative drugs.
Restrict over-the-counter (OTC) sales*	Results from studies of overdoses are conflicting.	Three studies from Canada and the UK.	No studies of psychoactive substances. Some evidence that OTC restrictions prevent health problems with analgesics.
Require prescription (versus OTC availability) *	Scattered research provides support for some effect.	Studies from several countries, but only one concerning psychoactive substances.	Changing a drug between OTC and prescription states has varying effects on sales. In some systems, the consumer pays more for an OTC drug.

Intervention	Effectiveness[a]	Amount of research support and cross-national testing[b]	Comments
Authoritative advice to physicians*	Some evidence of effects on prescribing or warning of newly determined adverse effects, when an alternative is available	Six studies from Canada, the UK, Australia, and the USA.	Some evidence that advice to physicians changes prescribing behaviour, but no studies of psychopharmaceuticals.
Enforcing prescription guidelines	Guidelines enforcement changed prescribing behaviour in one large US effort	Only one US study.	
Prescription restrictions, registers, monitoring*	Good evidence that prescription registers and monitoring reduces prescription of targeted drugs and reduces adverse events from the drugs.	Many studies from a variety of European and North American countries.	Although prescription of targeted drugs are reduced, substitution of drugs that are equally or even more harmful may result.
Restrict list of prescribers*	The few studies show some effect.	One Iranian study shows strong effects on adverse drug reactions.	Often applied but little evaluated (e.g. prescribers typically restricted for all forms of OST).
Withdraw prescription availability*	Good evidence for reducing prescribing and use of the drug.	Studies across a variety of European countries.	Substituted medications may carry additional risks.
Profile patients	No evidence.	No research.	

Enforcement of laws affecting physicians and patients	No evidence.	No research.	Law enforcement officials believe that Prescription Monitoring Programmes have eliminated diversion.
Controls on administering opiate substitution therapy (OST)*	Some effects in reducing overdoses from tighter controls on OST administration.	Studies in Australia, Denmark, the UK, and the USA.	Some evidence for reduced diversion.

* Interventions found to be effective in more than one country.

[a] This column describes the effectiveness level (good, some, no evidence) of each intervention and then specifies what outcomes the evidence supports (target behaviours or target conditions). In other words, the effectiveness column rates each intervention by how well it achieves what it aspires to achieve.

[b] This column combines the amount of research support (large, small, no studies) and cross-national testing (are there any studies in low or middle income (LAMI) countries). The column uses basic wording of large, small, or no research support, and then comments on the amount and quality of studies in LAMI countries.

[c] This column presents information on populations, dosages, unintended consequences, and effect size.

References

Aaserud M., Dahlgren A.T., Kösters J.P., Oxman A.D., Ramsay C., and Sturm H. (2006) Pharmaceutical policies: effects of reference pricing, other pricing, and purchasing polices [review]. *Cochrane Database of Systematic Reviews.* Issue 2, article no.: CD005979. DOI: 10.1002/14651858.CD005979.

ACC. See Australian Crime Commission.

Aceijas C. and Rhodes T. (2007) Global estimates of prevalence of HCV infection among injecting drug users. *International Journal of Drug Policy* **18**, 352–8.

Aceijas C., Friedman S.R., Cooper H.L., Wiessing L., Stimson G.V., and Hickman M. (2006) Estimates of injecting drug users at the national and local level in developing and transitional countries, and gender and age distribution. *Sexually Transmitted Infections* **82** (Suppl 3), 10–7.

Aceijas C., Stimson G.V., Hickman M., and Rhodes, T. (2004) Global overview of injecting drug use and HIV infection among injecting drug users. *AIDS* **18**, 2295–303.

Agrawal A. and Lynskey M.T. (2006) The genetic epidemiology of cannabis use, abuse and dependence. *Addiction* **101**, 801–12.

Aidala A., Cross J., Stall R., Harre D., and Sumartojo E. (2005) Housing status and HIV risk behaviors: implications for prevention and policy. *Archives of General Psychiatry* **9**, 251–65.

Aldington S., Williams M., Nowitz M., Weatherall M., Pritchard A., McNaughton A., Robinson G. and Beasley R. (2007) The effects of cannabis on pulmonary structure, function and symptoms. *Thorax* **62**, 1058–63.

Allott R., Paxton R., and Leonard R. (1999) Drug education: a review of British Government policy and evidence of effectiveness. *Health Education Research Theory and Practice* **14**, 491–505.

Alter M.J. (2006) Epidemiology of viral hepatitis and HIV co-infection. *Journal of Hepatology* **44**, S6–9.

Alva M. (2007) Big pharma's Rx for growth. *Investors Business Daily* 28 December. Available at: http://www.investors.com/editorial/IBDArticles.asp?artsec=23&issue=20071228.

Amato L., Davoli M., Perucci C.A., Ferri M., Faggiano F., and Mattick R.P. (2005) An overview of systematic reviews of the effectiveness of opiate maintenance therapies: available evidence to inform clinical practice and research. *Journal of Substance Abuse Treatment* **28**, 321–30.

Amon J.J., Garfein R.S., Adleh-Grant L., Armstrong G.L., Ouellet L.J., Latka M.H., Viahov D., Strathdee S.A., Hudson S.M., Kerndt P., Des Jarlais D., and Williams I.T. (2008) Prevalence of hepatitis C virus infection among injection drug users in the United States, 1994–2004. *Clinical Infectious Diseases* **46**, 1852–8.

Amundsen E.J. (2006) Measuring effectiveness of needle and syringe exchange programmes for prevention of HIV among IDUs. *Addiction* **101**, 161–3.

Anderson M. and Prout L.H. (1985) The real Miami vice?. *Newsweek* 11 November, 32.

Anderson S. (2006) Community pharmacy and the rise of welfare in Great Britain 1900 to 1986. In: *People and places: Proceedings of the 37th International Congress for the History of Pharmacy, 22–25 June 2005.* pp. 21–8. Leicester, UK: British Society for the History of Pharmacy. Available at: http://www.associationhq.org.uk/BSHPWebsite/Congress/ISHPCongress2005.pdf (accessed 20 May 2009).

Angell M. (2004) The truth about the drug companies. *New York Review of Books* 51(12), July 15. Available at: http://www.nybooks.com/articles/17244 (accessed 15 May 2009).

Anonymous (1965) Drug abuse control amendments of 1965. *New England Journal of Medicine* **273**, 1222–3.

Anonymous (2007) List of pharmaceutical companies. [Source: Top 50 Pharmaceutical companies. *MedAdNews* Sept. 2007] Available at: http://en.wikipedia.org/wiki/List_of_pharmaceutical_companies (accessed 15 May 2009).

Anthony R. and Fries A. (2004) Empirical modeling of narcotics trafficking from farm gate to street. *Bulletin on Narcotics* **56**, 1–48.

Applbaum K. (2006) Educating for global mental health: the adoption of SSRIs in Japan. In: Petryna A., Lakoff A. and Kleinman, A. (eds) *Global pharmaceuticals: ethics, markets, practices.* pp. 85–110. Durham, NC: Duke University Press.

Asia Pacific News (2009) *Australia set to outlaw motorcycle crime gangs.* 8 April. Available at: http://www.monstersandcritics.com/news/asiapacific/news/article_1469631.php/Australia_set_to_outlaw_motorcycle_crime_gangs_. (accessed 14 May 2009).

Auriacombe M., Pascale F., and Tignol, J. (2001) Deaths attributable to methadone versus buprenorphine in France [letter]. *Journal of the American Medical Association* **285**, 45.

Australian Crime Commission (2003) *Australian illicit drug report 2001/02.* Canberra, Australia: ACC.

Australian Crime Commission (2009) *Illicit drug data report 2006–2007, revised edition.* Canberra, Australia: ACC.

Australian Institute for Health and Welfare (2005) *2004 National drug strategy household survey: detailed findings.* Drug Statistics Series No 16. Canberra, Australia: Australian Institute for Health and Welfare.

Ayling J. (2005) Conscription in the war on drugs: recent reforms to the U.S. drug certification process. *International Journal of Drug Policy* **16**, 376–83.

Babor T.F., Campbell R., Room R., and Saunders J. (1994) *Lexicon of alcohol and drug terms.* Geneva, Switzerland: World Health Organization. Available at: http://whqlibdoc.who.int/publications/9241544686.pdf (accessed 15 May 2009).

Babor T.F., Stenius K., and Romelsjö A. (2008a) Alcohol and drug treatment systems in public health perspective: mediators and moderators of population effects. *International Journal of Methods in Psychiatric Research* **17** (suppl 1), S50–9.

Babor T.F., Stenius K., Savva S., and O'Reilly J. (eds) (2008b) *Publishing addiction science: a guide for the perplexed.* 2nd edn. Brentwood, UK: Multi-Science Publishing Company.

Baca C.T. and Grant K.J. (2005) Take-home naloxone to reduce heroin death. *Addiction* **100**, 1823–31.

Bachman J.G., Wallace J.M., O'Malley P.M., Johnston L.D., Kurth C.L., and Neighbors HW. (1991) Racial/ethnic differences in smoking, drinking, and illicit drug use among American high school seniors, 1976–89. *American Journal of Public Health* **81**, 372–7.

Bailey J.E., Barton P.L., Lezotte D., Lowenstein S.R., and Dart R.C. (2006) The effect of FDA approval of a generic competitor to OxyContin (oxycodone HCI controlled release) tablets on the abuse of oxycodone. *Drug and Alcohol Dependence* **84**, 182–7.

Baker A., Lewin T., Reichler H., Clancy R., Carr V., Garrett R., Sly K., Devir H., and Terry M. (2002) Evaluation of a motivational interview for substance use within psychiatric in-patient services. *Addiction* **97**, 1329–37.

Baker A., Lee N.K., Claire M., Lewin T.J., Grant T., and Pohlman S. (2005) Brief cognitive behavioural interventions for regular amphetamine users: a step in the right direction. *Addiction* **100**, 367–78.

Barnett P. (1999) The cost-effectiveness of methadone maintenance as a health care intervention. *Addiction* **94**, 479–88.

Barrio G., De la Fuente L., Royuela L., Díaz A., and Rodríguez-Artalejo F. (1998) Cocaine use among heroin users in Spain: the diffusion of crack and cocaine smoking. *Journal of Epidemiology and Community Health* **52**, 172–80.

Bashir K., King M., and Ashworth M. (1994) Controlled evaluation of brief intervention by general practitioners to reduce chronic use of benzodiazepines. *British Journal of General Practice* **44**, 408–12.

Basu D., Mattoo S.K., Malhotra A., Gupta N., and Malhotra R. (2000) A longitudinal study of male buprenorphine addicts attending an addiction clinic in India. *Addiction* **95**, 1363–72.

Bateman D.N., Good A.M., Afshari R., and Kelly C A. (2003) Effect of licence change on prescribing and poisons enquiries for antipsychotic agents in England and Scotland. *British Journal of Clinical Pharmacology* **55**, 596–603.

Bauman A. and Phongsavan P. (1999) Epidemiology of substance use in adolescence: prevalence, trends and policy implications. *Drug and Alcohol Dependence* **55**, 187–207.

Baumer E., Lauritsen J., Rosenfled R., and Wright R. (1998) The influence of crack cocaine on robbery, burglary, and homicide rates: a cross-city, longitudinal analysis. *Journal of Research in Crime and Delinquency* **35**, 316–40.

Beauvais F., Oetting E.R., and Edwards R.W. (1985) Trends in drug use of Indian adolescents living on reservations: 1975–1983. *American Journal of Drug and Alcohol Abuse* **11**, 209–29.

Beauvais F., Jumper-Thurman P., Helm H., Plested B., and Burnside M. (2004) Surveillance of drug use among American Indian adolescents: patterns over 25 years. *Journal of Adolescent Health* **34**, 493–500.

Beenstock M. and Rahav G. (2002) Testing gateway theory: do cigarette prices affect illicit drug use?. *Journal of Health Economics* **21**, 679–98.

Bejerot N. (1975) *Narkotika och narkomani* (Drugs and addiction). Stockholm, Sweden: Bonniers Grafiska Industrier AB.

Bennett T. and Holloway K. (2005) *Understanding drugs, alcohol and crime.* Maidenhead, UK: Open University Press.

Bennett T., Holloway K. and Farrington D. (2008) The statistical association between drug misuse and crime: A meta-analysis. *Aggression and Violent Behavior* **13**, 107–18.

Benson K. and Hartz A.J. (2000) A comparison of observational studies and randomized, controlled trials. *New England Journal of Medicine* **342**, 1878–86.

Berman P. and McLaughlin M.W. (1976) Implementation of educational innovations. *Educational Forum* **40**, 344–70.

Bernstein J., Bernstein E., Tassiopoilos K., Heeren T., Levenson S., and Hingson R. (2005) Brief intervention at a clinic visit reduced cocaine and heroin use. *Drug and Alcohol Dependency* **77**, 49–59.

Berridge V. (1999) *Opium and the people: opiate use and drug control policy in nineteenth and early twentieth century England.* Revised edn. London, UK: Free Association Books.

Berridge V. and Edwards G. (1981) *Opium and the people: opiate use in nineteenth-century England.* London, UK: St. Martin's Press.

Best D., Sidwell C., Gossop M., Harris J., Strang J. (2001a) Crime and expenditure amongst polydrug misusers seeking treatment. *British Journal of Criminology* **41**, 119–26.

Best D., Strang J., Beswick T., and Gossop M. (2001b) Assessment of a concentrated, high-profile police operation. *British Journal of Criminology* **41**, 738–45.

Best D., Gross S., Vingoe L., Witton J., and Strang, J. (2003) *Dangerousness of drugs: a guide to the risks and harms associated with substance use.* London, UK: UK Department of Health. Available at: http://www.dh.gov.uk/assetRoot/04/08/62/93/04086293.pdf (accessed 12 May 2009).

Bewley-Taylor D.R. (1999) *The United States and international drug control.* London, UK: Pinter.

Bewley-Taylor D.R. and Trace M. (2006) *The International Drug Control Board: watchdog or guardian of the conventions?* Report No. 7. Oxford, UK: The Beckley Foundation. Available at: http://www.internationaldrugpolicy.net/reports/BeckleyFoundation_Report_07.pdf (accessed 25 May 2009).

Biglan A., Ary D.V., Smolkowski K., Duncan T., and Black C. (2000) A randomised controlled trial of a community intervention to prevent adolescent tobacco use. *Tobacco Control* **9**, 24–32.

Binswanger I., Stern M., Deyo R., Heagerty P., Cheadle A., Elmore J., Koepsell T. (2007) Release from prison—a high risk of death for former inmates. *New England Journal of Medicine* **356**, 157–65.

Bishop M.T. and Vlasty R.J. (1993) The Illinois experience in achieving the medical/regulatory balance required to control prescription drug diversion. In: Cooper J.R., Czecowicz D.J., Molinari S.P., and Petersen R.C. (eds) *Impact of prescription drug diversion control systems on medical practice and patient care.* pp. 159–75. NIDA Research Monograph 131. Rockville, MD: National Institute on Drug Abuse.

Black J.K. (2005) *Latin America: its problems and its promise.* Boulder, CO: Westview Press.

Blane H.T. (1976) Issues in preventing alcohol problems. *Preventive Medicine* **5**, 176–86.

Bless R., Korf D.J., and Freeman M. (1995) Open drug scenes: a cross-national comparison of concepts and urban strategies. *European Addiction Research* **1**, 128–38.

Blomqvist J. (1998) *Beyond treatment? Widening the approach to alcohol problems and solutions.* Doctoral dissertation. Stockholm, Sweden: Stockholm University.

Blumstein A. and Cork D. (1996) Linking gun availability to youth gun violence. *Law and Contemporary Problems* **59**, 5–24.

Blumstein A., Rivara F., and Rosenfeld R. (2000) The rise and decline of homicide—and why. *Public Health* **21**, 505–41.

Bluthenhal R.N., Malik, M.R., Grau L.E., Singer M., Marshall P., and Heimer R. (2004) Sterile syringe access conditions and variations in HIV risk among drug injectors in three cities. *Addiction* **99**, 1136–46.

Boles S.M. and Miotto K. (2003) Substance use and violence: a review of the literature. *Aggression and Violent Behavior* **8**, 155–74.

Borches-Tempel S. and Kolte B. (2002) Cannabis consumption in Amsterdam, Bremen and San Francisco: a three-city comparison of long-term cannabis consumption. *Journal of Drug Issues* **32**, 395–412.

Botvin G.J. (2000) Preventing drug abuse in schools: social and competence enhancement approaches targeting individual-level etiologic factors. *Addictive Behaviors* **25**, 887–97.

Botvin G.J., Baker E., Filazzola A.D., and Botvin M. (1990) A cognitive-behavioral approach to substance abuse prevention: one-year follow-up. *Addictive Behaviors* **15**, 47–63.

Botvin G.J., Baker E., Dusenbury L., Botvin E., and Diaz T. (1995) Long term follow-up results of a randomized drug abuse prevention in a white middle class population. *Journal of the American Medical Association* **273**, 1106–12.

Botvin G.J., Griffin K.W., Diaz T., and Iffil-Williams M. (2001) Drug abuse prevention among minority adolescents: posttest and one-year follow-up of a school-based preventive intervention. *Prevention Science* **2**, 1–13.

Bouchard M. (2008) Towards a realistic method to estimate cannabis production in industrialized countries. *Contemporary Drug Problems* **35**(2/3), 291–320.

Bourgois P. (1996) *In search of respect: selling crack in el barrio*. Cambridge, UK: Cambridge University Press.

Bourgois P. (2003) *In search of respect: selling crack in El Barrio*. London, UK: Cambridge University Press.

Boyd C.J., McCabe S.E., and Teter C.J. (2006) Medical and nonmedical use of prescription pain medication by youth in a Detroit-area public school district. *Drug and Alcohol Dependence* **81**, 37–45.

Boyum D. (1992) *Reflections on economic theory and drug enforcement*. Doctoral dissertation. Cambridge, MA: Kennedy School of Government, Harvard University.

Boyum D. (1993) *Heroin and cocaine market structure*. Prepared for the Office of National Drug Control Policy. Cambridge, MA: Botec Analysis Corporation.

Boyum D. and Reuter P. (2001) Reflections on drug policy and social policy. In: Heymann P. and Brownsberger W. (eds) *Drug addiction and drug policy: the struggle to control dependence*. pp. 239–64. Cambridge, MA: Harvard University Press.

Boyum D. and Reuter P. (2005) *An analytic assessment of U.S. drug policy*. Washington, DC: American Enterprise Institute.

Braga A.A. and Pierce G.L. (2005) Disrupting illegal firearms markets in Boston: the effects of operation ceasefire on the supply of new handguns to criminals. *Criminology and Public Policy* **4**, 201–32.

Braga A.A., Kennedy D.M., Waring E.J., and Piehl A.M. (2001) Problem-oriented policing, deterrence, and youth violence: an evaluation of Boston's operation ceasefire. *Journal of Research in Crime and Delinquency* **38**, 195–225.

Bramley-Harker E. (2001) *Sizing the UK market for illicit drugs*. RDS Occasional Paper no. 74. London, UK: Home Office.

Bramness J.G., Skurtveit S., Furu K., Engeland A., Sakshaug S., and Rønning M. (2006) Endringer i salg og bruk av flunitrazepam etter 1999 (Changes in the sale and use of flunitrazepam in Norway after 1999). *Tidsskrift for den Norske Lægeforening* **126**, 589–90.

Brennan T.A., Rothman D.J., Blank L., Blumenthal D., Chimonas S.C., Cohen J.J., Goldman J., Kassirer J.P., Kimball H., Naughton J., and Smelser N. (2006) Health industry practices that create conflicts of interest: a policy proposal for academic medical centers. *Journal of the American Medical Association* **295**, 429–33.

Bretteville-Jensen A.L. (1999) Addiction and discounting. *Journal of Health Economics* **18**, 393–407.

Bretteville-Jensen A.L. (2005) *Økonomiske aspekter ved sprøytemisbrukeres forbruk av rusmidler: en analyse av intervjuer foretatt 1993–2004* (Economic aspects of injecting drug users' consumption of drugs: an analysis of interviews undertaken in the period 1993–2004). Oslo, Norway: National Institute for Alcohol and Drug Research.

Bretteville-Jensen A.L. (2006) Drug demand-initiation, continuation and quitting. *The Economist* **154**, 491–516.

Bretteville-Jensen A.L., Melberg H.O., and Jones A.M. (2008) Sequential patterns of drug use initiation: can we believe in the gateway theory? *The B.E: Journal of Economic Analysis and Policy* 8, article 1. Available at: http://www.bepress.com/bejeap/vol8/iss2/art1 (accessed 13 May 2009).

Brill H. and Hirose T. (1969) The rise and fall of a methamphetamine epidemic: Japan 1945–55. *Seminars in Psychiatry* **1**, 179–94.

Britten R.M. and Scott J. (2006) Community pharmacy services to drug misusers in the south west of England: results of the 2003–2004 postal survey. *International Journal of Pharmacy Practice* **14**, 235–41.

Brottsförebyggande rådet (2000) *The criminalisation of narcotic drug misuse—an evaluation of criminal justice system measures.* Stockholm, Sweden: BRÅ. Available at: http://www.bra.se/extra/faq/?action_question_show.228.0.=1&module_instance=2 (accessed 18 July 2007).

Brouwer K.C., Case P., Ramos R., Magis-Rodríguez C., Bucardo J., Patterson T.L., and Strathdee S.A. (2006) Trends in production, trafficking, and consumption of methamphetamine and cocaine in Mexico. *Substance Use and Misuse* **41**, 707–27.

Brown J.H. (2001) Youth, drugs and resilience education. *Journal of Drug Education* **31**, 83–122.

Brown M.H. (2005) Guns and drugs. *The Hartford Courant* **169**, 205, 24 July, pp. 1, 8.

Brown V. L. and Riley M.A. (2005) Social support, drug use, and employment among low-income women. *American Journal of Drug and Alcohol Abuse* **31**, 203–23.

Brownstein H.H., Baxi H.R.S., Goldstein P.J., and Ryan P.J. (1992) The relationship of drugs, drug trafficking, and drug traffickers to homicide. *Journal of Crime and Justice* **15**, 25–44.

Bruun K., Pan L., and Rexed I.(1975) *The gentlemen's club: international control of drugs and alcohol.* Chicago, IL: University of Chicago Press.

Buckmaster L. (2005) *Medication for attention deficit/hyperactivity disorder (ADHD): an analysis by federal electorate (200103).* Research Brief no. 2 200405. Canberra, Australia: Parliamentary Library. Available at: http://www.aph.gov.au/library/pubs/rb/2004-05/05rb02.htm (accessed 15 May 2009).

Buddenberg D. and Byrd W. (eds) (2006) *Afghanistan's drug industry: structure, functioning, dynamics and implications for counter-narcotics policy.* Vienna, Austria: UNODC and the World Bank. Available at: http://siteresources.worldbank.org/SOUTHASIAEXT/Resources/Publications/448813-1164651372704/UNDC.pdf (accessed 14 May 2009).

Budney A.J., Bickel W.K., and Amass L. (1998) Marijuana use and treatment outcome among opioid-dependent patients. *Addiction* **93**, 493–503.

Bureau of International Narcotics and Law Enforcement Affairs (2007) *International Narcotics Control Strategy Report, 2007.* Washington, DC: US State Department. Available at: http://www.state.gov/p/inl/rls/nrcrpt/2007/vol1/ (accessed 25 May 2009).

Burgess F. (2006) Pain treatment, drug diversion, and the casualties of war. *Pain Medicine* **7**, 474–5.

Burr A. (1983) The Piccadilly drug scene. *British Journal of Addiction* **78**, 5–19.

Burr A. (1984) The illicit non-pharmaceutical heroin market and drug scene in Kensington Market. *British Journal of Addiction* **79**, 337–343.

Bushway S., Caulkins J., and Reuter P. (2004) *Does state and local drug enforcement raise prices?.* Unpublished paper.

Busto U.E., Ruiz I., Busto M., and Gacitua A. (1996) Benzodiazepine use in Chile: impact of availability on use, abuse, and dependence. *Journal of Clinical Psychophramacology* **16**, 363–72.

Butzin C.A., Martin S.S., and Inciardi J.A. (2005) Treatment during transition from prison to community and subsequent illicit drug use. *Journal of Substance Abuse Treatment* **28**, 351–8.

Byrd W. and Ward C. (2004) *Drugs and development in Afghanistan.* Washington, DC: World Bank.

Caamaño F., Tomé-Otero M., and Takkouche B. (2006) Factors associated with the pharmacist counselling without dispensing. *Pharmacoepidemiology and Drug Safety* **15**, 428–31.

Cameron L. and Williams J. (2001) Cannabis, alcohol and cigarettes: substitutes or complements?. *Economic Record* **77**, 19–34.

Canty C., Sutton A., and James S. (2000) Models of community-based drug law enforcement. *Police Practice and Research* **2**, 171–87.

Carey B. (2007) Child studies may ease fears on misbehavior. *New York Times* 12 November. Available at: http://www.nytimes.com/2007/11/12/health/12cnd-kids.html (accessed 15 May 2009).

Carpenter T.G. (2005) *Mexico is becoming the next Colombia.* Cato Institute Foreign Policy Briefing No. 87. Available at: http://www.cato.org/pubs/fpbriefs/fpb87.pdf (accessed 31 July 2006).

Carstairs C. (2005) The stages of the international drug control system. *Drug and Alcohol Review* **24**, 57–65.

Carstairs C. (2006) *Jailed for possession: illegal drug use, regulation, and power in Canada, 1920–1961.* Toronto, Canada: University of Toronto Press.

Cartwright W.S. (2000) Cost–benefit analysis of drug treatment services: review of the literature. *Journal of Mental Health Policy and Economics* **3**, 11–26.

Catalano R.F., Gainey R.R., Fleming C.B., Haggerty K.P., and Johnson N.O. (1999) An experimental intervention with families of substance abusers: one year follow-up of the focus on families project. *Addiction* **94**, 241–54.

Caulkins J.P. (1990) *The distribution and consumption of illicit drugs: some mathematical models and their policy implications.* Doctoral dissertation. Cambridge, MA: Massachusetts Institute of Technology.

Caulkins J.P. (1994) *Developing price series for cocaine.* Santa Monica, CA: RAND.

Caulkins J.P. (1997) Modeling the domestic distribution network for illicit drugs. *Management Science* **43**, 1364–71.

Caulkins J.P. (1998) The cost-effectiveness of civil remedies: the case of drug control interventions. *Crime Prevention Studies* **9**, 219–37.

Caulkins J.P. (2002) *Law enforcement's role in a harm reduction regime.* Crime and Justice Bulletin Number 64. Sydney, Australia: New South Wales Bureau of Crime Statistics and Research.

Caulkins J.P. and Chandler S. (2006) Long-run trends in incarceration of drug offenders in the U.S. *Crime and Delinquency* **52**, 619–41.

Caulkins J.P. and MacCoun R. (2005) Analyzing illicit drug markets when dealers act with limited rationality. In: Parisi F. and Smith V.L. (eds) *The law and economics of irrational behavior.* pp. 315–338. Stanford, CA: Stanford University Press.

Caulkins J.P. and Pacula R. (2006) Marijuana markets: inferences from reports by the household population. *Journal of Drug Issues* **36**, 173–200.

Caulkins J.P. and Reuter P. (1998) What price data tell us about drug markets. *Journal of Drug Issues* **28**, 593–612.

Caulkins J.P. and Sevigny E. (2005) How many people does the US incarcerate for drug use, and who are they?. *Contemporary Drug Problems* **32**, 405–28.

Caulkins J.P., Larson R.C., and Rich T.F. (1993) Geography's impact on the success of focused local drug enforcement operations. *Socio-Economic Planning Sciences* **27**, 119–30.

Caulkins J.P., Rydell C.P., Schwabe W.L., and Chiesa J. (1997) *Mandatory minimum drug sentences: throwing away the key or the taxpayers' money?* MR-827-DPRC. Santa Monica, CA: RAND.

Caulkins J.P., Johnson B., Taylor A., and Taylor L. (1999) What drug dealers tell us about their costs of doing business. *Journal of Drug Issues* **29**, 323–40.

Caulkins J.P., with Chiesa J. and Everingham S.S. (2000) *Response to the National Research Council's assessment of RAND's controlling cocaine study*. Santa Monica, CA: RAND.

Caulkins J.P., Pacula R.L., Paddock S., and Chiesa J (2002) *School-based drug prevention: what kind of drug use does it prevent?*. Santa Monica, CA: RAND.

Caulkins J.P., Reuter P. and Taylor L. (2006) Can supply restrictions lower price? Violence, drug dealing and positional advantage. *Contributions to Economic Analysis and Policy* **5**, Issue 1, Article 3. Available at: http://www.bepress.com/bejeap/contributions/vol5/iss1/art3 (accessed 14 May 2009).

Centers for Disease Control and Prevention (2007) *Fact sheet: economic facts about U.S. tobacco use and tobacco production*. Available at: http://www.cdc.gov/tobacco/data_statistics/fact_sheets/economics/economic_facts.htm (accessed 14 May 2009).

Centralförbundet for alkohol-och narkotikaupplysning (2007) *Drogutvecklingen I Sverige 2007* (Drug trends in Sweden 2007). Stockholm, Sweden: CAN.

Ch'ien J.M.N. (1980) Hong Kong: a community-based voluntary program. In: Edwards G. and Arif A. (eds) *Drug problems in the sociocultural context: a basis for policies and programme planning*. pp. 114–20. Geneva, Switzerland: WHO.

Chabal C., Erjavec M.K., Jacobson L., Manario A., and Chaeny E. (1997) Prescription opiate abuse in chronic pain patients: clinical criteria, incidence, and predictors. *Clinical Journal of Pain* **13**, 150–5.

Chalmers T.C., Matta R.J., Smith H., Jr, and Kunzler A.-M. (1977) Evidence favouring the use of anticoagulants in the hospital phase of acute myocardial infarction. *New England Journal of Medicine* **297**, 1091–96.

Chaloupka F.J. and Laixuthai A. (1997) Do youths substitute alcohol and marijuana? Some econometric evidence. *Eastern Economic Journal* **23**, 253–76.

Chaloupka F.J., Grossman M., and Tauras J.A. (1999) The demand for cocaine and marijuana by youth. In: Chaloupka F.J., Grossman M., Bickel W.K., and Saffer H. (eds) *The economic analysis of substance use and abuse: an integration of economic and behavioral economic research*. pp. 133–56. Chicago, IL: University of Chicago Press.

Chassin L. and Ritter J. (2001) Vulnerability to substance use disorders in childhood and adolescence. In: Ingram R.E. and Price J.M. (eds) *Vulnerability to psychopathology: risk across the lifespan*. pp. 107–34. New York, NY: Guilford Press.

Chein I., Gerard D.L., Lee R.S., Rosenfeld E., and Wilner D.M. (1964) *The road to H: marcotics, delinquency, and social policy*. New York, NY: Basic Books.

Chermack S.T. and Blow F.C. (2002) Violence among individuals in substance abuse treatment: The role of alcohol and cocaine consumption. *Drug and Alcohol Dependence* **66**, 29–37.

Choudry N.K. and Avorn J. (2005) Over-the-counter statins. *Annals of Internal Medicine* **142**, 910–13.

Christie N. and Bruun K. (1969) Alcohol problems: the conceptual framework. In: Keller M. and Coffey T., eds. *Proceedings of the 28th International Congress on Alcohol and Alcoholism*, vol. 2. pp. 65–73. Highland Park, NJ: Hillhouse Press.

Christie N. and Bruun K. (1996) *Den gode fiende: narkotikapolitikk i Norden* (The good enemy: drug politics in the Nordic countries). 3rd edn. Oslo, Norway: Universitetsforlaget.

Christie P. and Ali R. (2000) Offences under the cannabis expiation notice scheme in South Australia. *Drug and Alcohol Review* **19**, 251–6.

Christo G. and Franey C. (1995) Drug users' spiritual beliefs, locus of control and the disease concept in relation to Narcotics Anonymous attendance and six-month outcomes. *Drug and Alcohol Dependence* **38**, 51–6.

Christo G. and Sutton S. (1994) Anxiety and self-esteem as a function of abstinence time among recovering addicts attending Narcotics Anonymous. *British Journal of Clinical Psychology* **33**, 198–200.

Cicero,T.J., Inciardi J.A., Adams E.H., Geller A., Senay E.C., Woody G.E., and Munoz A. (2005) Rates of abuse of tramadol remain unchanged with the introduction of new branded and generic products: results of an abuse monitoring system, 1994–2004. *Pharmacoepidemiology and Drug Safety* **14**, 851–9.

Clawson P. and Lee R. (1996) *The Andean cocaine industry*. New York, NY: St. Martin's Press.

Clements K.W. (2004) Three facts about marijuana prices. *Australian Journal of Agriculture and Resource Economics* **48**, 271–300.

CNN (2001) U.S. ranks international cooperation in drug war: Colombia, Mexico keep U.S. drug certification. *CNN.com/US*, 1 March. Available at: http://archives.cnn.com/2001/US/03/01/drug.assessment/index.html.

Collins D.J. and Lapsley H.M. (2002) *Counting the cost: estimates of the social costs of drug abuse in Australia 1998–99*. National Drug Strategy Monograph Series no. 49. Canberra, Australia: Commonwealth Department of Health and Ageing.

Compton W.M. and Volkow N.D. (2006) Major increases in opioid analgesic abuse in the United States: concerns and strategies. *Drug and Alcohol Dependence* **81**, 103–7.

Compton W.M., Stein J.B., Robertson E.B., Pintello D., Pringle B., and Volkow N.D. (2005a) Charting a course for health services research at the National Institute on Drug Abuse. *Journal of Substance Abuse Treatment* **29**, 167–72.

Compton W.M., Thomas Y.F., Conway K.P., and Colliver J.D. (2005b) Developments in the epidemiology of drug use and drug use disorders. *American Journal of Psychiatry* **162**, 1494–502.

Concato J., Shah N. and Horwitz R.I. (2000) Randomized, controlled trials, observational studies, and the hierarchy of research designs. *New England Journal of Medicine* **342**, 1887–92.

Connock M., Juarez-Garcia A., Jowett S., Frew E., Liu Z., Taylor R.J., Fry-Smith A., Day E., Lintzeris N., Roberts T., Burls A., and Taylor R.S. (2007) Methadone and buprenorphine for the management of opioid dependence: a systematic review and economic evaluation. *Health Technology Assessment* **11**, 1–190.

Conrad P. and Leiter V. (2008) From Lydia Pinkham to Queen Levitra: direct-to-consumer advertising and medicalisation. *Sociology of Health and Illness* **30**, 825–38.

Cook C. (2007) *Mexico's drug cartels.* Washington, DC: Congressional Research Service.

Cook P.J., Moore M.H., and Braga A. (2002) Gun control. In: Wilson J.Q. and Petersilla J. (eds) *Crime: public policies for crime control.* Oakland, CA: ICS Press.

Cook T.D., Shadish W.R., and Wong V.C. (2008) Three conditions under which experiments and observational studies produce comparable causal eximates: new findings from within-study comparisons. *Journal of Policy Analysis and Management* **27**, 724–50.

Coomber R. (1997) The adulteration of drugs: what dealers do, what dealers think. *Addiction Research* **5**, 297–306.

Coomber R. and Turnbull P. (2007) Arenas of drug transaction: adolescent cannabis transactions in England—social supply. *Journal of Drug Issues* **37**, 845–66.

Copeland J., Swift W., Roffman R., and Stephens R. (2001) A randomised controlled trial of brief interventions for cannabis use disorder. *Journal of Substance Abuse Treatment* **21**, 55–64.

Cormack M.A., Sweeney K.G., Hughes-Jones H., and Foot G.A. (1994) Evaluation of an easy, cost-effective strategy for cutting benzodiazepine use in general practice. *British Journal of General Practice* **44**, 5–8.

Corneil T., Kuyper L, Shoveller J., Hogg R., Li K., Spittal P., Schechter M., and Wood E. (2006) Unstable housing, associated risk behaviour, and increased risk for HIV infection among injection drug users. *Health & Place* **12**, 79–85.

Courtwright D.T. (1982) *Dark paradise: opiate addiction in America before 1940.* Cambridge MA: Harvard University Press.

Courtwright D.T. (2001) *Forces of habit: drugs and the making of the modern world.* Cambridge, MA: Harvard University Press.

Courtwright D.T. (2005) Mr. ATOD's wild ride: what do alcohol, tobacco, and other drugs have in common? *Social History of Alcohol and Other Drugs* **20**, 105–24.

Craib K., Spittal P., Wood E., Laliberte N., Hogg R., Li K., Heath K., Tyndall M., O' M., and Schechter, M. (2003) Risk factors for elevated HIV incidence among Aboriginal injection drug users in Vancouver. *Canadian Medical Association Journal* **168**, 19–24.

Crane B.D., Rivolo A.R., and Comfort G.C. (1997) *An empirical examination of counterdrug interdiction program effectiveness.* Alexandria, VA: Institute for Defense Analysis.

Crellin J.K. (2004) *A social history of medicines in the twentieth century: to be taken three times a day.* New York, NY: Pharmaceutical Products Press.

Crome I. and McArdle P. (2004) Prevention programmes. In: Crome I., Ghodse H., Gilvarry E., and McArdle P. (eds) *Young people and substance misuse,* pp. 15–30. London, UK: Gaskell.

Crothers T.D. (1902) *The drug habits and their treatment.* Chicago, IL: E.P. Englehard & Co.

Csémy L., Kubicka L., and Nociar A. (2002) Drug scene in the Czech Republic and Slovakia during the period of transformation. *European Addiction Research* **8**, 159–65.

Cuijpers P. (2003) Three decades of drug prevention research. *Drugs: Education, Prevention and Policy* **10**, 7–20.

Cunningham J.K. and Liu L.M. (2003) Impacts of federal ephedrine and pseudoephedrine regulations on methamphetamine related hospital admissions. *Addiction* **98,** 1229–37.

Cunningham J.K. and Liu L.M. (2005) Impacts of federal precursor chemical regulations on methamphetamine arrests. *Addiction* **100**, 479–88.

Currie J. (2005) *The marketization of depression: the prescribing of SSRI antidepressants to women*. Toronto, Ontario: Women and Health Protection. Available at: http://www.whp-apsf.ca/pdf/SSRIs.pdf (accessed 15 May 2009).

Curtis R. and Wendel T. (2007) You're always training the dog: strategic interventions to reconfigure drug markets. *Journal of Drug Issues* **37**, 867–92.

D'Amore J., Hung O., Chiang W., and Goldfrank L. (2001) The epidemiology of the homeless population and its impact on an urban emergency department. *Academic Emergency Medicine* **8**, 1051–5.

Darke S. and Hall W. (1997) The distribution of naloxone to heroin users. *Addiction* **92**, 1195–9.

Darke S. and Hall W. (2003) Heroin overdose: research and evidence-based intervention. *Journal of Urban Health* **80**, 189–200.

Darke S. and Ross J. (2001) The relationship between suicide and overdose among methadone maintenance patients in Sydney, Australia. *Addiction* **96**, 1443–53.

Darke S., Ross J., and Hall W. (1996) Overdose among heroin users in Sydney, Australia: I. Prevalence and correlates of non-fatal overdose. *Addiction* **91**, 405–11.

Darke S., Ross J., Zador D., and Sunjic S. (2000a) Heroin-related deaths in New South Wales, Australia, 1992–1996. *Drug and Alcohol Dependence* **60**, 141–50.

Darke S., Sims J., McDonald S., and Wickes W. (2000b) Cognitive impairment among methadone maintenance patients. *Addiction* **95**, 687–95.

Darke S., Ross J., Teesson M., and Lynskey M. (2003) Health service utilization and benzodiazepine use among heroin users: findings from the Australian Treatment Outcome Study (ATOS). *Addiction* **98**, 1129–35.

Darke S., Degenhardt L., and Mattik R. (2007) *Mortality amongst illicit drug users: epidemiology, causes and intervention*. Cambridge, UK: Cambridge University Press.

Dave D. (2006) The effects of cocaine and heroin price on drug-related emergency department visits. *Journal of Health Economics* **25**, 311–33.

Dave D. (2008) Illicit drug use among arrestees, prices and policy. *Journal of Urban Economics* **63**, 694–714.

Davies H.T.O., Crombie K., and Tavakoli M. (1998) When can odds ratios mislead?. *British Medical Journal* **316**, 989–91.

Davies R.B. (2005) *Mandatory minimum drug sentencing, drug purity, and a test of rational drug use*. Eugene, OR: University of Oregon Economics Department.

De Alarcon R. (1972) An epidemiological evaluation of a public health measure aimed at reducing the availability of methylamphetamine. *Psychological Medicine* **2**, 293–300.

Degenhardt L., Hall W., Warner-Smith M., and Lynskey M. (2004) Illicit drug use. In: Ezzati M., Lopez A.D., Rodgers A., and Murray C.J.L. (eds) *Comparative quantification of health risks. Global and regional burden of disease attributable to selected major risk factors*, pp. 1109–75. Geneva: World Health Organization.

Degenhardt L., Day C., Dietze P., Pointer S., Conroy E., Collins L., and Hall W. (2005a) Effects of a sustained heroin shortage in three Australian states. *Addiction* **100**, 908–20.

Degenhardt L., Reuter P., Collins L., and Hall W. (2005b) Evaluating explanations of the Australian 'heroin shortage'. *Addiction* **100**, 459–69.

Degenhardt L., Roxburgh A., van Beek I., Hall W.D., Robinson M.K.F., Ross J., and Mant A. (2008) The effects of the market withdrawal of temazapam gel capsules on benzodiazepine injecting in Sydney, Australia. *Drug and Alcohol Review* **27**, 145–51.

de Jong F.A., Engels F.K., Mathijssen R.H.J., van Zuylen L., and Verweij J. (2005) Medicinal cannabis in oncology practice: still a bridge too far?. *Journal of Clinical Oncology* **13**, 2886–91.

DeSimone J. (1998) *The relationship between marijuana prices at different market levels.* Working paper number 9915. Greenville, NC: Department of Economics, East Carolina University. Available at: http://www.ecu.edu/econ/wp/99/ecu9915.pdf.

DeSimone J. (2002) Illegal drug use and employment. *Journal of Labour Economics* **20**, 952–9.

DeSimone J. (2006) The relationship between illegal drug prices at different market levels. *Contemporary Economic Policy* **24**, 64–73.

DeSimone J. and Farrelly M.C. (2003) Price and enforcement effects on cocaine and marijuana demand. *Economic Inquiry* **41**, 98–115.

Des Jarlais D.C., Perlis T., Arasteh K., Torian L.V., Beatrice S., Milliken J., Mildvan D., Yancovitz S., and Friedman S.R. (2005) HIV incidence among injection drug users in New York City, 1990 to 2002: use of serologic test algorithm to assess expansion of HIV prevention services. *American Journal of Public Health* **95**, 1439–44.

De Wilde S., Carey I.M., Harris T., Richards N., Victor C., Hilton S.R., and Cook D.G. (2007) Trends in potentially inappropriate prescribing amongst older UK primary care patients. *Pharmacoepidemiology and Drug Safety* **16**, 658–67.

Diaz L. (2008) Mexico's death industry thrives on drug war killings. *Washington Post* 1 November. Available at: http://www.reuters.com/article/topNews/idUSTRE4A01QZ20081101 (accessed 2 June 2009).

Dijkgraaf M.G.W., van der Zanden B.P., de Borgie C.A.J.M., Blanken P., van Ree J.M., and van der Brink W. (2005) Cost utility analysis of co-prescribed heroin compared with methadone maintenance treatment in heroin addiction in two randomised trials. *British Medical Journal* **330**, 1297–303.

DiNardo J. (1993) Law enforcement, the price of cocaine, and cocaine use. *Mathematical and Computer Modeling* **17**, 53–64.

Disney E.R., Elkins I.J., McGue M., and Iacono W.G. (1999) Effects of ADHD, conduct disorder, and gender on substance use and abuse in adolescence. *American Journal of Psychiatry* **156**, 1515–21.

Dobkin C. and Nicosia N. (2005) *The war on drugs: methamphetamine, public health, and crime.* Working Paper. Santa Cruz, CA: University of California, Santa Cruz. Available at http://people.ucsc.edu/ cdobkin/Papers/Methamphetamine.pdf (accessed 19 May 2009).

Dodd E. (1993) OSTAR—Oklahoma Schedule II Abuse Reduction: an electronic point of sale diversion control system. In: Cooper J.R., Czecowicz D.J., Molinari S.P., and Petersen R.C. (eds) *Impact of prescription drug diversion control systems on medical practice and patient care*, pp. 151–8. NIDA Research Monograph 131. Rockville, MD: National Institute on Drug Abuse.

Dolan K., Rouen D., and Kimber J. (2004) An overview of the use of urine, hair, sweat and saliva to detect drug use. *Drug and Alcohol Review* **23**, 213–17.

Donnelly J. (1992) The United Nations and the global drug control regime. In: Smith P.H. (ed.) *Drug policy in the Americas.* pp. 282–304. Boulder, CO: Westview Press.

Donnelly N., Oldenburg B., Quine S., Macaskill P., Flaherty B., Spooner C., and Lyle D. (1992) Changes reported in drug prevalence among New South Wales secondary school students 1983–1989. *Australian Journal of Public Health* **16**, 50–57.

Donnelly N., Hall W., and Christie P. (1999) *The effects of the CEN scheme on levels and patterns of cannabis use in South Australia: evidence from national drug strategy household* *surveys 1985–1995*. Canberra, Australia: Commonwealth Department of Health and Family Services.

Donnelly N., Hall W., and Christie P. (2000) The effects of the Cannabis Expiation Notice scheme on levels and patterns of cannabis use in South Australia: evidence from national drug strategy household surveys 1985–95. *Drug and Alcohol Review* **19**, 265–9.

Dormitzer C.M., Gonzales G.B., Penna M., Bejerano J., Obando P., Sanchez M., Vittetoe K., Gutierrez U., Alfaro J., Meneses G., Diaz J.B., Herrera M., Hasbun J., Chisman A., Caris L., Chen C.-Y., and Anthony J.C. (2004) The PACARDO research project: youthful drug involvement in Central America and the Dominican Republic. *PanAmerican Journal of Public Health* **15**, 402–15.

Draguns J.G. (2004) From speculation through description toward investigation: a prospective glimpse at cultural research in psychotherapy. In: Gielen U.P., Fish J.M., and Draguns J.G. (eds) *Handbook of culture, therapy and healing*, pp. 369–87. Mahwah, NJ: Lawrence Erlbaum.

Drake J., Freedman P.S., Hawkins B.C., Horth C.E., Launchbury A.P., and Whateley-Smith C. (1991) Comparative pharmacokinetics of temazepam gelthix and liquid-filled soft gelatin capsules. *Journal of Clinical Pharmacy and Therapeutics* **16**, 345–51.

Dries-Daffner I., Landau S.C., Maderas N.M., and Taylor-McGhee B. (2007) Access to plan B emergency contraception in an OTC environment. *Journal of Nursing Law* **11**, 93–100.

Drummer O.H. (2005) Recent trends in narcotic deaths. *Therapeutic Drug Monitoring* **27**, 738–40.

Drummer O. H., Gerostamoulos J., Batziris H., Chu M., Caplehorn J., Robertson M.D., and Swann P. (2004) The involvement of drugs in drivers of motor vehicles killed in Australian road traffic crashes. *Accident Analysis and Prevention* **36**, 239–48.

Dusenbury L., Brannigan R., Falco M., and Hansen W. (2003) A review of research on fidelity of implementation: implications for drug abuse prevention in school settings. *Health Education Research* **18**, 237–56.

Dyer O. (2004) Seven doctors accused of over-prescribing heroin. *British Medical Journal* **328**, 483.

Eadie J.L. (1993) New York State's triplicate prescription program. In: Cooper J.R., Czecowicz D.J., Molinari S.P., and Petersen R.C. (eds) *Impact of prescription drug diversion control systems on medical practice and patient care*, pp. 176–93. NIDA Research Monograph 131. Rockville, MD: National Institute on Drug Abuse.

Edlund M.J., Sullivan M., Steffick D., Harris K.M., and Wells K.B. (2007) Do users of regularly prescribed opioids have higher rates of substance use problems than nonusers?. *Pain Medicine* **8**, 647–56.

Edmunds M., Hough M., and Urqufa N. (1996) *Tackling local drug markets*. Crime Detection and Prevention Series Paper 80. London, UK: Home Office Police Research Group.

Edwards G. (2004) *Matters of substance: drugs—and why everyone's a user*. New York, NY: St Martin's Press.

Edwards G (2005) *Matters of substance—drugs: is legalization the right answer—or the wrong question?*. London, UK: Penguin Books.

Edwards G. (ed.) (2002) *Addiction: evolution of a specialist field*. Oxford: Blackwell Publishing.

Edwards G., Arif A., and Hodgson, R. (1981) Nomenclature and classification of drug- and alcohol- related problems: a WHO memorandum. *Bulletin of the World Health Organization* **59**, 225–42.

Ekeberg O., Jacobsen D., Flaaten B., and Mack A. (1987) Effect of regulatory withdrawal of drugs and prescription recommendations on the pattern of self-poisonings in Oslo. *Acta Medica Scandinavica* **221**, 483–7.

Elekes Z. and Kovács L. (2002) Old and new drug consumption habits in Hungary, Romania and Moldova. *European Addiction Research* **8**, 166–9.

Ellickson P.L., Bell R.M., and Harrison E.R. (1993) Changing adolescent propensities to use drugs: results from Project ALERT. *Health Education Quarterly* **20**, 227–42.

Ellickson P.L., McCaffrey D.F., Ghosh-Dastidar B., and Longshore D.L. (2003) New inroads in preventing adolescent drug use: results from a large-scale trial of Project ALERT in middle schools. *American Journal of Public Health* **93**, 1830–6.

Emafo P. (2002) [Statement as president of the INCB to the 2002 substantive session of ECOSOC]. 24 July. Available at: http://www.incb.org/incb/en/speeches/ecosoc_02.html (accessed 25 May 2009).

EMCDDA. See European Monitoring Centre for Drugs and Drug Addiction.

Emmanuelli J. and Desenclos J-C. (2005) Harm reduction interventions, behaviors and associated health outcomes in France, 1996–2003. *Addiction* **100**, 1690–700.

English D.R., Knuiman M.W., Kurinczuk J.J., Lewin G.F., Ryan G.A., Holman C.D.J., Milne E., Winter M.G., Hulse G.K., Codde J.P., Bower C.I., Corti B., and De Klerk N. (1995) *The quantification of drug-caused morbidity and mortality in Australia 1995.* Canberra, Australia: Commonwealth Department of Human Services and Health.

Ennett S.T., Tobler N.S., Ringwalt C.L., and Flewelling R.L. (1994) How effective is drug abuse resistance education? A meta-analysis of Project DARE outcome evaluations. *American Journal of Public Health* **84**, 1394–401.

Erickson P.G. (1980) *Cannabis criminals: the social effects of punishment on drug users.* Toronto, Canada: Addiction Research Foundation.

Etheridge R.M., Craddock S.G., Hubbard R.L., and Rounds-Bryant J.L. (1999) The relationship of counseling and self-help participation to patient outcomes in DATOS. *Drug and Alcohol Dependence* **57**, 99–112.

European Monitoring Centre for Drugs and Drug Addiction (2003a) *Annual report: state of the drugs problem in the European Union and Norway.* Lisbon, Portugal: EMCDDA.

European Monitoring Centre for Drugs and Drug Addiction (2003b) *Drugs in focus: bimonthly briefing of the European Monitoring Centre for Drugs and Drug Addiction.* Lisbon, Portugal: EMCDDA.

European Monitoring Centre for Drugs and Drug Addiction (2003c) *The role of the quantity in the prosecution of drug offences.* ELDD Comparative Study. Available at: http://eldd.emcdda.europa.eu/index.cfm?fuseaction=public.Content&nnodeid=5175&sLanguageiso=EN (accessed 18 July 2007).

European Monitoring Centre for Drugs and Drug Addiction (2004) *2004 annual report: the state of the drugs problem in the European Union and Norway.* Lisbon, Portugal: EMCDDA. Available at: http://www.emcdda.europa.eu/publications/annual-report/2004 (accessed 13 May 2009).

European Monitoring Centre for Drugs and Drug Addiction (2005) *2005 annual report: the state of the drugs problem in Europe.* Lisbon, Portugal: EMCDDA. Available at: http://www.emcdda.europa.eu/publications/annual-report/2005 (accessed 13 May 2009).

European Monitoring Centre for Drugs and Drug Addiction (2006) *Annual report 2006: the state of the drugs problem in Europe.* Lisbon, Portugal: EMCDDA. Available at: http://www.emcdda.europa.eu/publications/annual-report/2006 (accessed 3 June 2009).

European Monitoring Centre for Drugs and Drug Addiction (2007) *2007 annual report: The state of the drugs problem in Europe.* Lisbon, Portugal: EMCDDA. Available at: http://www.emcdda.europa.eu/publications/annual-report/2007 (accessed 13 May 2009).

European Monitoring Centre for Drugs and Drug Addiction (2008) *Statistical bulletin 2008.* Lisbon, Portugal: EMCDDA. Available at: http://www.emcdda.europa.eu/stats08 (accessed 16 May 2009).

European Public Health Association (2004) *Direct-to-consumer advertising—for or against?* Update 61, 2 December. Available at: http://www.epha.org/a/533 (accessed 15 May 2009).

European Sourcebook on Crime and Criminal Justice (2003) 2nd edn. Meppel, The Netherlands: Boom Distribution Centre.

Evans-Whipp T., Beyers J.M., Lloyd S., Lafazia A.N., Toumbourou J.W., Arthur M.W., and Catalano R.F. (2004) A review of school drug policies and their impact on youth substance use. *Health Promotion International* **19**, 227–34.

Everingham S.S. and Rydell C.P. (1994) *Modeling the demand for cocaine.* RAND Drug Policy Research Center, MR-332-ONDCP/A/DPRC.

Ezzati M., Lopez A.D., Rodgers A., Murray C.J.L. (eds) (2004) *Comparative quantification of health risks: global and regional burden of disease attributable to selected major risk factors.* Geneva: World Health Organization.

Faggiano F., Vigna-Taglianti F.D., Versino E., Zambon A., Borraccino A., and Lemma P. (2005) School-based prevention for illicit drugs' use. *The Cochrane Database of Systematic Reviews.* Issue 2, article number CD003020. DOI: 10.1002/14651858.CD003020.pub2.

Fahey D.M. and Manian P. (2005) Poverty and purification: the politics of Gandhi's campaign for prohibition. *Historian* **67**, 489–506.

Falck R., Wang J., Carlson R., Eddy M., and Siegal H. (2002) The prevalence and correlates of depressive symptomatology among a community sample of crack-cocaine smokers. *Journal of Psychoactive Drugs* **34**, 281–8.

Falck R., Wang J., Siegal H., and Carlson R. (2004) The prevalence of psychiatric disorder among a community sample of crack cocaine users: an exploratory study with practical implications. *Journal of Nervous and Mental Disease* **192**, 503–7.

Families and Friends for Drug Law Reform (FFDLR) (2004) *Crime and illicit drugs: an information paper.* ISSN 1444-200. Australia: FFDLR. Available at: http://www.goldweb.com.au/ mcconnell/resources/Crime%20and%20Illicit%20drugs.htm#Ref%201.

Farnam R. (2005) Substance abuse in Iran: a brief overview. Presented in Istanbul at the International Conference on Delivery Systems for Substance Abuse Treatment. Available at: http://www.uclaisap.org/dssat2005/html/presentations.html (accessed 30 May 2009).

Farrell M., Ward J., Mattick W., Stimson G.V., des Jarlais D., Gossop M., and Strang J. (1994) Methadone maintenance treatment in opiate dependence: a review. *British Medical Journal* **309**, 997–1001.

Farrelly M., Bary J., Zarkin G., and Wendling B. (2001) The joint demand for cigarettes and marijuana: evidence from the National Household Survey on Drug Abuse. *Journal of Health Economics* **20**, 51–68.

Fass P. (1977) *The damned and the beautiful: American youth in the 1920s.* New York, NY: Oxford University Press.

Fawthrop T. (2005) Lao tribes suffer from drug crackdown. BBC News, 15 July. Available at http://news.bbc.co.uk/go/pr/fr/-/1/hi/world/asia-pacific/4673109.stm (accessed 9 May 2009).

Federal Bureau of Investigation (1999) *Uniform crime reports.* Washington DC: FBI. Available at: http://www.fbi.gov/ucr/ucr.htm (accessed 19 May 2009).

Fergusson D.M., Boden J.M., and Horwood L.J. (2006) Cannabis use and other illicit drug use: testing the cannabis gateway hypothesis. *Addiction* **101**, 556–69.

Ferri M.M.F., Davoli M., and Perucci C.A.A. (2005) Heroin maintenance for chronic heroin dependents. *Cochrane Database of Systematic Reviews*, issue 2, article number CD003410. DOI: 10.1002/14651858.CD003410.pub2.

Feucht T. and Keyser A. (1999) Reducing drug use in prisons: Pennsylvania's approach. *National Institute of Justice Journal* **241**, 10–15.

Fiellin D.A., O'Connor P.G., Chawarski M., Pakes J.P., Pantalon M.V., and Schottenfeld R.S. (2001) Methadone maintenance in primary care: a randomised controlled trial. *Journal of the American Medical Association* **286**, 1764–5.

Filion K.B., Delaney J.A.C., Brophy J.A., Ernst P., and Suissa S. (2007) The impact of over-the-counter simvastatin on the number of statin prescription in the United Kingdom: a view from the General Practice Research Database. *Pharmacoepidemiology and Drug Safety* **16**, 1–4.

Fiorentine R. (1999) After drug treatment: are 12-step programs effective in maintaining abstinence?. *American Journal of Drug and Alcohol Abuse* **25**, 93–116.

Fischer B. and Rehm J. (2007) Illicit opioid use in the 21st century: witnessing a paradigm shift?. *Addiction* **102**, 499–501.

Fischer B., Kendall P., Rehm J. and Room R. (1997) Charting WHO—goals for licit and illicit drugs for the year 2000: are we 'on track'?. *Public Health* **111**, 271–5.

Fischer B., Medved W., Gliksman L., Rehm J. (1999) Illicit opiates in Toronto: a profile of current users. *Addiction Research* **7**, 377–415.

Fischer B., Rehm J., and Blitz-Miller T. (2000) Injection drug use and preventive measures: a comparison of Canadian and Western European jurisdictions over time. *Canadian Medical Association Journal* **162**, 1709–13.

Fischer B., Haydon E., Rehm J., Krajden M., and Reimer J. (2004) Injection drug use and the hepatitis C virus: considerations for a targeted treatment approach—the case study of Canada. *Journal of Urban Health* **81**, 428–47.

Fischer B., Rehm J., Brissette S., Brochu S., Bruneau J., El-Guebaly N., Noël L., Tyndall M., Wild C., Mun P., and Baliunas D. (2005) Illicit opioid use in Canada: comparing social, health and drug use characteristics of untreated users in five cities (OPICAN Study). *Journal of Urban Health* **82**, 250–66.

Fischer B., Rehm J., Patra J. and Firestone Cruz M. (2006) Changes in illicit opioid use profiles across Canada. *Canadian Medical Association Journal* 175, 1385–7.

Fischer B., Oviedo-Joekes E., Blanken P., Haasen C., Rehm J., Schechter M.T., Strang J., and van den Brink W. (2007) Heroin-assisted treatment (HAT) a decade later: a brief update on science and politics. *Journal of Urban Health* **84**, 552–62.

Fischer B., Patra J., Firestone Cruz M., Gittins J., and Rehm J. (2008) Comparing heroin users and prescription opioid users in a Canadian multi-site population of illicit opioid users. *Drug and Alcohol Review* **27**, 625–32.

Fishman S.M., Papazian J.S., Gonzalez S., Riches P.S., and Gilson A. (2004) Regulating opioid prescribing through prescription monitoring programs: balancing drug diversion and treatment of pain. *Pain Medicine* **5**, 309–24.

Flaker V. (2002) Heroin use in Slovenia: a consequence or a vehicle of social changes. *European Addiction Research* **8**, 170–6.

Flay B.R., Graumlich S., Segawa E., Burns J.L., and Holliday M.Y., for the Aban Aya Investigators. (2004) Effects of two prevention programs on high-risk behaviors among African-American youth a randomized trial. *Archives of Pediatrics and Adolescent Medicine* **158**, 377–84.

Flynn P.M., Joe G.W., Broome K.M., Simpson D.D., and Brown B.S. (2003) Recovery from opioid addiction in DATOS. *Journal of Substance Abuse and Treatment* **25**, 177–86.

Food and Drug Administration (2006) *Legal requirements for the sale and purchase of drug products containing pseudoephedrine, ephedrine and phenylpropanolamine.* Silver Spring, MD: Center for Drug Evaluation and Research, US Food and Drug Administration. Available at: http://www.fda.gov/cder/news/methamphetamine.htm (accessed 20 May 2009).

Ford J.M. and Beveridge A.A. (2004) 'Bad' neighborhoods, fast food, 'sleazy' businesses, and drug dealers: relations between the location of licit and illicit businesses in the urban environment. *Journal of Drug Issues* **34**, 51–76.

Forman R.F. (2006) Narcotics on the net: the availability of websites selling controlled substances. *Psychiatric Services* **57**, 24–6.

Forster L.M., Tannhauser M., and Barros H.M. (1996) Drug use among street children in southern Brazil. *Drug and Alcohol Dependence* **43**, 57–62.

Forsyth A.J. and Barnard M. (1999) Contrasting levels of adolescent drug use between adjacent urban and rural communities in Scotland. *Addiction* **94**, 1707–18.

Fos P.J. and Fine D.J. (2000) *Designing health care for populations.* San Francisco, California: Jossey-Bass.

Fountain J., Griffiths P., Farrell M., Gossop M., and Strang J. (1999) Benzodiazepines in polydrug-using repertoires: the impact of the decreased availability of temazepam gel-filled capsules. *Drugs: Education, Prevention and Policy* **6**, 61–9.

Fountain J., Strang J., Gossop M., Farrell M., and Griffiths R. (2000) Diversion of prescription drugs by drug users in treatment: analysis of the UK market and new data from London. *Addiction* **95**, 393–406.

Foxcroft D.R., Lister-Sharp D.J., and Lowe G. (1997) Alcohol misuse prevention for young people: a systematic review reveals methodological concerns and lack of reliable evidence of effectiveness. *Addiction* **92**, 531–7.

Foxcroft D.R., Ireland D., Lister-Sharp D.J., Lowe G., and Breen R. (2003) Longer-term primary prevention for alcohol misuse in young people: a systematic review. *Addiction*, **98**, 397–411.

Freeman L. (2006) *State of siege: drug related violence and corruption in Mexico.* Washington, DC: Washington Office on Latin America. Available at: http://www.wola.org/media/publications/english/mexico/mexico_state_of_siege_06.06.pdf (accessed 17 July 2007).

Frei A. and Rehm J. (2002) Die Prävalenz psychischer Komorbidität unter Opiatabhängigen: eine Metaanalyse bisheriger Studien (The prevalence of psychiatric co-morbidity among opioid-dependent patients: a meta-analysis of studies). *Psychiatrische Praxis* **29**, 258–62.

Frei A., Greiner R.A., Mehnert A., and Dinkel R. (2000) Socioeconomic evaluation of heroin maintenance treatment: final report. In: Gutzwiller F. and Steffen T. (eds) *Cost-benefit analysis of heroin maintenance treatment. Medical prescription of narcotics,* vol 2. pp. 37–130. Basel: Karger Verlag.

French M.T., Roebuck M.C., and Kébreau Alexandre P. (2004) To test or not to test: do workplace drug testing programs discourage employee drug use?. *Social Science Research* **33**, 45–63.

Friedman S.R., Cooper H.L.F., Tempalski B., Keem M., Friedman R., Flom P.L., and DesJarlais D.C. (2006) Relationships of deterrence and law enforcement to drug-related harms among drug injectors in US metropolitan areas. *AIDS* **26**, 93–9.

Fudula P.J., Yu E., Macfadden W., Boardman C., and Chiang B.N. (1998) Effects of burprenorphine and naloxone on morphine-stabilized opioid addicts. *Drug and Alcohol Dependence* **50**, 1–8.

Fuentes J.R. (1998) *Life of a cell: managerial practice and strategy in Colombian cocaine distribution in the United States.* PhD dissertation. New York, NY: City University of New York.

Fung M., Thornton A., Mybeck K., Wu J.H.-H., Hornbuckle K., and Muniz E. (2001) Evaluation of the characteristics of safety withdrawals from worldwide pharmaceutical markets—1960 to 1999. *Drug Information Journal* **35**, 293–317.

Furr-Holden C.D.M., Ialongo N.S., Anthony J.C., Petras H., and Kellam S.G. (2004) Developmentally-inspired drug prevention middle school outcomes in a school-based randomized prevention trial. *Drug and Alcohol Dependence* **73**, 149–58.

Gable R.S. (2004) Comparison of acute lethal toxicity of commonly abused psychoactive substances. *Addiction* **99**, 686–96.

Galea S. and Vlahov D. (2002) Social determinants and the health of drug users: Socioeconomic status, homelessness, and incarceration. *Public Health Reports* **117** (Suppl. 1), S135–45.

Galea S., Ahern J., Tardiff K., Leon A., and Vlahov D. (2002) Drugs and firearm deaths in New York city, 1990–1998. *Journal of Urban Health* **79**, 70–86.

Gamarra E. (2002) *Has Bolivia won the war?: lessons from plan dignidad.* LACC Working Paper No. 3. (draft). Miami, FL: Latin American and Caribbean Center, Florida International University (draft). Available at: http://lacc.fiu.edu/research_publications/working_papers/WPS_003.pdf (accessed 19 May 2009).

Gates S., McCambridge J., Smith L.A., and Foxcroft D.R. (2006) Interventions for prevention of drug use by young people delivered in non-school settings. *Cochrane Database of Systematic Reviews.* Issue 1, article number CD005030. DOI: 10.1002/14651858.CD005030.pub2.

Gelber S. and Rinaldo D.W. (2005) *State substance abuse agencies and their placement within government: impact on organizational performance and collaboration in 12 states.* Final report to the Substance Abuse and Mental Health Services Administration. Berkeley, CA: The Avisa Group.

Gerritsen J.-W. (2000) *The control of fuddle and flash: a sociological history of the regulation of alcohol and opiates.* Leiden, The Netherlands: Brill.

Gerstein D.R. and Green L.W. (1993) *Preventing drug abuse: what do we know?.* Washington, DC: National Academy Press.

Gholami K., Shalviri G., Zarbakhsh A., Daryabari N., and Yousefian S. (2007) New guideline for tramadol usage following adverse drug reactions reported to the Iranian pharmacovigilance center. *Pharmacoepidemiology and Drug Safety* **16**, 229–37.

Godfrey C., Eaton G., McDougall C., and Culyer A. (2002) *The economic and social costs of class A drug use in England and Wales, 2000.* Home Office Research Study 249. London, UK: Home Office Research, Development and Statistics Directorate.

Godfrey C., Stewart D., and Gossop M. (2004) Economic analysis of costs and consequences of the treatment of drug misuse: 2-year outcome data from the National Treatment Outcome Research Study (NTORS). *Addiction* **99**, 697–707.

Godshaw G., Koppel R., and Pancoast R. (1987) *Anti-drug law enforcement efforts and their impact.* Bala Cynwyd, PA: Wharton Econometric Forecasting Associates.

Goldman B. (1998) The news on the street: prescription drugs on the black market. *Canadian Medical Association Journal* **159**, 149–50.

Goldstein P.J. (1985) The drugs/violence nexus: a tripartite conceptual framework. *Journal of Drug Issues* **15**, 493–506.

Goldstein P.J. (1999) Drug abuse and violence. In: *Proceedings of the inaugural symposium on crime and punishment in the United States*, pp. 87–98. Washington, DC: United States Sentencing Commission.

Goldstein, P.J., Lipton D.S., Preble E., Sobel I., Miller T., Abbott W., Paige W., and Soto F. (1984) The marketing of street heroin in New York City. *Journal of Drug Issues* **14**, 553–66.

Golub A.L. and Johnson B.D. (1999) Cohort changes in illegal drug use among arrestees in Manhattan: From the heroin injection generation to the blunts generation. *Substance Use and Misuse* **34**, 1733–63.

Golub A.L. and Johnson B.D. (2001) Variation in youthful risks of progression from alcohol and tobacco to marijuana and to hard drugs across generations. *American Journal of Public Health* **91**, 225–32.

Golub A.L. and Johnson B.D. (2005) The new heroin users among Manhattan arrestees: Variations by race/ethnicity and mode of consumption. *Journal of Psychoactive Drugs* **37**, 51–61.

Goode E. and Ben-Yehuda N. (1994) Moral panics: culture, politics, and social construction. *Annual Review of Sociology* **20**, 149–71.

Goodhand J. (2005) Frontiers and wars: the opium economy in Afghanistan. *Journal of Agrarian Change* **5**, 191–216.

Gorman D.M. (2002) The 'science' of drug and alcohol prevention: the case of the randomized trial of the Life Skills Training (LST) Program. *International Journal of Drug Policy* **13**, 21–6.

Gossop M. (1995) The treatment mapping survey: a descriptive study of drug and alcohol treatment responses in 23 countries. *Drug and Alcohol Dependence* **39**, 7–14.

Gossop M., Marsden J. and Stewart D. (1998) *NTORS at one year: the National Treatment Outcome Research Study—changes in substance use, health and criminal behaviours one year after intake.* London: UK Department of Health.

Gossop M., Marsden J., Stewart D., Lehmann P., and Strang J. (1999) Methadone treatment practices and outcome for opiate addicts treated in drug clinics and in general practice: results from the National Treatment Outcome Research Study. *British Journal of General Practitioners* **49**, 31–4.

Gossop M., Marsden J., Stewart D., and Treacy S. (2000) Routes of drug administration and multiple drug misuse: regional variations among clients seeking treatment at programmes throughout England. *Addiction* **95**, 1197–206.

Gossop M., Marsden J., and Stewart D. (2001) *NTORS after five years: changes in substance use, health and criminal behaviour during the five years after intake.* London, UK: National Addiction Centre.

Gossop M., Marsden J., Stewart D., and Kidd T. (2003) The National Treatment Outcome Research Study (NTORS): 4–5 year follow-up results. *Addiction* **98**, 291–303.

Gottfredson D.C., Najaka S.S., and Kearly B. (2003) Effectiveness of drug treatment courts: evidence from a randomized trial. *Criminology and Public Policy* **2**, 171–96.

Gotzsche P.C. and Olsen O. (2000) Is screening for breast cancer with mammography justifiable?. *Lancet* **355**, 129–34.

Gourlay D.L., Heit H.A., and Almahrez A. (2005) Universal precautions in pain medicine: a rational approach to the treatment of chronic pain. *Pain Medicine* **6**, 107–12.

Gramlich E. (1990) *A guide to cost-benefit analysis.* Englewood Cliffs, NJ: Prentice Hall.

Green P. and Purnell I. (1996) *Measuring the success of law enforcement agencies in Australia in targeting major drug offenders relative to minor drug offenders.* Report Series No. 127. Payneham, Australia: National Police Research Unit.

Greene S.L., Dargan P.I., Leman P., and Janes A.L. (2006) Paracetamol availability and recent changes in paracetamol poisoning: is the 1998 legislation limiting availability of paracetamol being followed?. *Postgraduate Medical Journal* **82**, 520–3.

Greenwald G. (2009) *Drug decriminalization in Portugal: lessons for fair and successful drug policies*, Washington, DC: Cato Institute.

Grogger J. and Willis M. (2000) The emergence of crack cocaine and the rise in urban crime rates. *Review of Economics and Statistics* **82**, S19–29.

Groseclose S.L., Weinstein B., Jones T.S., Valleroy L.A., Fehrs L.J., and Kassler W.J. (1995) Impact of increased legal access to needles and syringes on practices of injecting-drug users and police officer, Connecticut, 1992–1993. *Journal of Acquired Immune Deficiency Syndrome and Human Retrovirology* **10**, 82–9.

Grossman M. (2004) *Individual behaviors and substance abuse: the role of price.* NBER Working Paper No. 10948. Cambridge, MA: National Bureau of Economic Research.

Grossman M. (2005) Individual behaviors and substance use: the role of price. In: Lindgren B. and Grossman M. (eds) *Substance use: individual behaviors, social interactions, markets and politics*, pp. 15–40. Amsterdam, The Netherlands: Elsevier.

Grossman M. and Chaloupka F.J. (1998) The demand for cocaine by young adults: a rational addiction approach. *Journal of Health Economics* **17**, 427–74.

Gunne L-M. and Grönbladh L. (1981) The Swedish methadone maintenance program: a controlled study. *Drug and Alcohol Dependence* **7**, 249–56.

Haasen C., Verthein U., Degkwitz P., Berger J., Krausz M., and Naber D. (2007) Heroin-assisted treatment for opioid dependence. *British Journal of Psychiatry* **191**, 55–62.

Hafeiz H.B. (1995) Socio-demographic correlates and pattern of drug abuse in eastern Saudi Arabia. *Drug and Alcohol Dependence* **38**, 255–9.

Hagan H., Thiede H., Weiss N.S., Hopkins S.G., Duchin J.S., and Alexander E.R. (2001) Sharing of drug preparation equipment as a risk factor for hepatitis C. *American Journal of Public Health* **91**, 42–6.

Hagan H., Thiede H., and Des J. (2004) Hepatitis C virus infection among injection drug users: Survival analysis of time to seroconversion. *Epidemiology* **15**, 543–9.

Hall W.D. (2007) What's in a name?. *Addiction* **102**, 692.

Hall W.D. and Lynskey M. (2005) Is cannabis a gateway drug? Testing hypotheses about the relationship between cannabis use and the use of other illicit drugs. *Drug and Alcohol Review* **24**, 39–48.

Hall W.D, and Pacula R.L. (2003) *Cannabis use and dependence: public health and public policy.* Cambridge, UK: Cambridge University Press.

Hall W.D., Room R., and Bondy S. (1999) Comparing the health and psychological risks of alcohol, cannabis, nicotine and opiate use. In: Kalant H., Corrigal W., Hall W., and Smart R. (eds) *The health effects of cannabis*, pp. 477–508. Toronto, Canada: Addiction Research Foundation.

Hall W.D., Lynskey M., and Degenhardt L. (2000a) Trends in opiate-related deaths in the United Kingdom and Australia, 1985–1995. *Drug and Alcohol Dependence* **57**, 247–54.

Hall W.D., Ross J., Lynskey M., Law M., and Degenhardt L. (2000b) *How many dependent opioid users are there in Australia?* NDARC monograph no. 44. Sydney, Australia: National Drug and Alcohol Research Centre.

Hall W.D., Ross J.E., Lynskey M.T., and Degenhardt L.J. (2000c) How many dependent heroin users are there in Australia?. *Medical Journal of Australia* **173**, 528–31.

Hall W.D., Degenhardt L., and Lynskey M. (2001) *The health and psychological effects of cannabis use.* Monograph Series No. 44. Canberra: Commonwealth Department of Health and Ageing.

Hallfors D. and Godette D. (2002) Will the 'principles of effectiveness' improve prevention practice? Early findings from a diffusion study. *Health Education Research* **17**, 461–70.

Hamers F., Batter V., Downs A., Alix J., Cazein F., and Brunet J.-B. (1997) The HIV epidemic associated with injecting drug use in Europe: geographic and time trends. *AIDS* **11**, 1365–74.

Hammett T., Harmon M., and Rhodes W. (2002) The burden of infectious disease among inmates of and releasees from US correctional facilities, 1997. *American Journal of Public Health* **92**, 1789–94.

Hansen W.B., Johnson C.A., Flay B.R., Graham J.W., and Sobel J. (1988) Affective and social influences approaches to the prevention of multiple substance abuse among seventh grade students: results from project SMART. *Preventive Medicine* **17**, 135–54.

Hao W., Xiao S., Liu T., Young D., Chen S., Zhang D., Li C., Shi J., Chen G., and Yang K. (2002) The second National Epidemiological Survey on illicit drug use at six high-prevalence areas in China: prevalence rates and use patterns. *Addiction* **97**, 1305–15.

Hao W., Su Z., Xiao S., Fan C., Chen H., Liu T., and Young D. (2004) Longitudinal surveys of prevalence rates and use patterns of illicit drugs at selected high-prevalence areas in China from 1993 to 2000. *Addiction* **99**, 1176–80.

Harlow C.W. (2000) *Defense counsel in criminal cases.* Bureau of Justice Statistics Special Report NCJ 179023. Washington, DC: US Department of Justice. Available at: http://www.ojp.usdoj.gov/bjs/pub/pdf/dccc.pdf (accessed 14 May 2009).

Harrell A., Mitchell O., Merrill J., and Marlowe D. (2003) *Evaluation of breaking the cycle.* Washington, DC: Urban Institute.

Harris A.H.S., Humphreys K., Bowe T., Kivlahan D.R., and Finney J.W. (2009) Measuring the quality of substance use disorder treatment: evaluating the validity of the Department of Veterans Affairs continuity of care performance measure. *Journal of Substance Abuse Treatment* **36**, 294–305.

Harris K.M. and Edlund M.J. (2005) Self-medication of mental health problems: new evidence from a national survey. *Health Services Research* **40**, 117–34.

Harrison L.D. (2001) Understanding the differences in youth drug prevalence rates produced by the MTF, NHSDA, and YRBS studies. *Journal of Drug Issues* **31**, 665–94.

Hartnoll R.L., Mitcheson M.C., Battersby A., Brown G., Ellis M., Fleming P., and Hedley N. (1980) Evaluation of heroin maintenance in controlled trial. *Archives of General Psychiatry* **378**, 877–84.

Harwood, H., Fountain D., and Livermore G. (1998) *The economic costs of alcohol and drug abuse in the United States, 1992.* Washington, DC: US Department of Health and Human Services.

Hastings G. and McLean N. (2006) Social marketing, smoking cessation and inequalites. *Addiction* **101**, 303–4.

Havens J.R., Strathdee S.A., Fuller C.M., Ikeda R., Friedman S.R., Des Jarlais D.C., Morse P.S., Bailey S., Kerndt P., Garfein R.S.; Collaborative Injection Drug User Study Group. (2004) Correlates of attempted suicide among young injection drug users in a multi-site cohort. *Drug and Alcohol Dependence* **75**, 261–9.

Havens J., Walker R., and Leukefeld C. (2007) Prevalence of opioid analgesic injection among rural nonmedical opioid analgesic users. *Drug and Alcohol Dependence* **87**, 98–102.

Hawks D., Mitcheson M., Ogborne A., and Edwards G. (1969) Abuse of methylamphetamine. *British Medical Journal* **2**, 715–21.

Hawks D., Scott K., McBride N., Jones P., and Stockwell T. (2002) *Prevention of psychoactive substance use.* Geneva, Switzerland: World Health Organization.

Hawley M. (2002) Heroin shortage: the cause. *Platypus Magazine* **76**, 43–8.

Health Canada (2009) *Application for authorization to possess dried marihuana.* Ottawa, Canada: Drug & Health Products, Health Canada. Available at: http://www.hc-sc.gc.ca/dhp-mps/marihuana/how-comment/applicant-demandeur/forms_complete-eng.php (accessed 20 May 2009).

Hecht M.L., Marsiglia F.F., Elek E., Wagstaff D.A., Kulis S., and Dustman P. (2003) Culturally-grounded substance use prevention: an evaluation of the keepin' it REAL curriculum. *Prevention Science* **4**, 233–48.

Hesselbrock V.M. **and Hesselbrock M.N.** (2006) Are there empirically supported and clinically useful subtypes of alcohol dependence. *Addiction* **101** (suppl 1), 97–103.

Hibell B., Andersson B., Bjarnason T., Ahlström S., Balakireva O., Kokkevi A., and Morgan M. (2004) *The ESPAD report 2003: Alcohol and other drug use among students in 35 European countries.* Stockholm, Sweden: CAN. Available at: http://www.sedqa.gov.mt/pdf/information/reports_intl_espad2003.pdf (accessed 19 May 2009).

Hibell B., Guttormsson U., Ahlström S., Balakireva O., Bjarnasson T., Kokkevi A., and Kraus L. (2009) *The 2007 ESPAD Report: substance use among students in 35 European countries.* Stockholm, Sweden: CAN.

Higgins K., Percy A., and McCrystal P. (2004) Secular trends in substance use: the conflict and young people in Northern Ireland. *Journal of Social Issues* **60**, 485–506.

Hill E.M. and Newlin D.B. (2002) Evolutionary approaches to addiction: introduction. *Addiction* **97**, 375–379.

Hilts P.H. (1994) Is nicotine addictive? It depends on whose criteria you use: experts say the definition of addiction is evolving. *New York Times* 2 August, p. C3

Hoffman R.S., Wipfler M.G., Maddaloni M.A., and Weisman R.S. (1991) Has the New York State triplicate benzodiazepine prescription regulation influenced sedative-hypnotic overdoses?. *New York State Journal of Medicine* **10**, 436–9.

Hoffmeyer J.H., Klebak S., and Osler M. (1999) Tilsyn med laegers ordination af flunitrazepampr'parater i Kobenhavns amt og Frederiksberg kommune (Control of medical practitioners' prescription of flunitrazepam preparations in the county of Copenhagen and municipality of Frederiksberg). *Ugeskrift for Læger* **161**, 5429–32.

Howard M.O., Walker R.D., Suchinsky R.T., and Anderson B. (1996) Substance use and psychiatric disorders among American Indian veterans. *Substance Use and Misuse* **31**, 581–98.

Howley K. (2005) Locking up life-saving drugs. *Reason* August/September. Available at: http://www.reason.com/news/printer/33117.html (accessed 20 May 2009).

Hser Y.I., Hoffman V.**, Grella C.E., and Anglin M.D.** (2001) A 33-year follow-up of narcotics addicts. *Archives of General Psychiatry* **58**, 503–8.

Hser Y.I., Huang D., Teruya C., and Anglin M.D. (2003) Gender comparisons of drug abuse treatment outcomes and predictors. *Drug and Alcohol Dependence* **72**, 255–64.

Hser Y-I., Teruya C., Brown A.H., Huang D., Evans E. and Anglin M.D. (2007) Impact of California's Proposition 36 on the drug treatment system: treatment capacity and displacement. *American Journal of Public Health* **97**, 104–9.

Hughes C.E. and Stevens A. (2007) *The effects of decriminalization of drug use in Portugal.* Briefing Paper 14. London, UK: The Beckley Foundation Drug Policy Program. Available at: http://www.idpc.net/php-bin/documents/BFDPP_BP_14_EffectsOfDecriminalisation_EN.pdf.pdf (accessed 19 May 2009).

Hughes P. (1977) *Behind the wall of respect: community experiments in heroin addiction control.* Chicago, IL: Chicago University Press.

Hughes P.H., Barker N.W., Crawford G.A., and Jaffe J.H. (1972) The natural history of a heroin epidemic. *American Journal of Public Health* **62**, 995–1001.

Hulley S., Grady D., Bush T., Furberg C., Herrington D., Riggs B., and Vittinghoff E. (1998) Randomized trial of estrogen plus progestin for secondary prevention of coronary heart disease in postmenopausal women. *Journal of the American Medical Association* **280**, 605–13.

Hulse G.K., English D.R., Milne E., and Holman C.D.J. (1999) The quantification of mortality resulting from the regular use of illicit opiates. *Addiction* **94**, 221–9.

Human Rights Watch (2004) *Not enough graves: the war on drugs, HIV/AIDS, and violations of human rights.* Available at: http://hrw.org/reports/2004/thailand0704/thailand0704.pdf (accessed 14 May 2006).

Humeniuk R., Dennington V., Ali R., and WHO ASSIST Study Group (2008) *The effectiveness of a brief intervention for illicit drugs linked to the Alcohol, Smoking and Substance Involvement Screening Test (ASSIST) in primary health care settings: a technical report of phase III findings of the WHO assist randomized controlled trial.* Geneva, Switzerland: Department of Mental Health and Substance Abuse, World Health Organization.

Humphreys K. (2004) *Circles of recovery: self-help organisations for addictions.* Cambridge, UK: Cambridge University Press.

Humphreys K., Mavis B.E., and Stöffelmayr B.E. (1994) Are twelve step programs appropriate for disenfranchised groups? Evidence from a study of post-treatment mutual help group involvement. *Prevention in Human Services* **11**, 165–80.

Humphreys K., Mankowski E., Moos R.H., and Finney J.W. (1999) Do enhanced friendship networks and active coping mediate the effect of self-help groups on substance use?. *Annals of Behavioral Medicine* **21**, 54–60.

Humphreys K., Wagner T.H., and Gage M. (2009) *Why cost-offset studies do not convince medical centers to provide substance use disorder treatment.* Conference paper. Department of Veterans Affairs Health Services Research and Development (HSRD) 2009 National Meeting.

Hunt G. and Dong Sun A.X. (1998) The drug treatment system in the United States: a panacea for the drug war? In: Klingemann H. and Hunt G. (eds) *Treatment systems in an international perspective: drugs, demons and delinquents*, pp. 3–19. London, UK: Sage Publications.

Hurley S.F., Jolley D.J. and Kaldor J.M. (1997) Effectiveness of needle exchange programmes for prevention of HIV infection. *Lancet* **349**, 1797–1800.

Hurwitz W. (2005) The challenge of prescription drug misuse: a review and commentary. *Pain Medicine* **6**, 152–61.

INCB. See International Narcotics Control Board.

Inciardi J.A., Surratt H.L., Kurtz S.P., and Cicero T.J. (2007) Mechanisms of prescription drug diversion among drug-involved club- and street-based populations. *Pain Medicine* **8**, 171–83.

Independent Inquiry into the Misuse of Drugs Act 1971 (2000) *Drugs and the law*. London, UK: The Police Foundation. Available at: http://www.police-foundation.org.uk/site/police-foundation/latest/independent-inquiries/inquiry-into-the-misuse-of-drugs? (accessed 19 May 2009).

Integrated Substance Abuse Programs (2007) *Substance abuse and crime prevention act: final report*. Los Angeles, CA: UCLA Integrated Substance Abuse Programs. Available at: http://www.adp.cahwnet.gov/SACPA/PDF/SACPAEvaluationReport_Final2007Apr13.pdf (accessed 19 May 2009).

International Drug Policy Consortium (2007) *The 2007 commission on narcotic drugs*. IDPC Briefing Paper No. 5. Witley, UK: International Drug Policy Consortium. Available at: http://www.internationaldrugpolicy.net/reports/IDPC_Report_5.pdf (accessed 25 May 2009).

International Narcotics Control Board (2002) *Report of the International Narcotics Control Board for 2001*. New York, NY: United Nations. E/INCB/2001/1. Available at: http://www.incb.org/incb/en/annual_report_2001.html (accessed 25 May 2009).

International Narcotics Control Board (2006a) *Annual report, part four: statistical information on narcotic drugs*. New York, NY: United Nations.

International Narcotics Control Board (2006b) *Report of the International Narcotics Control Board for 2005*. Vienna, Austria: INCB. Available at: http://www.incb.org/pdf/e/ar/2005/incb_report_2005_full.pdf (accessed 20 May 2009).

International Narcotics Control Board (2007a) Part four: statistical information on narcotic drugs. In: *Narcotic drugs: estimated world requirements for 2007; statistics for 2005* (E/INCB/2006/2), pp. 67–289. New York, NY; United Nations. Available at: http://www.incb.org/pdf/e/tr/nar/2006/Narcotics_publication_2006_part4_en.pdf (accessed 15 May 2009).

International Narcotics Control Board (2007b) *Report of the International Narcotics Control Board for 2006*. (E/INCB/2006/1) New York, NY: United Nations. Available at: http://www.incb.org/incb/en/annual_report_2006.html (accessed 15 May 2009).

International Narcotics Control Strategy Report (2007) Washington DC: US Department of State to Congress. Available at: http://www.state.gov/p/inl/rls/nrcrpt/2007/ (accessed 19 May 2009).

Ives T.J., Chelminski P.R., Hammett-Stabler C.A., Malone R.M., Perhac J.S., Potisek N.M., Shilliday B.B., DeWalt D.A., and Pignone M.P. (2006) Predictors of opioid misuse in patients with chronic pain: a prospective cohort study. *BMC Health Services Research* **4**, 6–46.

Jacobs B. (1999) *Dealing crack: the social world of street corner selling*. Boston, MA: Northeastern University Press.

Jacobson M. (2004) Baby booms and drug busts: trends in youth drug use in the United States, 1975–2000. *Quarterly Journal of Economics* **119**, 1481–512.

Jagan L. (2003) Mixed progress for Yanhon's drug war. *Asia Times Online* 9 May. Available at: http://www.atimes.com/atimes/Southeast_Asia/EE09Ae01.html (accessed 14 May 2009).

Jankowiak W. and Bradburd D. (eds) (2003) *Drugs, labor, and colonial expansion*. Tucson, AZ: University of Arizona Press.

Jason L.A., Olson B.D., Ferrari J.R., and Lo Sasso A.T. (2006) Communal housing settings enhance substance abuse recovery. *American Journal of Public Health* **96**, 1727–9.

Johnson B.D. (2003) Patterns of drug distribution: implications and issues. *Substance Use and Misuse* **38**, 1789–806.

Johnson B.D., Goldstein P., Preble E., Schmeidler J., Lipton D., Spunt B., and Miller T. (1985) *Taking care of business: the economics of crime by heroin abusers.* Lexington, MA: D.C. Heath.

Johnson R.E., Chutuape M.A., Strain E.C., Walsch S.L., Stitzer M.L., and Bigelow G.E. (2000) A comparison of levomethadyl acetate, buprenorphine, and methadone for opioid dependence. *New England Journal of Medicine* **343**, 1290–7.

Johnston L.D., O'Malley P.M., and Bachman J.G. (1981) *Marijuana decriminalization: the impact on youth, 1975–1980.* Monitoring the Future Occasional Paper No. 13. Ann Arbor, MI: Institute for Social Research, University of Michigan.

Johnston L.D., O'Malley P.M., and Bachman J.G. (2003) Monitoring the Future: national results on adolescent drug use: Overview of key findings. *FOCUS* **1**, 213–34.

Johnston L.D., O'Malley P.M., Bachman J.G., and Schulenberg J.E. (2008) *Monitoring the Future national results on adolescent drug use: overview of key findings, 2007.* Bethesda, MD: National Institute on Drug Abuse. Advance data available at: http://www.drugabuse.gov/Newsroom/07/MTF2007Drug.pdf (accessed 15 May 2009).

Jonasson U. and Jonasson B. (2004) *Restrictions on the prescribing of dextropropoxyphene (DXP): effects on sales and cases of fatal poisoning.* Stockholm, Sweden: Rättsmedicinalverket (National Board of Forensic Medicine). Available at: http://www.rmv.se/pdf/dxp-report.pdf (accessed 20 May 2009).

Joranson D.E. and Gilson A.M. (2005) Drug crime is a source of abused pain medications in the United States. *Journal of Pain and Symptom Management* **30**, 299–301.

Joranson D.E. and Gilson A.M. (2006) Wanted: a public health approach to prescription opioid abuse and diversion. *Pharmacoepidemiology and Drug Safety* **15**, 632–4.

Kakko, J., Svanborg K.D., Kreek M.J., and Heilig M. (2003) 1-year retention and social function after buprenorphine-assisted relapse prevention treatment for heroin dependence in Sweden: a randomized, placebo-controlled trial. *Lancet* **361**, 662–8.

Kandall S.R. (1996) *Substance and shadow: a history of women and addiction in the United States—1850 to present.* Cambridge, MA: Harvard University Press.

Kandel D.B. and Davies M. (1996) High school students who use crack and other drugs. *Archives of General Psychiatry* **53**, 71–80.

Kandel D.B. and Yamaguchi K. (2002) Stages of drug involvement in the U.S. population. In: Kandel D.B. (ed.) *Stages and pathways of drug involvement*, pp. 65–89. Cambridge, UK: Cambridge University Press.

Kaplan E.H. and Heimer R. (1994) A circulation theory of needle exchange. *AIDS* **8**, 567–74.

Karam E., Melhem N., Mansour C., Maalouf W., Saliba S., and Chami A. (2000) Use and abuse of licit and illicit substances: prevalence and risk factors among students in Lebanon. *European Addiction Research* **6**, 189–97.

Kassirer J.P. (2005) *On the take: how medicine's complicity with big business can endanger your health.* Oxford, UK: Oxford University Press.

Kaukonen O. and Stenius K. (2005) Universalism under re-construction: from administrative coercion to professional subordination of substance misusers. In: Kildal N. and Kuhnle S. (eds) *Normative foundations of the welfare state: the Nordic experience*, pp. 130–148. London, UK: Routledge.

Kaya Y.C., Tugai Y., Filar J.A., Agrawal M.R., Ali R.L., Gowing L.R., and Cooke R. (2004) Heroin users in Australia: population trends. *Drug and Alcohol Review* 23, 107–16.

Keizer K., Lindenberg S., and Steg L. (2008) The spreading of disorder. *Science* **322**, 1681–5.

Kellam S., Reid J., and Balster R.L. (2008) Effects of a universal classroom behavior program in first and second grades on young adult outcomes. *Drug and Alcohol Dependence* **95**, Suppl 1, S1–104.

Kelling G.L. and Coles C.M. (1996) *Fixing broken windows: restoring order and reducing crime in our communities.* New York, NY: Free Press.

Kelly E., Darke S., and Ross J. (2004) A review of drug use and driving: epidemiology, impairment, risk factors and risk perceptions. *Drug and Alcohol Review* **23**, 319–44.

Kendler K.S., Karkowski L.M., Neale M.C., and Prescott C.A. (2000) Illicit psychoactive substance use, heavy use, abuse, and dependence in a US population-based sample of male twins. *Archives of General Psychiatry* **57**, 261–9.

Kenkel D., Mathios A.D., and Pacula RL. (2001) Economics of youth drug use, addiction and gateway effects. *Addiction* **96**, 151–64.

Kennedy D. (1991) *Closing the market: controlling the drug trade in Tampa.* Washington DC: National Institute of Justice.

Kennedy D.M. (1997) Pulling levers: chronic offenders, high-crime settings, and a theory of prevention. *Valparaiso University Law Review* **31**, 449–84.

Kerr T., Small W., and Wood E. (2005) The public health and social impacts of drug market enforcement: a review of the evidence. *International Journal of Drug Policy* **16**, 210–20.

Kerr T., Fairbairn N., Tyndall M., Marsh D., Li K., Montaner J., and Wood E. (2007) Predictors of non-fatal overdose among a cohort of polysubstance-using injection drug users. *Drug and Alcohol Dependence* **87**, 39–45.

Kessler R., Chiu W., Demler O., Merikangas K., and Walters E. (2005) Prevalence, severity, and comorbidity of 12-month DSM-IV disorders in the National Comorbidity Survey Replication. *Archives of General Psychiatry* **62**, 617–27.

Khantzian E.J. (1997) The self-medication hypothesis of substance use disorders: a reconsideration and recent applications. *Harvard Review of Psychiatry* **4**, 287–9.

Kiernan M., Toro P.A., Rappaport J., and Seidman E. (1989) Economic predictors of mental health utilization: a time-series analysis. *American Journal of Community Psychology* **17**, 801–20.

Killias M. and Aebi, M.F. (2000) The impact of heroin prescribing on heroin markets in Switzerland. *Crime Prevention Studies* **11**, 83–99.

Kilmer B. and Reuter P. (2009) Prime numbers: drug markets. *Foreign Policy.* In press.

Kim H.J., Chung W., and Lee S.G. (2004) Lessons from Korea's pharmaceutical policy reform: the separation of medical institutions and pharmacies for outpatient care. *Health Policy* **68**, 267–75.

Kimber J., Dolan K., van Beek I., Hedrich D. and Zurhold H. (2003) Drug consumption facilities: an update since 2000. *Drug and Alcohol Review* **22**, 227–33.

King S.M., Keyes M., Malone S.M., Elkins I., Legrand L.N., Iacono W.G., and McGue W. (2009) Parental alcohol dependence and the transmission of adolescent behavior disinhibition: a study of adoptive and non-adoptive families. *Addiction* **104**, 578–86.

Kirby K.N. and Petry N.M. (2004) Heroin and cocaine abusers have higher discount rates for delayed rewards than alcoholics or non-drug-using controls. *Addiction* **99**, 461–71.

Kleiman M.A.R. (1988) Crackdowns: the effects of intensive enforcement on retail heroin dealing. In: Chaiken M.R. (ed.) *Street-level drug enforcement: examining the issues*, pp. 3–34. Washington, DC: National Institute of Justice.

Kleiman M.A.R. (1992) *Against excess: drug policy for results.* New York, NY: Basic Books.

Kleiman M.A.R. (1997a) Coerced abstinence: a neopaternalist drug policy initiative. In: Mead L.M. (ed.) *The new paternalism: supervisory approaches to poverty*, pp. 182–219. Washington, DC: Brookings Institution.

Kleiman M.A.R. (1997b) The problem of replacement and the logic of drug law enforcement. *Drug policy analysis bulletin*, issue 3, article 3. Available at: http://www.fas.org/drugs/issue3.htm#3 (accessed 14 May 2009).

Kleiman M.A.R. (2009) *When brute force fails: how to have less crime and less punishment.* Princeton, NJ: Princeton University Press.

Klingemann H., Takala J.P., and Hunt G. (1992) *Cure, care or control: alcoholism treatment in sixteen countries.* Albany, NY: State University of New York Press.

Klingemann H., Takala J.P., and Hunt G. (1993) The development of alcohol treatment systems: an international perspective. *Alcohol Health and Research World* **3**, 221–7.

Klingemann H. and Hunt G. (eds) (1998) *Drug treatment systems in an international perspective. Drugs, demons, and delinquents.* London, UK: Sage Publications.

Klingemann H., Sobell L., Barker J., Blomqvist J., Cloud W., Ellinstad T., Finfgeld D., Granfield R., Hodgings D., Hunt G., Junker C., Moggi F., Peele S., Smart R., Sobell M., and Tucker J. (2001) *Promoting self-change from problem substance use: Practical implications for policy, prevention and treatment.* Dordrecht, The Netherlands: Kluwer Academic Publishers.

Kohn M. (1992) *Dope girls: the birth of the British drug underground.* London, UK: Lawrence & Wishart.

Kokkevi A., Terzidou M., Politikou K., and Stefanis C. (2002) Substance use among high school students in Greece: outburst of illicit drug use in a society under change. *Drug and Alcohol Dependence* **58**, 181–8.

Korf D.J. (2002) Dutch coffee shops and trends in cannabis use. *Addictive Behaviors* **27**, 851–66.

Kraft M.K., Rothbard A.B., Hadley T.R., McLellan A.T., and Asch D.A. (1997) Are supplementary services provided during methadone maintenance really cost-effective?. *American Journal of Psychiatry* 154, 1195–7.

Krajewski K. (1999) How flexible are the UN drug conventions?. *International Journal of Drug Policy* **10**, 329–38.

Kübler D. and Wälti S. (2001) Metropolitan governance and democracy: how to evaluate new tendencies? In: McLaverty P. (ed.) *Public participation and developments in community governance*, pp. 99–121. Aldershot, UK: Ashgate.

Kuehn B.M. (2007) Opioid prescriptions soar: increase in legitimate use as well as abuse. *Journal of the American Medical Association* **297**, 249–51.

Kuhns J.B. and Klodfelter T.A. (2009) Illicit drug-related psychopathological violence: the current understanding within a causal context. *Aggression and Violent Behaviour* **14**, 69–78.

Kuntsche E.N. (2004) Progression of a general substance use pattern among adolescents in Switzerland? Investigating the relationship between alcohol, tobacco, and cannabis use over a 12-year period. *European Addiction Research* **10**, 118–25.

Kuziemko I. and Levitt S.D. (2004) An empirical analysis of imprisoning drug offenders. *Journal of Public Economics* **88**, 2043–66.

Lagerspetz M. and Moskalewicz J. (2002) Drugs in the postsocialist transitions of Estonia, Latvia, Lithuania and Poland. *European Addiction Research* **8**, 177–83.

Lambo T.A. (1965) Medical and social problems of drug addiction in West Africa, with special emphasis on psychiatric aspects. *Bulletin on Narcotics* **17**, 3–13.

Larance B., Degenhardt L., Copeland J., and Dillon P. (2008) Injecting risk behaviour and related harm among men who use performance- and image-enhancing drugs. *Drug and Alcohol Review* **27**, 678–86.

Laven D.L. (ed.) (2006) Drug diversion and counterfeiting, Parts I and II. Two journal issues. *Journal of Pharmacy Practice* **18**, 135–81 and 191–254.

Lawal R.A., Adelekan M.L., Ohaeri J.U., and Orija O.B. (1998) Rehabilitation of heroin and cocaine abusers managed in a Nigerian psychiatric hospital. *East African Medical Journal* **75**, 107–12.

Lehto J. (1998) Equal access with optimum costs: issues of financing and managing drug treatment. In: Klingemann H. and Hunt G. (eds) *Drug treatment systems in an international perspective: drugs, demons, and delinquents*, pp. 269–80. London, UK: Sage Publications.

Lembke A., Humphreys K., and Moos R. (2009) Diagnosis, development and treatment of substance use disorders among adolescents and young adults. In: Steiner, H. (ed.) *Stanford University School of Medicine handbook of developmental psychiatry*. New York, NY: Jossey/Bass/Wiley. In press.

Lenton S., Christie P., Humeniuk R., Brooks A., Bennett P., and Heale P. (1999) *Infringement versus conviction: the social impact of a minor cannabis offence under a civil penalties system and strict prohibition in two Australian states.* National Drug Strategy Monograph No. 36. Canberra, Australia: Publications Productions Unit, Commonwealth Department of Health and Aged Care.

Lenton S., Heale P., Erickson P., Single E., Lang E., and Hawks D. (2000a) *The regulation of cannabis possession, use and supply*. Perth, Australia: National Drug Research Institute, Curtin University of Technology. Available at: http://espace.lis.curtin.edu.au/archive/00000377/01/M25_Regulation_Cannabis.pdf (accessed 25 May 2009).

Lenton S., Humeniuk R., Heale P., and Christie P. (2000b) Infringement versus conviction: the social impact of a minor cannabis offence in SA and WA. *Drug and Alcohol Review* **19**, 257–64.

Leri F., Bruneau J., and Stewart J. (2003) Understanding polydrug use: review of heroin and cocaine co-use. *Addiction* **98**, 7–22.

Levine H.G. (1981) The vocabulary of drunkenness. *Journal of Studies on Alcohol* **42**, 1038–51.

Levitt S. (2004) Understanding why crime fell in the 1990s: four factors that explain the decline and six that do not. *Journal of Economic Perspectives* **18**, 163–90.

Levitt S. and Venkatesh S.A. (2000) An economic analysis of a drug-selling gang's finances. *Quarterly Journal of Economics* **115**, 755–89.

Li X., Zhou Y., and Stanton B. (2002) Illicit drug initiation among institutionalized drug users in China. *Addiction* **97**, 575–82.

Ling W., Charuvastra C., Kaim S.C., and Klett C.J. (1976) Methadyl acetate and methadone as maintenance treatment for heroin addicts: a Veterans Administration cooperative study. *Archives of General Psychiatry* **33**, 709–20.

Lintzeris N. (2009) Prescription of heroin for the management of heroin dependence: current status. *CNS Drugs* **23**, 463–476.

Littlejohn C., Baldacchino A., Schifano F., and Deluca P. (2005) Internet pharmacies and online prescription drug sales: a cross-sectional study. *Drugs: Education, Prevention and Policy* **12**, 75–80.

Liu J.-L., Liu J.-T., Hammitt J.K., and Chou S-Y. (1999) The price elasticity of opium in Taiwan, 1914–1942. *Journal of Health Economics* **18**, 795–810.

Liu Z., Zhou W., Lian Z., Mu Y., Cai Z., and Cao J. (2001) The use of psychoactive substances among adolescent students in an area in the south-west of China. *Addiction* **96**, 247–50.

Liu Z., Lian Z., and Zhao C. (2006) Drug use and HIV/AIDS in China. *Drug and Alcohol Review* **25**, 173–5.

Longshore D., Reuter P., Derks J., Grapendal M., and Ebener P. (1998) Drug policies and harms: a conceptual framework. *European Addiction Research* **4**, 172–182.

Lundberg L. and Isacson D. (1999) The impact of over-the-counter availability of nasal sprays on sales, prescribing, and physician visits. *Scandinavian Journal of Primary Health Care* **17**, 1–45.

Luo R. and Cofrancesco J., Jr. (2006) Injection drug use and HIV transmission in Russia. *AIDS* **20**, 935–6.

Lussier J.P., Heil S.H., Mongeon J.A., Badger G.J., and Higgins S.T. (2006) A meta-analysis of voucher-based reinforcement therapy for substance use disorders. *Addiction* **101**, 192–203.

Luthar S.S. and D'Avanzo K. (1999) Contextual factors in substance use: a study of suburban and inner-city adolescents. *Development and Psychopathology* **11**, 845–67.

Lynskey M.T. and Hall W. (2001) Attention deficit hyperactivity disorder and substance use disorders: is there a causal link?. *Addiction* **96**, 815–22.

Lynskey M.T., Heath A.C., Bucholz K.K., Slutske W.S., Madden P.A., Nelson E.C., Statham D.J., and Martin N.G. (2003) Escalation of drug use in early-onset cannabis users vs co-twin controls. *Journal of the American Medical Association* **289**, 427–33.

MacAndrew C. and Edgerton R. (1969) *Drunken comportment.* Chicago, IL: Aldine.

MacCoun R.J. and Reuter P. (2001a) *Drug war heresies: learning from other vices, times and places.* Cambridge, UK: Cambridge University Press.

MacCoun R.J. and Reuter P. (2001b) Evaluating alternative cannabis regimes. *British Journal of Psychiatry* **178**, 123–8.

MacCoun R.J., Pacula R., Chiriqi J., Harris K., and Reuter P. (2008) *Do citizens accurately perceive differences in marijuana sanction risks? A test of a critical assumption in deterrence theory and the decriminalization debate.* JSP/Center for the Study of Law and Society Faculty Working Papers. Paper 64. Available at: http://repositories.cdlib.org/csls/fwp/6 (accessed 19 May 2009).

MacDonald S., Anglin-Bodrug K., Mann R.E., Erickson P., Hathaway A., Chipman M., and Rylett M. (2003) Injury risk associated with cannabis and cocaine use. *Drug and Alcohol Dependence* **72**, 99–115.

MacDonald Z., Collingwood J. and Gordon L. (2006). *Measuring the harm from illegal drugs using the Drug Harm Index: an update.* Home Office Online Report 08/06. London, UK: The Home Office.

Macleod J., Oakes R., Copello A., Crome I., Egger M., Hickman M., Oppenkowski T., Stokes-Lampard H., and Davey Smith G. (2004) Psychological and social sequelae of cannabis and other illicit drug use by young people: a systematic review of longitudinal, general population studies. *Lancet* **363**, 1579–88.

Magura S., Nwakeze P.C., Rosenblum A., and Joseph H. (2000) Substance misuse and related infectious diseases in a soup kitchen population. *Substance Use and Misuse* **35**, 551–83.

Maher L. and Dixon D. (2001) The cost of crackdowns: policing Cabramatta's heroin market. *Current Issues in Criminal Justice* **13**, 5–22.

Maher L., Dixon D., Hall W., and Lynskey M. (2002) Property crime and income generation by heroin users. *Australian and New Zealand Journal of Criminology* **35**, 187–202.

Mäkelä K., Arminen I., Bloomfield K., Eisenbach-Stangl I., Helmersson Bergmark K., Mariolini N., Ólafsdóttir H., Petersen J.H., Phillips M., Rehm J., Room R., Rosenqvist P., Rosovsky H., Stenius K., Swiatkiewicz G.,Woronowicz B. and Zieli ski A. (1996) *Alcoholics Anonymous as a mutual help movement: a study in eight societies.* Madison, WI: University of Wisconsin Press.

Manchikanti L., Cash K.A., Damron K.S., Manchukonda R., Pampati V., and McManus C.D. (2006a) Controlled substance abuse and illicit drug use in chronic pain patients: an evaluation of multiple variables. *Pain Physician* **9**, 215–25.

Manchikanti L., Manchukonda R., Damron K.S., Brandon D. McManus C.D. and Cash K. (2006b) Does adherence monitoring reduce controlled substance abuse in chronic pain patients?. *Pain Physician* **9**, 57–60.

Mandel J. (1987) Are lower penalties a green light for drug users?. *Journal of Psychoactive Drugs* **19**, 383–5.

Manderson D. (1987) *Proscription and prescription: Commonwealth government opiate policy 1905–1937.* National Campaign against Drug Abuse, Monograph Series No. 2. Canberra, Australia: Australian Government Publishing Service.

Manderson D. (1993) *From Mr Sin to Mr Big.* Melbourne, Australia: Oxford University Press.

Mandryk J.A., Mackson J.M., Horn F.E., Wutzke S.E., Badcock C.-A., Hyndman R.J., and Weekes L.M. (2006) Measuring change in prescription drug utilization in Australia. *Pharmacoepidemiology and Drug Safety* **15**, 477–84.

Mann R.E., Smart R., Anglin L., and Rush B. (1988) Are decreases in liver cirrhosis rates a result of increased treatment for alcoholism?. *British Journal of Addiction* **83**, 683–8.

Mann S. (1999) $150m opiates trade at risk. *The Age.* Melbourne, Australia, 18 December. Available at http://www.mapinc.org/drugnews/v99/n1378/a05.html (accessed 25 May 2009).

Manski C.F., Pepper J.V., and Thomas Y.F. (eds) (1999) *Assessment of two cost-effectiveness studies on cocaine control policy.* Washington, DC: National Academy Press.

Manski C.F., Pepper J.V., and Petrie C.V. (eds) (2001) *Informing America's policy on illegal drugs: what we don't know keeps hurting us.* Washington, DC: National Academy Press.

Manzoni P, Brochu S., Fischer B., and Rehm J. (2006) Determinants of property crime among illicit opiate users outside of treatment across Canada. *Deviant Behavior* **27**, 351–76.

Marijuana Policy Project (2008) *State by state medical marijuana laws: how to remove the threat of arrest.* Washington, DC: Marijuana Policy Project. Available at: http://www.mpp.org/legislation/state-by-state-medical-marijuana-laws.html (accessed 20 May 2009).

Marijuana Treatment Project Research Group. (2004) Brief treatments for cannabis dependence: findings from a randomized multisite trial. *Journal of Consulting and Clinical Psychology* **72**, 455–66.

Marmot M. (2004) *The status syndrome: how social standing affects our health and longevity.* New York, NY: Times Books.

Marsden J., Stillwell G., Barlow H., Boys A., Taylor C., Hunt N., and Farrell M. (2005) An evaluation of a brief motivational intervention among young ecstasy and cocaine users: no effect on substance and alcohol use outcomes. *Addiction* **101**, 1014–26.

Martyres R.F., Clodes D., and Burns J.M. (2004) Seeking drugs or seeking help? Escalating 'doctor shopping' by young heroin users before fatal overdose. *Medical Journal of Australia* **180**, 211–14.

Massari M. (2005) Ecstasy in the city: synthetic drug markets in Europe. *Crime, Law and Social Change* **44**, 1–18.

Matrix Knowledge Group (2007) *The illicit drug trade in the United Kingdom.* Home Office online report 20/07. London, UK: The Home Office.

Mazerolle L., Soole D., and Rombouts S. (2006) Street-level drug law enforcement: a meta-analytic review. *Journal of Experimental Criminology* **2**, 409–35.

McAllister W.B. (2000) *Drug diplomacy in the twentieth century: an international history.* New York, NY: Routledge.

McCabe S.E., Teter C.J., and Boyd C.J. (2006) Medical use, illicit use, and diversion of prescription stimulant medication. *Journal of Psychoactive Drugs* **38**, 43–56.

McCabe S.E., Cranford J.A., Boyd C.J., and Teter C.J. (2007) Motives, diversion and routes of administration associated with nonmedical use of prescription opioids. *Addictive Behavior* **32**, 562–75.

McCoy C.B., McCoy H.V., Lai S., Yu Z., Wang X., and Meng J. (2001) Reawakening the dragon: changing patterns of opiate use in Asia, with particular emphasis on China's Yunnan province. *Substance Use and Misuse* **36**, 49–69.

McGeorge J. and Aitken C.K. (1997) Effects of cannabis decriminalization in the Australian capital territory on university students' patterns of use. *Journal of Drug Issues* **27**, 785–93.

McKegany N. (2005) *Random drug testing of schoolchildren: a shot in the arm or a shot in the foot for drug prevention?* York, UK: Joseph Rowntree Foundation.

McKinlay J.B. (1992) Health promotion through healthy public policy: the contribution of complementary research methods. *Canadian Journal of Public Health* **83** (Suppl.), 11S–9S.

McLellan A.T., Arndt I.O., Metzger D.S., Woody G.E., and O'Brien C.P. (1993) The effects of psychosocial services in substance abuse treatment. *Journal of the American Medical Association* **269**, 1953–9.

McLellan A.T., Lewis D.C., O'Brien C.P., and Kleber H. (2000) Drug dependence, a chronic medical illness: implications for treatment, insurance and outcomes evaluation. *Journal of the American Medical Assciation* **284**, 1689–95.

McLellan A.T., Carise D., and Kleber H.D. (2003) Can the national addiction treatment infrastructure support the public's demand for quality care?. *Journal of Substance Abuse Treatment* **25**, 117–21.

McLellan A.T., McKay J.R., Forman R., Cacciola J., and Kemp J. (2005) Reconsidering the evaluation of addiction treatment: from retrospective follow-up to concurrent recovery monitoring. *Addiction* **100**, 447–58.

Meara E. and Frank R. (2005) Spending on substance abuse treatment: how much is enough?. *Addiction* **100**, 1240–8.

Medawar C. and Hardon A. (2004) *Medicines out of control? Antidepressants and the conspiracy of goodwill.* Amsterdam, The Netherlands: Aksant.

Medina-Mora M.E., Borges G., Fleiz C., Benjet C., Rojas E., Zambrano J., Villatoro J., and Aguilar-Gaxiola S. (2006) Prevalence and correlates of drug use disorders in Mexico. *Revista Panamericana de Salud Pública (Pan American Journal of Public Health)* **19**, 265–76.

Meier B. (2007) Narcotic maker guilty of deceit over marketing. *New York Times* 11 May. Available at: http://www.nytimes.com/2007/05/11/business/11drug.html (accessed 15 May 2009).

Merikangas K.R., Mehta R.L., Molnar B.E., Walters E.E., Swendsen J.D., Aguilar-Gaziola S., Bijl R., Borges G., Caraveo-Anduaga J.J., DeWit D.J., Kolody B., Vega W.A., Wittchen H.U., and Kessler R.C. (1998a) Comorbidity of substance use disorders with mood and anxiety disorders: results of the International Consortium in Psychiatric Epidemiology. *Addictive Behaviors* **23**, 893–907.

Merikangas K.R., Stolar M., Stevens D.E., Goulet J., Preisig M.A., Fenton B., Zhang H., O' S.S., and Rounsaville B.J. (1998b) Familial transmission of substance use disorders. *Archives of General Psychiatry* 55, 973–9.

Meyer R.E. (1986) *Psychopathology and addictive disorders.* New York, NY: Guilford.

Michna E., Ross E.L., Hynes W.L., Nedeljkovic S.S., Soumekh S., Janfaza D., Palombi D., and Jamison R.N. (2004) Predicting aberrant drug behavior in patients treated for chronic pain: importance of abuse history. *Journal of Pain and Symptom Management* **28**, 250–8.

Midford R., McBride N., and Munro G. (1998) Harm reduction in school education: developing an Australian approach. *Drug and Alcohol Review* **17**, 319–27.

Millar T., Gemmell I., Hay G., Heller R.F., and Donmall M. (2006) How well do trends in incidence of heroin use reflect hypothesised trends in prevalence of problem drug use in the North West of England?. *Addiction Research and Theory* **14**, 537–49.

Miller C.L., Johnston C., Spittal P.M., Li K., LaLiberté N., Montaner J.S.G., and Schechter M.T. (2002) Opportunities for prevention: hepatitis C prevalence and incidence in a cohort of young injection drug users. *Hepatology* **36**, 737–42.

Mills W. (1985) Cape smoke: alcohol issues in the Cape Colony in the nineteenth century. *Contemporary Drug Problems* **12**, 221–47.

Mingardi G. (2001) Money and the international drug trade in Sao Paolo. *International Social Science Journal* **53**, 379–86.

Minozzi S., Amato L., Vecchi S., Davoli M., Kirchmayer U., and Verster A. (2006) Oral naltrexone maintenance treatment for opioid dependence. *Cochrane Database of Systematic Reviews*, issue 1, article number CD001333. DOI: 10.1002/14651858.CD001333.pub2.

Miron J.A. (2003a) *A critique of estimates of the economic costs of drug abuse.* Manuscript. Boston, MA: Department of Economics, Boston University.

Miron J.A. (2003b) *Bringing honest cost-benefit analysis to U.S. drug policy: a critique of estimates of the economic costs of drug abuse.* New York: Drug Policy Alliance. Available at: http://www.drugpolicy.org/docUploads/Miron_Report.pdf (accessed 13 May 2009).

Mitcheson M., Edwards G., Hawks D., and Ogborne A. (1976) Treatment of methylamphetamine users during the 1968 epidemic. In: Edwards G., Russell M.A.H., Hawks D., and MacCafferty M. (eds) *Drugs and drug dependence*, pp. 155–62. London, UK: Saxon House Publishers.

Model K.E. (1993) The effect of marijuana decriminalization on hospital emergency room drug episodes: 1975–1978. *Journal of the American Statistical Association* **88**, 737–47.

Mokri A. (2005) Substance abuse treatment and HIV in Iran. Presented in Istanbul at the International Conference on Delivery Systems for Substance Abuse Treatment. Available at: http://www.uclaisap.org/dssat2005/html/presentations.html (accessed 30 May 2009).

Monshouwer K., Smit F., de Graaf R., van Os J., and Vollebergh W. (2005) First cannabis use: does onset shift to younger ages? Findings from 1988 to 2003 from the Dutch National School Survey on Substance Use. *Addiction* **100**, 963–70.

Moore M.H. (1973) Policies to achieve discrimination on the effective price of heroin. *American Economic Review* **63**, 270–7.

Moore T.J. (2005) *What is Australia's 'drug budget'? The policy mix of illicit drug-related government spending in Australia.* DPMP Monograph Series. Fitzroy, Australia: Turning Point Alcohol and Drug Centre.

Moore T.J. and Caulkins J.P. (2005) How studies of the cost-of-illness of substance abuse can be made more useful for policy analysis. Paper presented at the 27th Australian Health Economists Conference, September.

Moore T.J., Caulkins J.P., Ritter A., Dietze P., Monagle S., and Pruden J. (2005) *Heroin markets in Australia: current understanding and future possibilities.* DPMP Monograph Series. Fitzroy, Australia: Turning Point Alcohol and Drug Centre.

Moravek J. (2008) Problem drug use, marijuana, and European projects: how epidemiology helped Czech drug reformers. *Central European Journal of Public Policy* **2**, 26–39.

Morgan O. and Majeed A. (2005) Restricting paracetamol in the United Kingdom to reduce poisoning: a systematic review. *Journal of Public Health* **27**, 12–18.

Morgan P. (1983) Alcohol, disinhibition, and domination: a conceptual analysis. In: Room R. and Collins G. (eds) *Alcohol and disinhibition: nature and meaning of the link*, pp. 405–20. Research Monograph No. 12, DHHS Publication No. (ADM) 83-1246. Rockville, MD: National Institute on Alcohol Abuse and Alcoholism,

Morral A.R., McCafrey D.F., and Paddock S.M. (2002) Evidence does not favor marijuana gateway effects over a common-factor interpretation of drug use initiation: responses to Anthony, Kenkel & Mathios and Lynskey. *Addiction* **97**, 1509–10.

Morrato E.H. and Staffa J.A. (2007) Effectiveness of risk management plans: a case study of pemoline using pharmacy claims data. *Pharmacoepidemiology and Drug Safety* **16**, 104–12.

Moskalewicz J. (2002) Drugs in countries of Central and Eastern Europe. *European Addiction Research* **8**, 157–8.

Mugford S. (1993) Harm reduction: does it lead where its proponents imagine? In: Heather N., Wodak A., Nadelmann E., and O'Hare P. (eds) *Psychoactive drugs and harm reduction: from faith to science*, pp. 21–33. London, UK: Whurr Publishers.

Munn C. (2000) The Hong Kong opium revenue, 1845–1885. In: Brook T. and Wakabayashi B.T. (eds) *Opium regimes: China, Britain and Japan, 1839–1952*, pp. 105–26. Berkeley, CA: University of California Press.

Murray C.J.L. and Lopez A.D. (eds) (1996) *The global burden of disease: a comprehensive assessment of mortality and disability from diseases, injuries and risk factors in 1990 and projected to 2020.* Boston: Harvard School of Public Health on behalf of the World Health Organization and the World Bank.

Musto D. (1973) *The American disease: origins of narcotic control.* New Haven, CT: Yale University Press.

Nadelmann E. (1993) *Cops across borders: the internationalization of U.S. criminal law enforcement.* University Park, PA: Pennsylvania State University Press.

Nagin D.S. (1998) Criminal deterrence research: a review of the evidence and a research agenda for the outset of the 21st century. In: Tonry M. (ed.) *Crime and justice: an annual review of research*, vol. 23, pp. 1–42. Chicago, IL: University of Chicago Press.

NAOMI Study Team (2008) *Reaching the hardest to reach—treating the hardest-to-treat: summary of the primary outcomes of the North American opiate medication initiative (NAOMI).* Available at: http://www.naomistudy.ca/documents.html (accessed 15 May 2009).

Narcotics Control Bureau, India (2003) *Narcotics Annual Report 2002.* Delhi, India: Narcotics Control Bureau.

Natarajan M. and Hough M. (eds) (2000) *Illegal drug markets: from research to policy.* Crime Prevention Studies Vol. 11. Monsey, NY: Criminal Justice Press.

National Institute for Health Care Management (2002) *Prescription drug expenditures in 2001: another year of escalating costs.* 6 Mat revision. Washington, DC: NIHCM. Available at: http://www.nihcm.org/~nihcmor/pdf/spending_2001.pdf (accessed 15 May 2009).

National Institute of Justice (2003) *2000 arrestee drug abuse monitoring: annual report.* NCJ 193013. Washington DC: US Department of Justice.

National Institute of Justice (2004) *Drug and alcohol use and related matters among arrestees, 2003.* Washington, DC: US Department of Justice. Available at: http://www.ncjrs.gov/nij/adam/ADAM2003.pdf (accessed 10 January 2009).

National Institute on Drug Abuse (2008) Monitoring the Future survey, overview of findings 2007. Bethesda, MD: NIDA. Available at: http://www.drugabuse.gov/newsroom/07/MTF07Overview.html#one (accessed 15 May 2009).

National Research Council (2005) Improving evaluation of anti-crime programs. Washington, DC: National Academy Press.

National Research Council and Institute of Medicine (2009) *Preventing mental, emotional and behavioral disorders among young people: progress and possibilities.* O'Connell M.E., Boat T., and Warner K.E., eds. Washington, DC: The National Academies Press.

National Swedish Police Board [Rikspolisstyrelsen] (2003) *Regional report.* POL-420-2705/02.

Navarro M. (1996) Marijuana farms are flourishing indoors, producing a more potent drug. *The New York Times*, 24 November: Section 1: 18.

Neeleman J. and Farrell M. (1997) Fatal methadone and heroin overdoses: time trends in England and Wales. *Journal of Epidemiology and Community Health* **51**, 435–7.

Neill M., Christie P., and Cormack S. (1991) *Trends in alcohol and other drug use by South Australian school children, 1986–1989.* Adelaide, Australia: Drug and Alcohol Services Council South Australia.

Nerad J. and Neradova L. (1991) Alcohol and drug problems in Czechoslovakia. *Journal of Substance Abuse Treatment* **8**, 83–8.

Neumark Y.D., Grotto I., and Kark J.D. (2004) Twenty-year trends in illicit drug use among young Israelis completing military duty. *Addiction* **99**, 641–8.

New York Times (1998) Mexico Adds to Sentence in Drug Corruption Case. 7 June, New York edition: Section 1: 14.

Newman R.G. and Whitehill W.B. (1979) Double-blind comparisons of methadone and placebo maintenance treatments of narcotic addicts. *Lancet* **2**, 485–8.

Newman R.K. (1995) Opium smoking in late imperial china. *Modern Asian Studies* **29**, 765–94.

Nicholas S., Kershaw C., and Walker A. (eds) (2007) *Home office statistical bulletin: Crime in England and Wales 2006/07*, 4th edn. London, UK: Home Office.

NIJ. See National Institute of Justice.

Nordt C. and Stohler R. (2006) Incidence of heroin use in Zurick, Swizerland; a treatment case register analysis. *Lancet* **367**, 1830–34.

Norwegian Institute for Alcohol and Drug Research (2008) *Illicit drug use statistics among 15–20-year-olds.* Oslo, Norway: SIRUS (Norwegian Institute for Alcohol and Drug Research).

Novins D.K., Beals J., and Mitchell C.M. (2001) Sequences of substance use among American Indian adolescents. *Journal of the American Academy of Child and Adolescent Psychiatry* **40**, 1168–74.

Nutt D.J., King L.A., Saulsbury B., and Blakemore C. (2007) Development of a rational scale to assess the harm of the drugs of potential misuse. *Lancet* **369**, 1047–53.

O'Connell M.E., Boat T., and Warner K.E. (eds) (2009) *Preventing mental, emotional and behavioral disorders amongst young people: progress and possibilities.* Washington, DC: National Academies Press.

O'Donnell J.A. (1969) *Narcotic addicts in Kentucky.* Chevy Chase, MD: National Institute of Mental Health (US Government Printing Office).

O'Driscoll P., McGough J., Hogan H., Thiede H., Critchlow C., and Alexander R. (2001) Predictors of accidental fatal drug overdose among a cohort of injection drug users. *American Journal of Public Health* **92**, 984–7.

Obot I.S. (2004) Assessing Nigeria's drug control policy, 1994–2000. *International Journal of Drug Control Policy* **15**, 17–26.

Obot I.S. (1990) Substance abuse, health and social welfare in Africa: an analysis of the Nigerian experience. *Social Science and Medicine* **31**, 699–704.

Obot I.S. (1992) Ethical and legal issues in the control of drug abuse and drug trafficking: the Nigerian case. *Social Science and Medicine* **35**, 481–93.

Obot I.S. and Anthony J.C. (2000) School dropout and injecting drug use in a national sample of white non-Hispanic American adults. *Journal of Drug Education* **30**, 145–52.

Ochoa K., Hahn J., Seal K., and Moss A. (2001) Overdosing among young injection drug users in San Francisco. *Addictive Behaviors* **26**, 453–60.

Office of National Drug Control Policy (1997) *The national drug control strategy, 1997: FY 1998 budget strategy.* Washington, DC: ONDCP. Available at: http://www.ncjrs.gov/htm/tables.htm#table3 (accessed 31 July 2006).

Office of National Drug Control Policy (2001a) *National drug control strategy: 2001 annual report.* Washington, DC: ONDCP.

Office of National Drug Control Policy (2001b) *What America's users spend on illicit drugs.* Washington, DC: Executive Office of the President.

Office of National Drug Control Policy (2004a) *The economic costs of drug abuse in the United States, 1992–2002.* Publication No. 207303. Washington, DC: Executive Office of the President.

Office of National Drug Control Policy (2004b) *The price and purity of illicit drugs: 1981 through the 2nd quarter of 2003.* Washington, DC: ONDCP.

Office of National Drug Control Policy (2006) *Certification for major illicit drug producing and transit countries.* ONDCP fact sheet. Available at: http://www.whitehousedrugpolicy.gov/publications/international/factsht/cert_major_illct.html (accessed 25 May 2009).

Office of the Auditor General of Canada (2001) *2001 December report of the Auditor General of Canada.* Ottawa, Canada: Office of the Auditor General of Canada. Available from: http://www.oag-bvg.gc.ca/internet/English/parl_oag_200112_e_1134.html (accessed 12 May 2009).

Office of the Inspector General, Audit Division (2007) *The Drug Enforcement Administration's international operations.* Audit Report 07-19 (redacted—public version). Washington, DC: US Department of Justice. Available at: http://www.usdoj.gov/oig/reports/DEA/a0719/final.pdf (accessed 25 May 2009).

Oliver R.G. and Hetzel B.S. (1972) Rise and fall of suicide rates in Australia: relation to sedative availability. *Medical Journal of Australia* **2**, 919–23.

Oliver R.G. and Hetzel B.S. (1973) An analysis of recent trends in suicide rates in Australia. *International Journal of Epidemiology* **2**, 91–101.

Omoluabi P.F. (1995) A review of the incidence of nonprescription psychoactive substance use/misuse in Nigeria. *Substance Use and Misuse* **30**, 445–58.

ONDCP. See Office of National Drug Control Policy.

Orwin R., Cadell D., Chu A., Kalton G., Maklan D., Morin C., Piesse A., Sridharan S., Steele D., Taylor K., and Tracy E. (2006) *Evaluation of the national youth anti-drug media campaign: 2004 report of findings.* Washington, DC: National Institute on Drug Abuse.

Owen D. (1934) *British opium policy in China and India.* New Haven, CT: Yale University Press (reprint 1968).

Pacula R.L. (1998) Does increasing the beer tax reduce marijuana consumption?. *Journal of Health Economics* **17**, 557–86.

Pacula R.L., Grossman M., Chaloupka F.J., O'Malley P.M., and Farrelly M.C. (2001) Marijuana and youth. In: Gruber J. (ed.) *Risky behavior among youths: an economic analysis.* pp. 271–326, Chicago, IL: University of Chicago Press.

Pacula R.L., Chriqui J.F., and King J. (2003) *Decriminalization in the United States: what does it mean?* National Bureau of Economic Research Working Paper No. 9690. Cambridge, MA: NBER.

Pacula R.L., Chriqui J.F. and King J. (2004) *Marijuana decriminalization: what does it mean in the United States?* NBER Working Paper No. 9690. Santa Monica, CA: RAND. Available at: http://www.rand.org/pubs/working_papers/2004/RAND_WR126.pdf (accessed 19 May 2009).

Paglia A. and Room R. (1999) Preventing substance abuse problems among youth: a literature review and recommendations. *Journal of Primary Prevention* **20**, 3–50.

Palm Beach County Sheriff's Office (2001) Prescription fraud. Palm Beach, FL: PBSO, Drug Division Unit. Available at: http://www.pbso.org/oldpbso/PBSO_Org/Law_Enforcement/Drug_Diversion/drug_diversion.htm (accessed 20 May 2009).

Pan L. (1975) *Alcohol in colonial Africa.* Helsinki, Finland: Finnish Foundation for Alcohol Studies.

Paoli L. (2000) *Drug markets in Frankfurt and Milan.* Freiburg, Germany: Max Plank Institute.

Paoli L. (2003) *Mafia brotherhoods.* London, UK: Oxford University Press.

Paoli L., Rabkov I., Greenfield V., and Reuter P. (2007) Tajikistan: the rise of a narco-state. *Journal of Drug Issues* **37**, 951–79.

Paoli L., Greenfield V.A., and Reuter P. (2009a) *The world heroin market: Can supply be cut?* Oxford, UK: Oxford University Press.

Paoli L., Greenfield V.A., Charles M., and Reuter P. (2009b) The global diversion of pharmaceutical drugs. India: the third largest illicit opium producer? *Addiction* **104**, 347–54.

Parker H., Bury C., and Egginton R. (1998) *New heroin outbreaks amongst young people in England and Wales.* Crime detection and prevention series. Paper 92. London, UK: Home Office, Police Research Group.

Parker H., Newcombe R., and Bakx K. (1987) The new heroin users: prevalence and characteristics in Wirral, Merseyside. *British Journal of Addiction* **82**, 147–57.

Parry C.D., Bhana A., Plüddemann A., Myers B., Siegfried N., Morojele N.K., Flisher A.J., and Kozel N.J. (2002) The South African Community Epidemiology Network on Drug Use (SACENDU): description, findings (1997–99) and policy implications. *Addiction* **97**, 969–76.

Parry C.D.H., Myers B., Morojele N.K., Flisher A.J., Bhana A., Donson H., and Plüddemann A. (2004) Trends in adolescent alcohol and other drug use: findings from three sentinel sites in South Africa (1997–2001). *Journal of Adolescence* **27**, 429–40.

Patterson K.M., Holman C.D., English D.R., Hulse G.K., and Unwin E. (1999) First-time hospital admissions with illicit drug problems in indigenous and non-indigenous Western Australians: an application of record linkage to public health surveillance. *Australian and New Zealand Journal of Public Health* **23**, 460–3.

Paulozzi L., Bundnitz D., and Xi Y. (2006) Increasing deaths from opioid analgesics in the United States. *Pharmacoepidemiology and Drug Safety* **15**, 618–627.

Pearson G. and Hobbs D. (2001) *Middle market drug distribution.* Home Office Research Study no. 227. London, UK: The Home Office.

Peles E., Schreiber S., Gordon J., and Adelson M. (2005) Significantly higher methadone dose for methadone maintenance treatment (MMT) patients with chronic pain. *Pain* **113**, 340–6.

Perkonigg A., Lieb R., and Wittchen H.-U. (1998) Substance use, abuse and dependence in Germany: a review of selected epidemiological data. *European Addiction Research* **4**, 8–17.

Perry C.L., Komro K.A., Veblen-Mortensen S., Bosma L.M., Farbakhsh K., Munson K.A., Stigler M.H., and Lytle L.A. (2003) A randomized controlled trial of the middle and junior high school DARE and DARE plus programs. *Archives of Pediatrics and Adolescent Medicine* **157**, 178–84.

Phillips C.D., Hubbard R.L., Dunteman G., Fountain D.L., Czechowicz D., and Cooper J.R. (1995) Measuring program performance in methadone treatment using in-treatment outcomes: an illustration. *Journal of Mental Health Administration* **22**, 214–25.

Pietschmann T. (2004) Price-setting behavior in the heroin market. *Bulletin on Narcotics* **56**, 105–39.

Pijlman F.T.A., Rigter S.M., Hoek J., Goldschmidt H.M.J., and Niesink R.J.M. (2005) Strong increase in total delta-THC in cannabis preparations sold in Dutch coffee shops. *Addiction Biology* **10**, 171–180.

Pimlott N.J., Hux J.E., Wilson L.M., Kahan M., Li C., and Rosser W.W. (2003) Educating physicians to reduce benzodiazepine use by elderly patients: a randomized controlled trial. *Canadian Medical Association Journal* **168**, 835–9.

Plunkett M. and Mitchell C.M. (2000) Substance use rates among American Indian adolescents: regional comparisons with Monitoring the Future high school seniors. *Journal of Drug Issues* **30**, 575–91.

Pocock S.J. and Elbourne D.R. (2000) Randomized trials or observational tribulations?. *New England Journal of Medicine* **342**, 1907–9.

Pollack H.A. (2001) Cost-effectiveness of harm reduction in preventing hepatitis C among injection drug users. *Medical Decision Making* **21**, 357–67.

Popova S., Rehm J., and Patra J. (2006) Illegal drug-attributable mortality and potential years of life lost in Canada 2002: conclusions for prevention and policy. *Contemporary Drug Problems* **33**, 343–66.

Porter C.J.W. and Armstrong J.R. (2004) Burns from illegal drug manufacture: case series and management. *Journal of Burn Care and Rehabilitation* **25**, 314–18.

Porter L., Argandoña M., and Curran W.J. (1999) *Drug and alcohol dependence policies, legislation and programmes for treatment and rehabilitation.* Geneva, Switzerland: WHO.

Poshyachinda V., Ch'ien J.M.N., Suwaki H., Robinson D., and Willie, R. (1982) Treatment is a cultural process and social act. *UNESCO Courier* **35**, 20–4.

Power R. (1994) Drug trends since 1968. In: Strang J. and Gossop M. (eds) *Heroin addiction and the British system*, pp. 29–41. Oxford, UK: Oxford University Press.

Poznyak V.B., Pelipas V.E., Vievski A.N., and Miroshnichenko L. (2002) Illicit drug use and its health consequences in Belarus, Russian Federation and Ukraine: impact of transition. *European Addiction Research* **8**, 184–9.

Preble E. and Casey J.J. (1969) Taking care of business: the heroin user's life on the street. *International Journal of the Addictions* **4**, 1–24.

Prendergast M.L., Podus D., Chang E., and Urada D. (2002) The effectiveness of drug abuse treatment: a meta-analysis of comparison group studies. *Drug and Alcohol Dependence* **67**, 53–73.

Prendergast M.L., Podus D., Finney J.W., Greenwell L., and Roll, J. (2006) Contingency management for treatment of substance use disorders: a meta-analysis. *Addiction* **101**, 1546–60.

Preston J. (1997). Mexico's drug czar busted. *The New York Times*, 23 February: Section 4: 2.

Prezelj I. and Gaber M. (2005) *Smuggling as a threat to national and international security: Slovenia and the Balkan route.* Athena Papers Series No 5. Garmisch-Partenkirchen, Germany: PfP Consortium of Defense Academies and Security Studies Institutes.

Prior M.J., Cooper K., Cummins P., and Bowen D. (2004) Acetaminophen availability increases in Canada with no increase in the incidence of reports of inpatient hospitalizations with acetaminophen overdose and acute liver toxicity. *American Journal of Therapeutics* **11**, 443–52.

QUERI Substance Abuse Module Executive Committee. (2001) Treatment for opiate dependence. *VA Practice Matters* **6**, 1–6.

Rajkumar A. and French M. (1997) Drug abuse, crime costs, and the economic benefits of treatment. *Journal of Quantitative Criminology* **13**, 291–323.

Ramsay M. and Percy A. (1997) A national household survey of drug misuse in Britain: a decade of development. *Addiction* **92**, 931–7.

Ramstedt M. (2006) What drug policies cost: Estimating drug policy expenditures in Sweden, 2002. *Addiction* **101**, 330–8.

Rasmussen D.W. and Benson B.L. (1994) *The economic anatomy of a drug war.* Lanham, MD: Rowman and Littlefield.

Rawson R., Marinelli-Casey P., Anglin M.D., Dickow A., Frazier Y., Gallagher C., Galloway G., Herrell J., Huber A., McCann M., Obert J., Pennell S., Reiber C., Vandersloot D., and Zweben J. (2004) A multi-site comparison of psychosocial approaches for the treatment of methamphetamine dependence. *Addiction* **99**, 708–17.

Rehm J. and Room R. (2005) The global burden of disease attributable to alcohol, tobacco and illicit drugs (2005). In: Stockwell T., Gruenewald P., Toumbourou T., and Loxley W. (eds) *Preventing harmful substance use: the evidence base for policy and practice*, pp. 25–41. Chichester, UK: Wiley.

Rehm J., Geschwend P., Steffen T., Gutzwiller F., Dobler-Mikola A., and Uchtenhagen A. (2001) Feasibility, safety, and efficacy of injectable heroin prescription for refractory opioid addicts: a follow-up study. *Lancet* **358**, 1417–23.

Rehm J., Room R., van den Brinkt W., and Kraus L. (2005) Problematic drug use and drug use disorders in EU countries and Norway: an overview of the epidemiology. *European Neuropsychopharmacology* **15**, 389–97.

Rehm J., Baliunas D., Brochu S., Fischer B., Gnam W., Patra J., Popova S., Sarnocinska-Hart A., and Taylor B. (2006) *The costs of substance abuse in Canada 2002.* Ottawa, Canada: Canadian Centre on Substance Abuse.

Reinarman C. (2009) Cannabis policies and user practices: market separation, price, potency, and accessibility in Amsterdam and San Francisco. *International Journal of Drug Policy* **20**, 28–37.

Resnik D.B. (2007) *The price of truth: how money affects the norms of science.* Oxford, UK, Oxford University Press.

Reuter P. (1983) *Disorganized crime: the economics of the visible hand.* Cambridge, MA: MIT Press.

Reuter P. (2001) Why does research have so little impact on American drug policy?. *Addiction* **96**, 373–6.

Reuter P. (2006) What drug policies cost: estimating government drug policy expenditures. *Addiction* **101**, 315–322.

Reuter P. and Caulkins J.P. (2004) Illegal lemons: price dispersion in the cocaine and heroin markets. *UN Bulletin on Narcotics* **56**, 141–65.

Reuter P. and Kleiman M. (1986) Risks and prices: An economic analysis of drug enforcement. *Crime and Justice: An Annual Review* **9**, 128–79.

Reuter P. and MacCoun R.J. (1992) Street drug markets in inner-city neighbourhoods. In: Steinberg J.B., Lyon D.W., and Vaiana M.E. (eds) *Urban America.* Santa Monica, CA: RAND.

Reuter P. and MacLean-Abaroa R. (2008) *Drug control in Bolivia.* Draft. Available at: http://www.puaf.umd.edu/faculty/reuter/Working%20Papers/Publications.htm.

Reuter P. and Pollack H. (2006) How much can treatment reduce national drug problems?. *Addiction* **101**, 341–7.

Reuter P. and Ronfeldt D. (1992) Quest for integrity: the Mexican–U.S. drug issue in the 1980s. *Journal of Interamerican Affairs* **34**, 89–153.

Reuter P. and Stevens A. (2007) *An analysis of UK drug policy.* London, UK: Drug Policy Commission.

Reuter P. and Trautmann F. (eds) (2009) *A report on global illicit drugs markets, 1998–2007.* The Netherlands: European Commission.

Reuter P., Crawford G., and Cave J. (1988) *Sealing the borders; the effects of increased military participation in drug interdiction.* Santa Monica, CA: RAND.

Reuter P., MacCoun R., and Murphy P. (1990) *Money from crime: a study of the economics of drug dealing in Washington, D.C.* Santa Monica, CA: RAND.

Rhee S.H., Hewitt J.K., Young S.E., Corley R.P., Crowley T.J., and Stallings M.C. (2003) Genetic and environmental influences on substance initiation, use, and problem use in adolescents. *Archives of General Psychiatry* **60**, 1256–64.

Rhodes,W.R., Hyatt R., and Scheiman P. (1994) The price of cocaine, heroin, and marijuana, 1981–1993. *Journal of Drug Issues* **24**, 383–402.

Rhodes T., Ball A., Stimson G.V., Kobyshcha Y., Fitch C., Pokrovsky V., Bezruchenko-Novachuk M., Burrows D., Renton A., and Andrushchak L. (1999) HIV infection associated with drug injecting in the newly independent states, eastern Europe: the social and economic context of epidemics. *Addiction* **94**, 1323–36.

Richard J. and Reidenberg M. (2005) The risk of disciplinary action by state medical boards against physicians prescribing opioids. *Journal of Pain and Symptom Management* **29**, 206–12.

Rigter H. (2006) What drug policies cost: drug policy spending in the Netherlands in 2003. *Addiction* **101**, 323–9.

Riley K.J. (1997) *Crack, powder cocaine, and heroin: drug purchase and use patterns in six U.S. cities.* Washington, DC: National Institute of Justice and Office of National Drug Control Policy.

Ritter A. and Di Natale R. (2005) The relationship between take-away methadone policies and methadone diversion. *Drug and Alcohol Review* **24**, 347–52.

Robins L.N. and Slobodyan S. (2003) Post-Vietnam heroin use and injection by returning US veterans: clues to preventing injection today. *Addiction* **98**, 1053–60.

Robins L.N., Davis D.H., and Nurco D.N. (1974) How permanent was Vietnam drug addiction?. *American Journal of Public Health* **64** (Suppl), 38–43.

Robinson J. (2001) *Prescription games: money, ego and power inside the global pharmaceutical industry.* London, UK: Simon & Schuster.

Rocheleau A.M. and Boyum D. (1994) *Measuring heroin availability in three cities.* Washington, DC: Office of National Drug Control Policy.

Roe S. and Becker J. (2005) Drug prevention with vulnerable young people: a review. *Drugs: Education, Prevention and Policy* **12**, 85–99.

Roizen R. (1991) *The American discovery of alcoholism, 1933–1939.* Doctoral dissertation. Berkeley, CA: University of California, Berkeley. Available at: http://www.roizen.com/ron/disshome.htm (accessed 25 May 2009).

Room R. (1975) Normative perspectives on alcohol use and problems. *Journal of Drug Issues* **5**, 358–68.

Room R. (1980) Treatment-seeking populations and larger realities. In: Edwards G. and Grant M. (eds) *Alcoholism treatment in transition*, pp. 205–24. London, UK: Croom Helm.

Room R. (1984) A 'reverence for strong drink': the lost generation and the elevation of alcohol in American culture. *Journal of Studies on Alcohol* **45**, 540–6.

Room R. (1989) Drugs, consciousness and self-control: popular and medical conceptions. *International Review of Psychiatry* **1**, 63–70.

Room R. (1999) The rhetoric of international drug control. *Substance Use and Misuse* **34**, 1689–707.

Room R. (2000) Control systems for psychoactive substances. In: Ferrence R., Slade J., Room R., and Pope M. (eds) *Nicotine and public health*, pp. 36–61. Washington, DC: American Public Health Association.

Room R. (2001) Intoxication and bad behaviour: understanding cultural differences in the link. *Social Science and Medicine* **53**, 189–98.

Room R. (2002a) 'Nobody likes coercion': current themes and issues in the international drug control system. *Nordic Alcohol and Drug Studies Engl. suppl* **19**, 83–9.

Room R. (ed.) (2002b) *The effects of Nordic alcohol policies: what happens to drinking when alcohol controls change?* NAD Publication 42. Helsinki, Finland: Nordic Council for Alcohol and Drug Research. Available at: http://www.nad.fi/pdf/NAD_42.pdf (accessed 19 May 2009).

Room R. (2005a) Stigma, social inequality and alcohol and drug use. *Drug and Alcohol Review* **24**, 143–55.

Room R. (2005b) Symbolism and rationality in the politics of psychoactive substances. In: Lindgren B. and Grossman M. (eds) *Substance use: individual behaviour, social interactions, markets and politics*, pp. 331–46. Advances in Health Economics and Health Services Research, vol. 16. Amsterdam, The Netherlands: Elsevier.

Room R. (2005c) Trends and issues in the international drug control system—Vienna 2003. *Journal of Psychoactive Drugs* **37**, 373–83.

Room R. (2006) The dangerousness of drugs. *Addiction* **101**, 166–8.

Room R. and Paglia A. (1999) The international drug control system in the post-Cold War era: managing markets or Fighting a war?. *Drug and Alcohol Review* **18**, 305–16.

Room R., Fischer B., Hall W., Lenton S., and Reuter P. (2008) *Cannabis policy: moving beyond stalemate*. Beckley Park, UK: Beckley Foundation. Available at: http://www.beckleyfoundation.org/pdf/BF_Cannabis_Commission_Report.pdf (accessed 19 May 2009).

Roques B. (chair) (1999) *La dangerosité de drogues: rapport au Secrétariat d'Etat à la Santé* (The dangerousness of drugs: report to the State Secretariat for Health). Paris, France: La Documentation Française-Odile Jacob.

Rose G. (1985) Sick individuals and sick populations. *International Journal of Epidemiology* **14**, 32–8.

Rose G. (1992) *The strategy of preventive medicine*. Oxford, UK: Oxford University Press.

Rose N. (2007) Psychopharmaceuticals in Europe. In: Knapp M., McDaid D., Mossialos E., and Thornicroft G. (eds) *Mental health policy and practices across Europe: the future direction of mental health care*, pp. 146–187. Maidenhead, UK: Open University Press.

Rosenblum A., Joseph H., Fong C., Kipnis S., Cleland C., and Portenoy R.K. (2003) Prevalence and characteristics of chronic pain among chemically dependent patients in methadone maintenance and residential treatment facilities. *Journal of the American Medical Association* **289**, 2370–8.

Rosenqvist P. and Kurube N. (1992) Dissolving the Swedish alcohol treatment system. In: Klingemann H., Takala J.P., and Hunt G. (eds) *Cure, care or control: alcoholism treatment in sixteen countries*, pp. 65–86. Albany, NY: State University of New York Press.

Rosenqvist P. and Stenius K. (1986) Nya målgrupper för alkoholistvården (New target groups for alcohol treatment). *Alkoholpolitik-Tidskrift för nordisk alkoholforskning* **3–4**, 215–19.

Ross J., Teesson M., Darke S., Lynskey M., Ali R., Ritter A., and Cooke R. (2004) *Twelve month outcomes of treatment for heroin dependence: findings from the Australian Treatment Outcome Study (ATOS)*. NDARC Technical Report No. 196. Sydney, Australia: National Drug and Alcohol Research Centre, University of New South Wales.

Ross-Degnan D., Soumerai S., Fortess E.E., and Gurwitz J.H. (1993) Examining product risk in context: market withdrawal of zomepirac as a case study. *Journal of the American Medical Association* **270**, 1937–42.

Roughead E.E., Semple S.J., and Vitry A.I. (2005) Pharmaceutical care services: a systematic review of published studies, 1990 to 2003, examining effectiveness in improving patient outcomes. *International Journal of Pharmacy Practice* **13**, 53–70.

Roy K., Hay G., Andragetti R., Taylor A., Goldberg D., and Wiessing L. (2002) Monitoring hepatitis C virus infection among injecting drug users in the European Union: a review of the literature. *Epidemiology and Infection* **129**, 577–585.

Royal College of Psychiatrists and Royal College of Physicians (2000) *Drugs: dilemmas and choices*. London, UK: Gaskell.

Ruhm C.J. (2000) Are recessions good for your health?. *Quarterly Journal of Economics* **115**, 617–50.

Rush B. (1996) Alcohol and other drug problems and treatment systems: a framework for research and development. *Addiction* **91**, 629–42.

Ryan J.M., Kidder S.W., Daiello L.A., and Tariot P.N. (2002) Psychopharmacologic interventions in nursing homes: What do we know and where should we go?. *Psychiatric Services* **53**, 1407–13.

Rydell C.P. and Everingham S.S. (1994) *Controlling cocaine: supply versus demand programs*. MR-331-ONDCP/A/DPRC. Santa Monica, CA: RAND.

Sacks H., Chalmers T.C., and Smith H., Jr. (1982) Randomized versus historical controls for clinical trials. *American Journal of Medicine* **72**, 233–40.

Saffer H. and Chaloupka F.J. (1999a) Demographic differentials in the demand for alcohol and illicit drugs. In: Chaloupka F.J., Grossman M., Bickel W.K., and Saffer H. (eds) *The economic analysis of substance use and abuse: an integration of econometric and behavioral economic research*, pp. 187–211. Chicago, IL: University of Chicago Press.

Saffer H. and Chaloupka F.J. (1999b) The demand for illicit drugs. *Economic Inquiry* **37**, 401–11.

Saffer H., Chaloupka F.J., and Dave D. (2001) State drug control spending and illicit drug participation. *Contemporary Economic Policy* **19**, 150–61.

Sajan A., Corneil T., and Grzybowski S. (1998) The street value of prescription drugs. *Canadian Medical Association Journal* **159**, 139–42.

Saltz R.F. (2005) What is 'evidence' and can we provide it? In: Stockwell T., Gruenwald P.J., Toumbourou J.W., and Loxley W. (eds) *Preventing harmful substance use: the evidence base for policy and practice*, pp. 313–23. Chichester, UK: John Wiley & Sons.

SAMHSA. See Substance Abuse and Mental Health Services Administration.

Samii A.W. (2003) Drug abuse, Iran's thorniest problem. *Brown Journal of World Affairs* **9**, 283–99.

Sampson R. J. and Raudenbush S.W. (1999) Systematic social observation of public spaces: a new look at disorder in urban neighborhoods. *American Journal of Sociology* **105**, 603–51.

Samuels D. (2008) Dr. Kush: how medical marijuana is transforming the pot industry. *New Yorker* July 28. Available at: http://www.newyorker.com/reporting/2008/07/28/080728fa_fact_samuels (accessed 20 May 2009).

Sarason S. (1978) The nature of problem solving in social action. *American Psychologist* **33**, 370–80.

Saveland W. and Bray D.F. (1981) Trends in cannabis use among American states with different and changing legal regimes, 1972–1977. *Contemporary Drug Problems* **10**, 335–61.

Saxe L., Kadushin C., Beveridge A., Livert D., Tighe E., Rindskopf D., Ford J., and Brodsky A. (2001) The visibility of illicit drugs: implications for community-based drug control strategies. *American Journal of Public Health* **91**, 1987–94.

Schaepe H. (1999) INCB position on shooting galleries [letter to Father John M. George, Chaplain, CFC Waverley Community, 20 August]. Available at: http://www.endeavourforum.org.au/March2001-08a.htm.

Schinke S.P., Tepavac L.O., and Cole K.C. (2000) Preventing substance use among native American youth: three-year results. *Addictive Behaviors* **25**, 387–97.

Schmid H. (2001) Cannabis use in Switzerland: the role of attribution of drug use to friends, urbanization and repression. *Swiss Journal of Psychology* **60**, 99–107.

Schrad M.L. (2007) *The prohibition option: transnational temperance and national policymaking in Russia, Sweden and the United States.* Doctoral dissertation. Madison, WI: University of Wisconsin.

Schweich T. (2008) 'Is Afghanistan a narco-state?' *New York Times Magazine* July 27, New York edition, MM45. Available at: http://www.nytimes.com/2008/07/27/magazine/27AFGHAN-t.html (accessed 25 May 2009).

Science. (1990) Still flying blind in the war on drugs. *Science* **250**, 28.

Scott M.S. (2003) *The benefits and consequences of police crackdowns.* US Department of Justice Problem-Oriented Guides for Police, No. 1. Washington DC: United States Government Printing Office.

Seaman S., Brettle R., and Gore S. (1998) Mortality from overdose among injecting drug users recently released from prison: database linkage study. *British Medical Journal* **316**, 426–8.

Sees K.L., Delucchi K.L., Masson C., Rosen A., Clark H.W., Robillard H., Banys P., and Hall, S. (2000) Methadone maintenance versus 180-day psychosocially enriched detoxification for treatment of opioid dependence: a randomized controlled trial. *Journal of the American Medical Association* **283**, 1303–10.

Sevigny E.L. and Caulkins J.P. (2004) Kingpins or mules? An analysis of drug offenders incarcerated in federal and state prisons. *Criminology and Public Policy* **3**, 401–34.

Shepard C.W., Finelli L., and Alter M.J. (2005) Global epidemiology of hepatitis C virus infection. *Lancet Infectious Diseases* **5**, 558–67.

Sheridan J. and Butler R. (2008) *Prescription drug misuse: issues for primary care. Final report of findings.* Auckland, NZ: School of Pharmacy, University of Auckland. Available at: http://www.ndp.govt.nz/moh.nsf/pagescm/7540/$File/prescription-drug-misuse-primary-care-2008v2.pdf (accessed 14 May 2009).

Shih Y.-C.T., Pasad M., and Luce B.R. (2002) The effect on social welfare of a switch of second-generation antihistamines from prescription to over-the-counter status: a microeconomic analysis. *Clinical Therapeutics* **24**, 701–16.

Shrestha N.M. (1992) Alcohol and drug abuse in Nepal. *British Journal of Addiction* **87**, 1241–8.

Shrestha S., Smith M.W., Broman K.W., Farzadegan H., Vlahov D., and Strathdee S.A. (2006) Multi-person-use of syringes among injection drug users in a needle exchange program: a gene based molecular epidemiological analysis. *Journal of Acquired Immune Deficiency Syndrome* **43**, 335–43.

Shults R.A., Elder R.W., Sleet D.A., Nichols J.L., Alao M.O., Carande-Kulis V.G., Zaza S., Sosin D.M., Thompson R.S., and the Task Force on Community Prevention Services. (2001) Reviews of evidence regarding interventions to reduce alcohol-impaired driving. *American Journal of Preventive Medicine* **21**(Suppl. 1), 66–88.

Sibbald B. (2002) Medical marijuana program 'a sham': lawyer. *Canadian Medical Association Journal* **167**, 1153.

Simkin S., Hawton K., Sutton L., Gunnell D., Bennewith O., and Kapur N. (2005) Co-proxamol and suicide: preventing the continuing of overdose deaths. *Quarterly Journal of Medicine* **98**, 159–70.

Simoni-Wastila L. and Tompkins C. (2001) Balancing diversion control and medical necessity: the case of prescription drugs with abuse potential. *Substance Use and Misuse* **36**, 1275–96.

Simpson D.D., Wexler H.K. and Inciardi J.A. (eds) (1999) Drug treatment outcomes for correctional settings, Part I. *Prison Journal* **79** (special issue). 291–371.

Singer N. (2008) No mug? Drug makers cut out goodies for doctors. *New York Times* December 31, New York edition, A1.

Single E., Collins D., Easton B., Harwood H., Lapsley H., and Maynard A. (1996) *International guidelines for estimating the costs of substance abuse.* Ottawa: Canadian Centre on Substance Abuse.

Single E.W. (1981) The impact of marijuana decriminalization. In: Israel Y., Glaser F.B., Kalant H., Popham R.E., Schmidt W., and Smart R.G. (eds) *Research advances in alcohol and drug problems,* vol. 6, pp. 405–24. New York, NY: Plenum Press.

Single E.W. (1989) The impact of marijuana decriminalization: an update. *Journal of Public Health Policy* **10**, 456–66.

Singleton N., Murray R., and Tinsley L. (eds) (2004) *Measuring different aspects of problem drug use: methodological developments.* London, UK: Home Office.

Siqueira L.M. and Brook J.S. (2003) Tobacco use as a predictor of illicit drug use and drug-related problems in Colombian youth. *Journal of Adolescent Health* **32**, 50–7.

Skog O.-J. (1992) The validity of self-reported drug use. *Addiction* **87**, 539–48.

Skogan W. (1990) *Disorder and decline: Crime and the spiral of decay in American cities.* Berkeley, CA: University of California Press.

Skretting A. (2007) *Trends in adolescents' alcohol and drug use: 1968-2007.* Oslo, Norway: SIRUS (Norwegian Institute for Alcohol and Drug Research).

Slater M.D., Kelly K.J., Edwards R.W., Thurman P.J., Plested B.A., Keefe T.J., Lawrence F.R., and Henry K.L. (2006) Combining in-school and community-based media efforts: Reducing marijuana and alcohol uptake among younger adolescents. *Health Education Research* **21**, 157–67.

Sloboda Z. (2002) Changing patterns of 'drug abuse' in the United States: connecting findings from macro- and microepidemiologic studies. *Substance Use and Misuse* **37**, 1229–51.

Smart R.G. and Mann R.E. (2000) The impact of programs for high-risk drinkers on population levels of alcohol problems. *Addiction* **95**, 37–52.

Smart R.G. and Murray G.F. (1983) Drug abuse and affluence in five countries: a study of economic and health conditions, 1960–1975. *Drug and Alcohol Dependence* **11**, 297–307.

Smart R.G. and Ogborne A.C. (2000) Drug use and drinking among students in 36 countries. *Addictive Behaviors* **25**, 455–60.

Smith L., Watson M., Gates S., Ball D., and Foxcroft D.R. (2008) Meta-analysis of the association of the Taq1A polymorphism with the risk of alcohol dependency: a HuGE gene–disease association review. *American Journal of Epidemiology* **167**, 125–38.

Smith M.L., Glass G.V., and Miller T.I. (1980) *The benefits of psychotherapy.* Baltimore, MD: Johns Hopkins University Press.

Snow D.L., Tebes J.K., Arthur M.W., and Tapasak R.C. (1992) Two-year follow-up of a social–cognitive intervention to prevent substance use. *Journal of Drug Education* **22**, 101–14.

Snowdon M. and Roy-Byrne P. (1998) Mental illness and nursing home reform: OBRA-87 ten years later. *Psychiatric Services* **49**, 229–33. Available at: http://ps.psychiatryonline.org/cgi/content/full/49/2/229 (accessed 20 May 2009).

Solivetti L.M. (2001) *Drug use criminalization v. decriminalization: an analysis in the light of the Italian experience.* Bern, Switzerland: Swiss Federal Office of Public Health.

Solomon K.R., Anadon A., Cerdeira A.L., Marshall J., and Sanin L-H. (2005) *Environmental and human health assessment of the aerial spray program for coca and poppy control in Colombia*. Washington, DC: OAS/CICAD.

SourceWatch (2008) *Direct-to-consumer advertising: the campaign to overturn Europe's ban.* Madison, WI: Center for Media and Democracy. Available at: http://www.sourcewatch.org/index.php?title=Direct-to-consumer_advertising:_The_Campaign_To_Overturn_Europe%27s_Ban (accessed 15 May 2009).

Spear H.B. (1975) The British experience. *John Marshall Journal of Practice and Procedure* **9**, 67–98.

Spelman W. (2000) What recent studies do (and don't) tell us about imprisonment and crime. In: Tonry M. (ed.) *Crime and justice: a review of research*, Vol. **27**, pp. 419–94. Chicago, IL: University of Chicago Press.

Spooner C., McPherson M., and Hall W. (2004) *The role of police in preventing and minimising illicit drug use and its harms.* NDLERF Monograph Series No. 2. Hobart, Tasmania: National Drug Law Enforcement Research Fund.

Spoth R., Redmond C., Shin C., and Azevedo K. (2004) Brief family intervention effects on adolescent substance initiation: school-level growth curve analyses 6 years following baseline. *Journal of Consulting and Clinical Psychology* **72**, 535–42.

Spoth R.L., Clair S., Shin C., and Redmond C. (2006) Long-term effects of universal preventive interventions on methamphetamine use among adolescents. *Archives of Pediatrics and Adolescent Medicine* **160**, 876–82.

Stafford J., Degenhardt L., Black E., Bruno R., Buckingham K., Fetherston J., Jenkinson R., Kinner S., Newman J., and Weekley J. (2006) *Australian drug trends 2005: findings from the Illicit Drug Reporting System (IDRS)*. NDARC Monograph No 59. Sydney, Australia: National Drug and Alcohol Research Centre, University of New South Wales.

Stanton M.D. and Shadish W.R. (1997) Outcome, attrition, and family-couples treatment for drug abuse: a meta-analysis and review of the controlled, comparative studies. *Psychological Bulletin* **122**, 170–91.

Stares P.B. (1996) *Global habit: the drug problem in a borderless world.* Washington, DC: Brookings Institution.

Staulcup H., Kenward K., and Frigo D. (1979) A review of federal primary alcoholism prevention projects. *Journal of Studies on Alcohol* **40**, 943–68.

Steentoft A., Teige B., Ceder G., Vuori E., Kristinsson J., Simonsen K.W. Holmgren P., Wethe G., and Kaa E. (2001) Fatal poisoning in drug addicts in the Nordic countries. *Forensic Science International* **123**, 63–9.

Steentoft A., Teige B., Holmgren P., Vuori E., Kristinsson J., Hansen A., Ceder G., Wethe G., and Rollmann D. (2006) Fatal poisoning in Nordic drug addicts in 2002. *Forensic Science International* **160**, 148–56.

Stenius K. (1999) *Privat och offentligt I svensk alkoholistvard. Arbetsfordelning, samverkan och stynring under 1900-talet.* (Division of labour, co-operation and management principles during the 20th century). Lund, Sweden: Arkiv forlag.

Stenius K., Romelsjö A., and Storbjörk J. (2005) *Decentralisation and integration of addiction treatment: does it make any difference?* Paper presented at the 31st KBS Annual Epidemiology Symposium, Riverside, CA.

Stephens R.S., Roffman R.A., and Curtin L. (2000) Comparison of extended versus brief treatment for marijuana use. *Journal of Consulting and Clinical Psychology* **68**, 898–908.

Stewart D., Gossop M., Marsden J., and Rolfe A. (2000) Drug misuse and acquisitive crime among clients recruited to the National Treatment Outcome Research Study (NTORS). *Criminal Behaviour and Mental Health* **10**, 10–20.

Storr C.L., Arria A.M., Workman R.L., and Anthony J.C. (2004) Neighborhood environment and opportunity to try methamphetamine ('ice') and marijuana: evidence from Guam in the Western Pacific Region of Micronesia. *Substance Use and Misuse* **39**, 253–76.

Storti C.C. and De Grauwe P. (2009) Globalization and the price decline of illicit drugs. *International Journal of Drug Policy* **20**, 48–61.

Stoudemire A. and Smith D.A. (1996) OBRA regulations and the use of psychotropic drugs in long-term care facilities: impact and implications for geropsychiatric care. *General Hospital Psychiatry* **18**, 77–94.

Strain E.C., Bigelow G.E., Liebson I.A., and Stitzer M.L. (1999) Moderate- vs high-dose methadone in the treatment of opioid dependence: a randomized trial. *Journal of the American Medical Association* **281**, 1000–5.

Strang J. and Gossop M. (eds) (2005) *Heroin addiction and 'the British system': Volume 2—treatment and policy responses.* London, UK: Routledge.

Strang J., Sheridan J., and Barber N. (1996) Prescribing injectable and oral methadone to opiate addicts: Results from the 1995 national survey of community pharmacies in England and Wales. *British Medical Journal* **313**, 270–2.

Strang J., McCambridge J., Best D., Beswick T., Bearn J., Rees S., and Gossop M. (2003) Loss of tolerance and overdose mortality after inpatient opiate detoxification: follow up study. *British Medical Journal* **326**, 959–60.

Strang J., Manning V., Mayet S., Ridge G., Best D., and Sheridan J. (2007) Does prescribing for opiate addiction change after national guidelines? Methadone and buprenorphine prescribing to opiate addicts by general practitioners and hospital doctors in England, 1995–2005. *Addiction* **102**, 761–70.

Strathdee S., Patrick D., Archibald C., Ofner M., Cornelisse P., Rekart M., Schechter M., and O'Shaughnessy M. (1997) Social determinants predict needle-sharing behaviour among injection drug users in Vancouver, Canada. *Addiction* **92**, 1339–47.

Strathdee S., Galai N., Mahboobeh S., Vlahov D., Lisette J., and Kenrad N. (2001) Sex differences in risk factors for HIV seroconversion among injection drug users: a 10-year perspective. *Archives of Internal Medicine* **161**, 1281–8.

Streatfeild D. (2003) *Cocaine: an unauthorized biography*. New York, NY: Picador.

Streltzer J. (2005) Analgesia and opiate addicts—a response. *American Journal on Addictions* **14**, 396.

Stuart R.B., Guire K., and Krell M. (1976) Penalty for the possession of marijuana: an analysis of some of its concomitants. *Contemporary Drug Problems* **5**, 553–63.

Substance Abuse and Mental Health Services Administration (2006a) How young adults obtain prescription pain relievers for nonmedical usage. *The NSDUH report*. Issue 39. Available at: http://www.oas.samhsa.gov/2k6/getPain/getPain.htm (accessed 15 May 2009).

Substance Abuse and Mental Health Services Administration (2006b) *Treatment Episode Data Set (TEDS). Highlights—2005. National admissions to substance abuse treatment services.* DASIS Series: S-36, DHHS Publication No. (SMA) 07-4229, Rockville, MD: SAMHSA. Available at: http://oas.samhsa.gov/teds2k5/TEDSHi2k5Tbl4.htm (accessed 18 July 2007).

Substance Abuse and Mental Health Services Administration (2007) *Results from the 2006 national survey on drug use and health: national findings.* NSDUH Series H-32, DHHS Publication No SMA 07-4293. Rockville, MD: SAMHSA.

Sue S. (1998) In search of cultural competence in psychotherapy and counseling. *American Psychologist* **53**, 440–8.

Sussman S., Dent C.W., Stacy A.W., and Craig S. (1998) One-year outcomes of project towards no drug abuse. *Preventive Medicine* **27**, 632–42.

Swensen G. (1988) Opioid drug deaths in Western Australia: 1974–1984. *Drug and Alcohol Review* **7**, 181–5.

Swensen G. (2007) *Statutory review of cannabis control act 2003.* Report to the Minister for Health: Main report. Perth, Australia: Drug and Alcohol Office.

Tanaka-Matsumi J., Higginbotham H.N., and Chang R. (2002) Cognitive-behavioral approaches to counseling across cultures: a functional analytic approach for clinical applications. In: Pedersen P.B., Draguns J.G., Lonner W.J., and Trimble J.E. (eds) *Counseling across cultures*, pp. 337–53. Thousand Oaks, CA: Sage.

Tang Y-L. and Hao W. (2007) Improving drug treatment in China. *Addiction* **102**, 1057–63.

Tarricone R. (2006) Cost-of-illness analysis: what room in health economics?. *Health Policy* **77**, 51–63.

Taylor A. (1993) *Women drug users: an ethnography of a female injecting community.* Oxford, UK: Clarendon Press.

Teesson M., Hodder T., and Buhrich N. (2000) Substance use disorders among homeless people in inner Sydney. *Social Psychiatry and Psychiatric Epidemiology* **35**, 451–6.

Thom B. (1999) *Dealing with drink: alcohol and social policy: from treatment to management.* London, UK: Free Association Books.

Thorpe L.E., Ouellet L.J., Hershow R., Bailey S.L., Williams I.T., Williamson J., Monterroso E.R., and Garfein R.S. (2002) Risk of hepatitis C virus infection among young adult injection drug users who share injection equipment. *American Journal of Epidemiology* **155**, 645–53.

Thoumi F.E. (2003) *Illegal drugs, economy and society in the Andes.* Baltimore, MD: Johns Hopkins University Press.

Tiet Q.Q., Byrnes H.F., Barnett P., and Finney J.W. (2006) A practical system for monitoring the outcomes of substance use disorder patients. *Journal of Substance Abuse Treatment* **30**, 337–47.

Timko C., DeBenedetti A., and Billow R. (2006) Intensive referral to 12-step self-help groups and six-month substance use disorder outcomes. *Addiction* **101**, 678–88.

TNI. See Transnational Institute.

Tobin K. and Latkin C. (2003) The relationship between depressive symptoms and nonfatal overdose among a sample of drug users in Baltimore, Maryland. *Journal of Urban Health* **80**, 220–9.

Towns C.B. (1915) *Habits that handicap: the menace of opium, alcohol, and tobacco and the remedy.* New York, NY: The Century Co.

Tragler G., Caulkins J.P., and Feichtinger G. (2001) Optimal dynamic allocation of treatment and enforcement in illicit drug control. *Operations Research* **49**, 352–62.

Transnational Institute (2003) *Drugs and conflict in Burma (Myanmar): dilemmas for policy responses.* Drugs & Conflict Debate Paper 9. Amsterdam, The Netherlands: Transnational Institute.

Transnational Institute (2008) *Rewriting history: a response to the 2008 World Drug Report.* Drug Policy Briefing No. 26. Amsterdam, The Netherlands: Transnational Institute. Available at: http://www.ungassondrugs.org/images/stories/brief26.pdf (accessed 25 May 2009).

[Treaties] (2002) *The united nations drug control treaties.* Paris, France: Senlis Council.

Trimbos Institute (2006) *Prevention and reduction of health-related harm associated with drug dependence: an inventory of policies, evidence and practices in the EU relevant to the implementation of the Council Recommendation of 18 June 2003.* Utrecht, The Netherlands: Trimbos Institute.

Trygstad T.K., Hansen R.A., and Wegner S.E. (2006) Evaluation of product switching after a state Medicaid program began covering loratadine OTC one year after market availability. *Journal of Managed Care Pharmacy* **12**, 108–20.

Tyner E.A. and Fremouw W.J. (2008) The relation of methamphetamine use and violence: a critical review. *Aggression and Violent Behavior* **13**, 285–97.

Tyrrell I. (1991) *Women's world, women's empire: the Woman's Christian Temperance Union in international perspective, 1880–1930.* Chapel Hill, NC: University of North Carolina Press.

Uchtenhagen A., Ali R., Berglund M., Eap C., Farrell M., Mattick R., McLellan T., Rehm J., and Simpson S. (2004) *Methadone as a medicine for the management of opioid dependence and HIV/AIDS prevention.* Geneva, Switzerland: World Health Organization.

Uchtenhagen A., Ladjevic T., and Rehm J. (2007) *WHO guidelines for psychosocially assisted treatment of persons dependent on opioids: Background document.* Geneva, Switzerland: World Health Organization. Available at: http://www.who.int/substance_abuse/activities/background_paper.pdf (accessed 20 May 2009).

Uchtenhagen A., Stamm R., Huber J., and Vuille R. (2008) A review of systems for continued education and training in the substance abuse field. *Substance Abuse* **29**, 95–102.

UNAIDS (2006) *2006 report on the global AIDS epidemic.* Geneva, Switzerland: Joint UN Programme on HIV/AIDS. Available at: http://www.unaids.org/en/KnowledgeCentre/HIVData/GlobalReport/2006/default.asp (accessed 8 July 2009).

UNIDCP. See United Nations International Drug Control Programme.

United Nations. (1953) The surprising extinction of the charas traffic. *Bulletin on Narcotics* **1**, 1–14.

United Nations (1973) *Commentary on the single convention on narcotic drugs, 1961.* New York, NY: United Nations.

United Nations (1976) *Commentary on the protocol amending the single convention on narcotic drugs, 1961.* New York, NY: United Nations. Available at: http://www.drugtext.org/library/legal/treat/1971commentary/default.htm (accessed 25 May 2009).

United Nations (2001) *Protocol against the illicit manufacturing of and trafficking in firearms, their parts and components and ammunition, supplementing the United Nations convention against transnational organized crime.* General Assembly Resolution 55/255. A/RES/55/255. New York, NY: United Nations. A/RES/55/255. Available at: http://www.unodc.org/pdf/crime/a_res_55/255e.pdf (accessed 25 May 2009).

United Nations International Drug Control Programme (1997) *World drug report.* Oxford, UK: Oxford University Press.

United Nations International Drug Control Programme (2007) *World drug report 2007.* Vienna, Austria: United Nations Office on Drugs and Crime. Available at: http://www.unodc.org/india/world_drug_report_2007.html (accessed 25 May 2009).

United Nations International Drug Control Programme (2008) *World drug report 2008.* Vienna, Austria: United Nations Office on Drugs and Crime. Available at: http://www.unodc.org/unodc/en/data-and-analysis/WDR-2008.html (accessed 25 May 2009).

United Nations Office on Drugs and Crime (2000) *Global illicit drug trends 2000.* Vienna, Austria: UNODC. Available at: http://www.unodc.org/pdf/report_2000-09-21_1.pdf (accessed 14 May 2009).

United Nations Office on Drugs and Crime (2003a) *Global illicit drug trends.* Vienna, Austria: UNODC. Available at: http://www.unodc.org/unodc/en/data-and-analysis/global_illicit_drug_drug_trends.html (accessed 14 May 2009).

United Nations Office on Drugs and Crime (2003b) *The opium economy in Afghanistan: an international problem.* New York, NY: UNODC. Available at: http://www.unodc.org/pdf/publications/afg_opium_economy_2003.pdf (accessed 19 May 2009).

United Nations Office on Drugs and Crime (2003c) *Caribbean drug trends 2001–2002.* Bridgetown, Barbados: UNODC. Available at: http://www.scribd.com/doc/341545/01582caribbean-drugtrends-20012002 (accessed 19 May 2009).

United Nations Office on Drugs and Crime (2004) *Afghanistan: opium survey, 2004.* Vienna, Austria: UNODC. Available at: http://www.unodc.org/pdf/afg/afghanistan_opium_survey_2004.pdf (accessed 14 May 2009).

United Nations Office on Drugs and Crime (2005) *World drug report 2005.* Vienna, Austria: UNODC. Available at: http://www.unodc.org/unodc/en/data-and-analysis/WDR-2005.html (accessed 14 May 2009).

United Nations Office on Drugs and Crime (2006) *World drug report 2006.* Vienna, Austria: UNODC. Available at: http://www.unodc.org/unodc/en/data-and-analysis/WDR-2006.html (accessed 14 May 2009).

United Nations Office on Drugs and Crime (2007) *World drug report 2007.* Vienna, Austria: UNODC. Available at: http://www.unodc.org/unodc/en/data-and-analysis/WDR-2007.html (accessed 14 May 2009).

United Nations Office on Drugs and Crime (2008) *2008 World drug report.* Vienna, Austria: UNODC. Available at: http://www.unodc.org/documents/wdr/WDR_2008/WDR_2008_eng_web.pdf (accessed 14 May 2009).

United Nations Office on Drugs and Crime with the World Bank (2007) *Crime, violence and development: trends, costs, and policy options in the Caribbean.* Vienna and Washington, DC: UNODC/World Bank. Available at: http://www.unodc.org/pdf/research/Cr_and_Vio_Car_E.pdf (accessed 19 May 2009).

United States Department of State (2008) *International narcotics control strategy report.* Washington, DC: US Department of State. Available at: http://www.state.gov/p/inl/rls/nrcrpt/index.htm (accessed 19 May 2009).

United States Drug Enforcement Administration (2008) Marijuana. In: *National drug threat assessment 2009*, pp. 17–23. Washington, DC: National Drug Intelligence Center, US Department of Justice. Available at: http://www.usdoj.gov/dea/concern/18862/ndic_2009.pdf (accessed 14 May 2009).

UNODC. See United Nations Office on Drugs and Crime.

Uribe S. (2004) Development of the Colombian heroin industry: 1990–2003. Report submitted for the project *Modeling the world heroin market: Assessing the consequences of changes in Afghanistan production.* Mimeo.

USDEA. See United States Drug Enforcement Administration.

US Department of State, Bureau for International Narcotics and Law Enforcement Affairs (2003) *International narcotics control strategy report.* Washington, DC: US Government Printing Office. Available at: http://www.state.gov/p/inl/rls/nrcrpt/2002/index.htm (accessed 25 May 2009).

US Department of State, Bureau for International Narcotics and Law Enforcement Affairs (2008) *International narcotics control strategy report.* 2 vols. Washington, DC: US Government Printing Office. Available at: http://www.state.gov/p/inl/rls/nrcrpt/2008/index.htm (accessed 25 May 2009).

US General Accounting Office (1993) *Needle exchange programs: research suggests promise as an AIDS prevention strategy.* Report HRD-93-60. Washington, DC: United States GAO.

US General Accounting Office (1995) *Nonprescription drugs: value of a pharamcist-controlled class has yet to be demonstrated.* GAO/PEMD-95-12. Washington, DC: United States GAO. Available at: http://www.gao.gov/archive/1995/pe95012.pdf (accessed 20 May 2009).

US General Accounting Office (2002) *Prescription drugs: state monitoring programs provide useful tool to reduce diversion.* Washington, DC: US Government Printing Office.

US House of Representatives, Committee on Government Reform (2005) *The national drug control strategy for 2005 and the national drug control budget for fiscal year 2006.* Report #109-172. Washington, DC: Government Printing Office.

VandenBos G.R. (2007) *APA dictionary of psychology.* Washington, DC: American Psychological Association.

van den Brink W., Hendriks V.M., Blanken P., Koeter M.W.J., van Zwieten B.J., and van Ree J.M. (2003) Medical prescription of heroin to treatment resistant heroin addicts: two randomised controlled trials. *British Medical Journal* **327**, 310–12.

van Ours J.C. (1995) The price elasticity of hard drugs: the case of opium in the Dutch East Indies, 1923–1938. *Journal of Political Economy* **103**, 261–79.

van Ours J.C. (2003) Is cannabis a stepping-stone for cocaine?. *Journal of Health Economics* **22**, 539–54.

van Romunde L.K.J., Pepperlinkhuizen L., and Stronks D.L. (1992) Het aantal opnamen in Nederlandse ziekenhuizen voor barbituraatvergiftiging in de periode 1981–1989 en die voor vergiftiging met sedativa en hypnotica, en benzodiazepinen (The number of admissions to Dutch hospitals for barbiturate poisoning in the period 1981–1989 and those for poisoning with sedatives and hypnotics and benzodiazepines). *Nederlands Tijdschrift voor Geneeskunde* **136**, 1615–17.

Vargas R. (2002) The anti-drug policy, aerial spraying of illicit crops and their social, environmental, and political impacts in Colombia. *Journal of Drug Issues* **32**, 11–60.

Verstraete A.G. and Pierce A. (2001) Workplace drug testing in Europe. *Forensic Science International* **121**, 2–6.

Vick K. (2005) AIDS crisis brings radical change in Iran's response to heroin use. *Washington Post* 5 July, A09. Available at: http://www.washingtonpost.com/wp-dyn/content/article/2005/07/04/AR2005070401182.html (accessed 28 May 2009).

Victorri-Vigneau C., Basset G., Bourin M., and Jolliet P. (2003) Impacts de la nouvelle réglementation du flunitrazépam sur la consommation d'hypnotiques (Impacts of the new flunitrazepam regulations on the consumption of hypnotics). *Therapie* **58**, 425–30.

Vienna NGO Committee (2009) *Beyond 2008 Vienna: global summary report.* Vienna, Austria: Vienna NGO Committee. Available at: http://www.vngoc.org/images/uploads/file/GlobalSummaryReportBeyond2008(1).pdf (accessed 25 May 2009).

Voas R.B., Holder H.D., and Greunewald P.J. (1997) The effect of drinking and driving interventions on alcohol-involved traffic crashes within a comprehensive community trial. *Addiction* **92**, S221–36.

Wagner A.K., Soumerai S.B., Zhang F., Mah C., Simoni-Wastila L., Cosler L., Fanning T., Gallagher P., and Ross-Degnan D. (2003) Effects of state surveillance on new post-hospitalization benzodiazepine use. *International Journal for Quality in Health Care* **15**, 423–31.

Wagner F.A. and Anthony J.C. (2002) From first drug use to drug dependence: developmental periods of risk for dependence upon marijuana, cocaine, and alcohol. *Neuropsychopharmacology* **26**, 479–88.

Walker W.O., III (1992) International collaboration in historical perspective. In: Smith P.H. (ed.) *Drug policy in the Americas*, pp. 265–81. Boulder, CO: Westview Press.

Wall R., Rehm J., Fischer B., Brands B., Gliksman L., Stewart J., Medved W., and Blake J. (2000) Social costs of untreated opiate use. *Journal of Urban Health* **77**, 688–722.

Wallace J.M., Jr, Bachman J.G., O'Malley P.M., Johnston L.D., Schulenberg J.E., and Cooper S.M. (2002) Tobacco, alcohol, and illicit drug use: racial and ethnic differences among U.S. high school seniors, 1976–2000. *Public Health Reports* **117** (Suppl 1), S67–75.

Walsh J. (2004) *Are we there yet? Measuring success in the war on drugs in Latin America* A WOLA briefing series. Washington, DC: Washington Office on Latin America.

Walters S.T., Foy B.D., and Castro R.J. (2002) The agony of ecstasy: responding to growing MDMA use among college students. *Journal of American College Health* **51**, 139–41.

Ward C., Mansfield D., Oldham P. and Byrd W. (2007) *Afghanistan: economic incentives and development initiative to reduce opium production.* London, UK: Department for International Development and The World Bank.

Warner L.A., Kessler R.C., Hughes M., Anthony J.C., and Nelson C.B. (1995) Prevalence and correlates of drug use and dependence in the United States: results from the national comorbidity survey. *Archives of General Psychiatry* **52**, 219–29.

Warner-Smith M., Darke S., Lynskey M., and Hall W. (2001) Heroin overdose: causes and consequences. *Addiction* **96**, 1113–25.

Weatherburn D. and Lind B. (1997) The impact of law enforcement activity on a heroin market. *Addiction* **92**, 557–69.

Weatherburn D. and Lind B. (1999a) Street level drug law enforcement and entry into methadone maintenance treatment. *Addiction* **96**, 577–87.

Weatherburn D. and Lind B. (1999b) *Heroin harm minimisation: do we really have to choose between law enforcement and treatment?* Crime and Justice Bulletin 46. Sydney, Australia: New South Wales Bureau of Crime Statistics and Research.

Weekes L.M., Mackson J.M., Fitzgerald M., and Phillips S.R. (2005) National prescribing service: creating an implementation arm for national medicines policy. *British Journal of Clinical Pharmacology* **59**, 112–16.

Weick K.E. (1984) Small wins: redefining the scale of social issues. *American Psychologist* **39**, 40–9.

Weintraub M., Singh S., Byrne L., Maharaj K., and Guttmacher L. (1993) Consequences of the 1989 New York state triplicate benzodiazepine prescription regulations. In: Cooper J.R., Czecowicz D.J., Molinari S.P., and Petersen R.C. (eds) *Impact of prescription drug diversion control systems on medical practice and patient care*, pp. 279–93. NIDA Research Monograph 131. Rockville, MD: National Institute on Drug Abuse. Available at: http://www.nida.nih.gov/pdf/monographs/download131.html (accessed 20 May 2009).

Weiss R.D., Griffin M.L., Gallop R., Onken L.S., Gastfriend D.R., Daley D., Crits-Christoph P., Bishop S., and Barber J.P. (2000) Self-help group attendance and participation among cocaine dependent patients. *Drug and Alcohol Dependence* **60**, 169–77.

Wendel T. and Curtis R. (2000) The heraldry of heroin: 'dope stamps' and the dynamics of drug markets in New York City. *Journal of Drug Issues* **30**, 225–60.

West S.L. and O'Neal, K.K. (2004) Project D.A.R.E. outcome effectiveness revisited. *American Journal of Public Health* **94**, 1027–9.

Wexler H.K., Melnick G., Lowe L., and Peters J. (1999) Three-year reincarceration outcomes for Amity in-prison therapeutic community and aftercare in California. *Prison Journal* **79**, 321–36.

White D. and Pitts M. (1998) Educating young people about drugs: a systematic review. *Addiction* **93**, 1475–87.

White W. (1998) *Slaying the dragon: the history of addiction treatment and recovery in America.* Bloomington, IL: Chestnut Hill Health Systems.

WHO. See World Health Organization.

Wiessing L., Likatavicius G., Klempová D., Hedrich D., Nardone A., and Griffiths P. (2009) Associations between availability and coverage of HIV-prevention measures and subsequent incidence of diagnosed HIV infection among injection drug users. *American Journal of Public Health* **99**, 1049–52.

Wild C. (2006) Social control and coercion in addiction treatment: towards evidence-based policy and practice. *Addiction* **101**, 40–9.

Wild T.C., el-Guebaly N., Fischer B., Brissette S., Brochu S., Bruneau J., Noël L., Rehm J., Tyndall M., and Mun P. (2005) Comorbid depression among opiate users: results from a multisite Canadian study. *Canadian Journal of Psychiatry* **50**, 512–18.

Wilkins C., Reilly J. and Casswell S. (2006) Cannabis 'tinny' houses in New Zealand: implications for the use and sale of cannabis and other illicit drugs in New Zealand. *Addiction* **100**, 971–80.

Williams J. (2003) The effects of price and policies on cannabis consumption. *Health Economics* **13**, 123–37.

Williams J., Pacula R.L., Chaloupka F.J., and Wechsler H. (2006) College students' use of cocaine. *Substance and Misuse* **41**, 489–509.

Willis J. (2002) *Potent brews: a social history of alcohol in East Africa 1850–1999.* Nairobi, Kenya: British Institute in East Africa.

Wilson J.Q. and Kelling G.L. (1982) Broken windows: the police and neighborhood safety. *Atlantic Monthly* **249**(3), 29–38.

Windle M. and Wiesner M. (2004) Trajectories of marijuana use from adolescence to young adulthood: predictors and outcomes. *Development and Psychopathology* **16**, 1007–27.

Winstock A.R., Wolff K., and Ramsey J. (2001) Ecstasy pill testing: harm minimization gone too far?. *Addiction* **96**, 1139–48.

Wodak A. (2007) Health exchange and prevention of HIV: the evidence for effectiveness is beyond dispute. *Addiction* **102**, 161.

Wood E., Spittal P.M., Small W., Kerr T., Li K., Hogg R.S., Tyndall M.W., Montaner J.S.G., and Schechter M.T. (2004) Displacement of Canada's largest public illicit drug market in response to a police crackdown. *Canadian Medical Association Journal* **170**, 1551–6.

Wood E., Tyndall M., Zhang R., Stoltz J-A., Lai C., Montaner J., and Kerr T. (2006) Attendance at supervised injecting facilities and use of detoxification services. *New England Journal of Medicine* **354**, 2512–13.

Wood J. (1997) *Report of the royal commission into the New South Wales police service.* Sydney, Australia: Royal Commission into the New South Wales Police Service.

Woody G.E., McLellan A.T., Luborsky L., and O'Brien C.P. (1995) Psychotherapy in a community methadone programs: a validation study. *American Journal of Psychiatry* **152**, 1302–8.

World Bank and Department for International Development (2008) *Afghanistan: economic incentives and development initiatives to reduced opium production* Washington, DC: World Bank.

World Health Organization (1992) *The ICD-10 classification of mental and behavioural disorders: clinical descriptions and diagnostic guidelines.* Geneva, Switzerland: World Health Organization.

World Health Organization (1993) *Programme on substance abuse: assessing the standards of care in substance abuse treatment.* Geneva, Switzerland: WHO.

World Health Organization (1998) *The world health report 1998: Life in the 21st century. A vision for all.* Geneva, Switzerland: World Health Organization.

World Health Organization (2000) *Guidelines for the WHO review of dependence-producing psychoactive substances for international control.* WHO/EDM/QSM/2000.5. Geneva, Switzerland: World Health Organization.

World Health Organization (2002) *World health report 2002.* Geneva, Switzerland: WHO. Available at: http://www.who.int/whr/2002/en/ (accessed 25 May 2009).

World Health Organization (2004) *Neuroscience of psychoactive substance use and dependence.* Geneva, Switzerland: WHO. Available at: http://www.naabt.org/documents/Neuroscience%20of%20psychoactive.pdf (accessed 25 May 2009).

World Health Organization (2006) *Towards universal access by 2010: how WHO is working with countries to scale-up HIV prevention, treatment, care and support.* Geneva, Switzerland: WHO. Available at: http://www.who.int/hiv/pub/advocacy/universalaccess/en/index.html (accessed 8 July 2009).

World Health Organization (2007) *Improving access to medications controlled under international drug conventions.* Access to Controlled Medications Programme, Briefing Note. Geneva, Switzerland: WHO. Available at: http://www.who.int/medicines/areas/quality_safety/access_to_controlled_medications_brnote_english.pdf (accessed 25 May 2009).

Wu Z., Detels R., Zhang J., Li V., and Li J. (2002) Community-based trial to prevent drug use among youth in Yunnan, China. *American Journal of Public Health* **92**, 1952–7.

Yamaguchi R., Johnston L.D., and O'Malley P.M. (2003) *Drug testing in schools: Policies, practices, and association with student drug use.* Youth, Education & Society, Occasional Paper 2. Ann Arbor, MI: University of Michigan. Available at: http://www.rwjf.org/files/research/YESOccPaper2.pdf (accessed 16 May 2009).

Yawnghwe C.T. (2005) Shan state politics: the opium–heroin factor. In: Jelsma M., Kramer T., and Vervest P. (eds) *Trouble in the triangle: opium and conflict in Burma,* pp. 23–32. Chiang Mai: Silkworm.

Yongming Z. (2000) Nationalism, identity, and state-building: the antidrug crusade in the People's Republic, 1949–1952. In: Brook T. and Wakabayashi B.T. (eds) *Opium regimes: China, Britain and Japan, 1839–1952,* pp. 380–403. Berkeley, CA: University of California Press.

Young J.H. (1961) *The toadstool millionaires: a social history of patent medicines in America before federal regulation.* Princeton NJ: Princeton University Press.

Zabransky T., Mrav ik V., Gajdošikova H., and Miovsky M. (2001) *PAD: impact analysis project of new drugs legislation (summary final report).* Prague, Czech Republic: Office of the Czech Governmment, Secretariat of the National Drug Commission. Available at: http://www.ak-ps.cz/client/files/PAD_en.pdf (accessed 19 May 2009).

Zacny J., Bigelow G., Compton P., Foley K., Iguchi M., and Sannerud C. (2003) College on Problems of Drug Dependence taskforce on prescription opioid non-medical use and abuse: position statement. *Drug and Alcohol Dependence* **69**, 215–32.

Zaric G.S., Barnett P., and Brandeau M. (2000) HIV transmission and the cost-effectiveness of methadone maintenance. *American Journal of Public Health* **90**, 1100–11.

Ziegler P.P. (2005) Addiction and the treatment of pain. *Substance Use and Misuse* **40**, 1945–54.

Zimmer L. (1987) *Operation pressure point: the disruption of street-level drug trade on New York's lower east side*. Occasional Papers from The Center for Research in Crime and Justice. New York, NY: New York University School of Law.

Zlotnick C., Robertson M. J., and Tam T. (2002) Substance use and labor force participation among homeless adults. *American Journal of Drug and Alcohol Abuse* **28**, 37–53.

Zullich S.G., Grasela T.H., Jr, Fiedler-Kelly J.B., and Gengo F.M. (1992) Impact of triplicate prescription program on psychotropic prescribing patterns in long-term care facilities. *Annals of Pharmacotherapy* **26**, 539–46.

Glossary of terms, abbreviations, and acronyms[1]

Abuse liability The propensity of a particular psychoactive substance to be susceptible to abuse, defined in terms of the relative probability that use of the substance will result in social, psychological, or physical problems for an individual or for society. Under international drug control treaties (*see* international drug conventions) the World Health Organization is responsible for determining the abuse liability and dependence potential, as distinct from therapeutic usefulness, of controlled substances.

Abuse potential See abuse liability.

Betel nut Betel chewing is widely practised in some parts of Asia and the Pacific islands. Betel (or areca) nut, the large seed of an Asian palm tree *Areca catechu*, is wrapped in the leaf of the betel pepper tree, *Piper betle*, to which is added a pinch of burnt lime and flavourings. In contact with saliva, the mixture releases arecoline, an anticholinergic CNS stimulant, somewhat similar to nicotine. Betel chewing can produce dependence, and habitual use often results in health problems, particularly diseases of the mouth, including cancer. There have been few official efforts to control use.

Charas The name given to hand-made hashish in Afghanistan, Pakistan, Nepal, and India. It is made from the extract of the cannabis plant (*Cannabis sativa*).

Chasing the dragon A slang phrase of Cantonese origin referring to the smoke inhaled from heated morphine, heroin, or opium that has been placed on a piece of foil. The 'chasing' occurs as the user keeps the liquid moving in order to prevent it from coalescing into a single, unmanageable mass. Such ingestion may pose less immediate danger to the user than injecting heroin.

Cochrane review Cochrane reviews explore the evidence for and against the effectiveness and appropriateness of medical treatments (e.g. medications, surgery, education, etc.) in specific circumstances. These systematic reviews and meta-analyses are designed to facilitate the choices that doctors, patients, policymakers, and others face in health care decisions.

---

[1] Most definitions in this glossary were adapted from:

Babor T.F., Campbell R., Room R., and Saunders J. (1994) *Lexicon of alcohol and drug terms.* Geneva, Switzerland: World Health Organization.

VandenBos G.R. (2007) *APA dictionary of psychology.* Washington, DC: American Psychological Association.

Wikipedia Available at: http://en.wikipedia.org/wiki/Main_Page.

Confounding, confounder A distortion of results that occurs when the apparent effects of a variable of interest actually result entirely or in part from an extraneous variable that is associated with the factor under investigation.

Contingency management The regulation of rewards in the management of drug patients in a therapy programme. This usually takes the form of giving small amounts of money or gift vouchers when urine screen results show that no recent drug use has occurred.

Conventions, international drug See international drug conventions.

Criminalization The process leading up to and including the finding of guilt for a criminal offence, as well as the consequences following the designation of a criminal label.

Cross-sectional studies Investigations that use an experimental design and research methods to obtain an estimate of the frequency and characteristics of a disease or disorder in a population at a particular point in time. Unlike time series analysis, cross-sectional analysis relates to how variables affect each other at the same time and period. This type of data can be used to assess the prevalence of acute or chronic conditions in a population. However, since exposure and disease status are measured at the same point in time, it may not always be possible to distinguish whether the exposure preceded or followed the disease. In a cross-sectional survey, a specific group is looked at to see if a substance or activity, say cannabis smoking, is related to the health effect being investigated, for example lung cancer.

Decriminalization Removal of criminal penalties

Depenalization Reduction in severity of penalties without necessarily removing the entire criminal penalty. An example would be elimination of a prison term. Decriminalization is a subform of depenalization.

Dependence potential The propensity of a substance, as a consequence of its pharmacological effects on physiological or psychological functions, to give rise to dependence on that substance. Dependence potential is determined by those intrinsic pharmacological properties that can be measured in animal and human drug testing procedures.

Diversion The use of prescription drugs for recreational purposes. Drug diversion can also be defined as the diversion of licit drugs for illicit purposes. Frequently diverted psychopharmaceuticals are opioids and pseudoephedrine (an ingredient used to produce methamphetamine). Finally, drug diversion may refer to programmes available to first-time drug law offenders that 'divert' them from the criminal system to a programme of education and rehabilitation.

Drug misuse The use of illegal drugs or the use of medicines in a way not recommended by a physician or the drug manufacturer. Some illegal drugs have been categorized as prescription-only, meaning that they may only be used legally if prescribed by a doctor and are illegal to use, possess, or supply in any other circumstances.

Drug use disorder See substance use disorder.

Economic evaluation (CBA, CEA) A systematic determination of the costs associated with the implementation of a programme's services, which can take the form of cost–benefit analysis (CBA—a comparison of the monetary value of costs and benefits of different programmes) and cost–effectiveness analysis (CEA—the cost of achieving a unit of programme outcome).

EMCDDA See European Monitoring Centre for Drugs and Drug Addiction.

European Monitoring Centre for Drugs and Drug Addiction (EMCDDA) Established in Lisbon, Portugal in 1993, the EMCDDA is a clearinghouse of drug-related information in the EU. It provides the European Union (EU) and its Member States with a factual overview of European drug problems and a common information framework to support the drugs debate. The EMCDDA consists of over 90 specialists representing some 20 nationalities. It offers policymakers a scientific evidence base for drawing up drug laws and strategies and helps professionals and researchers pinpoint best practice and new areas for analysis.

Ethnographic research The descriptive study of communities, groups, or cultures based on direct observation and some degree of active participation or first-hand familiarity with community life. This method has been used to study social and cultural aspects of drug use and misuse.

Experimental study Research based on randomized experiments with the objective of drawing causal inferences.

Evaluation research The application of scientific principles, methods, and theories to identify, describe, conceptualize, measure, and control those factors that are important to the development of effective human service delivery systems.

INCB See International Narcotics Control Board.

International Narcotics Control Board (INCB) An independent and quasi-judicial control organ that monitors the implementation of the United Nations drug control treaties. This includes responsibility for ensuring that the licit (medical) market is supplied, and that illicit drug trafficking is suppressed.

Incidence The rate of occurrence of new cases of an event (e.g. drug use) or condition (e.g. drug dependence). See also prevalence.

International drug conventions Drug-related treaties signed by member states of the United Nations. The three major international drug control treaties are the Single Convention on Narcotic Drugs (1961), the Convention on Psychotropic Substances (1971), and the Convention against the Illicit Traffic in Narcotic Drugs and Psychotropic Substances (1988). An important purpose of the first two treaties is to codify internationally applicable control measures in order to ensure the availability of narcotic drugs and psychotropic substances for medical and scientific purposes, and to prevent their diversion into illicit channels. They also include general provisions on illicit trafficking and drug abuse.

Khat The leaves and buds of an East African plant, *Catha edulis*, which are chewed or brewed as a beverage. Used also in parts of the Eastern Mediterranean and North Africa, khat is a mild stimulant containing an active principle, cathinone, similar to amphetamine. Heavy use can result in dependence and physical and mental problems resembling those produced by other stimulants.

Lifetime prevalence The proportion of people who have ever used a substance.

Mediator An intervening or intermediate factor (e.g. intoxication) that occurs in a causal pathway running from a risk factor (e.g. alcohol consumption) to a health or social problem (e.g. an accidental injury). It causes variation in the problem indicator, and variation within itself is caused by the risk factor.

Meta-analytical review, meta-analysis Statistical analysis in which data from several different studies are selected and re-analysed together. The approach is particularly useful when there is a specific question to answer and at least a few relatively strong studies that come to different conclusions.

Naloxone An opiate antagonist that blocks the ability of heroin to occupy receptor sites; a morphine-derived opioid antagonist that prevents the binding of opioids to opioid receptors, having primary activity at the mu receptor. Like other opioid antagonists, it can quickly reverse the effects of opioid overdose and is useful in emergency settings to reverse respiratory depression.

Natural experiment The investigation of change within and in relation to its naturally occurring context, as when a policy is implemented in one community but not in a comparable community. The term implies that the researcher had no influence on the occurrence of the change.

Natural recovery The ability to overcome addiction without treatment. Other terms used to describe this phenomenon are self-change and spontaneous remission.

Observational studies Research that draws inferences about the effect of a treatment where the assignment of subjects into a treated group versus a control group is outside the control of the investigator. This is in contrast to controlled experiments, such as randomized controlled trials, where each subject is randomly assigned to a treated group or a control group before the start of the treatment.

ONDCP See Office of National Drug Control Policy.

Office of National Drug Control Policy (ONDCP) A component of the Executive Office of the President of the USA, established in 1988. The principal purpose of ONDCP is to establish policies, priorities, and objectives for the US drug control programme. The goals of the programme are to reduce illicit drug use, manufacturing, and trafficking; drug-related crime and violence; and drug-related health consequences. By law, the Director of ONDCP also evaluates, coordinates, and oversees both the international and the domestic antidrug efforts of executive branch agencies.

OxyContin The brand name of a time-release formula of oxycodone produced by the pharmaceutical company Purdue Pharma. Oxycodone is an opioid analgesic medication synthesized from opium-derived thebaine. It was developed in 1916 in Germany as one of several new semi-synthetic opioids with several benefits over the older traditional opiates and opioids, morphine, heroin, and codeine. Currently it is best known as the main active ingredient in a number of oral medications commonly prescribed for the relief of moderate to severe pain.

Pharmaceutical drug, pharmaceutical A drug that is manufactured, prepared, dispensed, or sold for medical use.

Precursor chemical A chemical that is used in the production of heroin or methamphetamine.

Prevalence The total number of cases (e.g. of a disease or disorder) existing in a given population at a given time (point prevalence) or during a specified period (period prevalence). See also incidence.

Psychoactive drugs A group of drugs that have significant effects on psychological processes, such as thinking, perception, and emotion. Psychoactive drugs include those deliberately taken to produce an altered state of consciousness (e.g. hallucinogens, opioids, inhalants, and cannabis) and therapeutic agents designed to ameliorate a mental condition (e.g. antidepressants, sedatives, and antipsychotics). Psychoactive drugs are often referred to as psychotropic drugs (or psychotropics) in clinical contexts.

Psychoactive pharmaceuticals See psychopharmaceutical drugs.

Psychoactive substance See psychoactive drugs.

Psychopharmaceutical drugs Drugs that are manufactured, prepared, dispensed, or sold for use in medicine to relieve pain or other mental distress. In the context of this book, psychopharmaceuticals are drugs with abuse liability and dependence potential that are used outside of a medical prescription in order to experience their psychoactive effects.

Psychopharmaceuticals See psychopharmaceutical drugs.

Psychotropics See psychoactive drugs.

Qualitative research Research that employs non numeric information to produce findings not arrived at by statistical procedures or other quantitative means (e.g. case studies).

Quasi-experimental Lacking complete control over the scheduling of experimental stimuli that makes true experiments possible (see natural experiment). A quasi-experimental design does not include random assignment. The causal certainty of a quasi-experimental design is lower than that of a true experimental design.

Randomized clinical trial A study design in which research participants are randomly allocated to one or more intervention conditions to determine which one would be of greatest benefit. Randomization is done to eliminate error from self-selection or other kinds of systematic basis.

Randomized controlled trial See randomized clinical trial.

Regression toward the mean An example of bias due to the unreliability of measurement instruments, such that earlier measurements that were extremely deviant from a sample mean will tend, on retesting, to result in a value closer to the sample mean than the original value.

SAMHSA See Substance Abuse and Mental Health Services Administration.

Substance Abuse and Mental Health Services Administration (SAMHSA) An agency of the United States Federal Government that funds and administers programmes that support state and community efforts to support prevention and early intervention programmes and to improve the quality, availability, and range of substance abuse treatment, mental health, and recovery support services.

Substance use disorders A group of psychiatric disorders related to alcohol or other drug use. ICD-10 section F10–F19, 'Mental and behavioural disorders due to psychoactive substance use', contains a wide variety of disorders of different severity and clinical form, all having in common the use of one or more psychoactive substances, which may or may not have been medically prescribed. The substances specified are alcohol, opioids, cannabinoids, sedatives or hypnotics, cocaine, other stimulants including caffeine, hallucinogens, tobacco, and volatile solvents. The clinical states that may occur (though not necessarily with all psychoactive substances) include acute intoxication, harmful use, dependence syndrome, withdrawal syndrome (state), withdrawal state with delirium, psychotic disorder, late-onset psychotic disorder, and amnesic syndrome.

Time-series analysis A statistical procedure that allows inferences to be drawn from two series of repeated measurements made on the same individuals or organization over time. Where the emphasis is on understanding causal relations, the key question is how a change on one series correlates with a change on the other (with other factors controlled).

UNODC See United Nations Office on Drugs and Crime.

United Nations Office on Drugs and Crime (UNODC) The administrative body for the United Nations' programmes in both the drug area and the crime area.

WHO See World Health Organization.

World Health Organization (WHO) A United Nations agency established in 1948 to protect and promote the health of member states through public health measures and relevant policy research. In addition to the WHO's headquarters in Geneva, there are six regional offices. Under international drug control treaties, the WHO is responsible for determining the abuse liability and dependence potential of psychoactive substances, as distinct from therapeutic usefulness.

Index